T0099988

THE FAULT IN OUR SARS

COVID-19 in the Biden Era

Rob Wallace

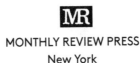

MONTHLY REVIEW PRESS
New York

Library of Congress Cataloging-in-Publication data
available from the publisher

ISBN paper: 978-158367-993-7
ISBN cloth: 978-158367-994-4

Typeset in Minion Pro and Brown

MONTHLY REVIEW PRESS, NEW YORK
monthlyreview.org

5 4 3 2 1

In memory of Andrea Garcia,
Deanna Reber, and Hawanya Henley Finch

A secure and pleasant vessel, carrying inside it a disaster retold.
—OLGA RAVIN (2018)

When the ship arrives in Naples, Godard quotes, unattributed, Curzio Malaparte's novel The Skin: *"The plague had broken out in Naples on 1 October 1943." The plague is the Americans, who arrived that day, along with their American freedom, the presence or promise of which turns every woman, Malaparte chides, into a prostitute, and every man into a scheming wretch.* The Skin *celebrates, perversely and relentlessly, the desperation of Neapolitans, their double-edged gratitude to their American "liberators." Naples, Malaparte declares, "the only city in the world that did not founder in the colossal shipwreck of ancient civilisation," has survived only to face genuine ruin when the Americans arrive with their health, cheer, clean morals, tight-fitting uniforms and deep contradictions. But as Godard shows us, in his majestic views of the [now sunk]* Concordia *as an unearthly, glistening iceberg, pure and whole, the plague can be beautiful.*
—RACHEL KUSHNER (2015)

"Seems to me," said Coyle, "whoever did this knew your systems inside out."
"Yes, they did." And our miserable cost-cutting souls too.
—RICHARD MORGAN (2007)

\

Contents

Introduction

Since the pandemic, the desire for a straight, white smile has only grown, says Sydney cosmetic dentist, Dr Gamer Verdian. "There has definitely been a rise in smile makeovers and veneers since COVID."

—Natalie Reilly (2022)

FROM THE VERY BEGINNING of the pandemic, many of my COVID commentaries took the broad view, connecting a variety of political economies to viral dynamics.[1]

The world's governments, we learned together, treat the capitalism that helped spring the virus out of commoditized forests as realer than the ecologies and epidemiologies upon which the global system depends. To protect that mirage of a difference, each new variant that has since emerged is strangely presented as the beginning of COVID's end, resetting the next round of denialism, instead of alerting us that in reality we are caught in a loop-de-loop of viral evolution.

Each "surprise" that the virus refuses to cooperate with such hopium, acting in its own interests instead of ours, also serves to protect the system from the implications of its refusal to act.[2] These surprises—pretending we don't know what we know—are themselves an ideological project. The logic of fantasy remains stuck to the logic of production.[3] The business of governing a system in decline, after all, is about managing expectations. All is well, get back to work, until, suddenly, it isn't, as it always was. From SARS-CoV-2's vantage, the resulting public health dithering and half-measures serve the virus as both escape hatch out of our control efforts and selection pressure to evolve around those campaigns.[4] A combo that can lead to the worst of epidemiological outcomes.

If we wish to avoid this trap, we have to deploy a full-spectrum intervention that drives SARS-2 under its rate of replacement. This requires us to reject not only the Global North's business bipartisanism country-to-country, but also the core model of our economy, around which our civilization is organized. That's no small matter, but with climate change and other pandemics also on the wing, perhaps our sole option out. Slovenian philosopher Alenka Zupančič makes the critical point, as Slavoj Žižek replays it: "If reacting to the pandemic in full solidarity would cause greater damage to our society and economy than the pandemic itself, is this not an indication that something is terribly wrong?"[5]

The something terribly wrong isn't a mysterious affliction, political theorist Angela Mitripoulos explains, but the very mechanics around which global circuits of capital wheel:

[The pandemic] is a moment in which what it takes to live, to be healthy and flourish, vividly clashes with capitalist mystique of economic productivity, of the idealized household and the metrics of the Gross National Product. . . .

On the one hand, [pandemic preparation] policies were highly amenable to a merger of insurance with financial speculation—as with catastrophe bonds. On the other hand, manufacturers had scaled back on production of [personal protection equipment and prophylaxes before the outbreak] because they did not think that the products would find a market. The problem is less the absence of preparation or just-in-time systems than that preventative and life-saving equipment is a commodity. In that regard, the claims of economic nationalism around PPE supply-chains has far less to do with ensuring that needs are met than with mercantilism and facilitating the monopolistic carving-up of global markets through the combined action of states and corporations.[6]

ALL PAINFULLY OBVIOUS, save to the true believers. But it's that spectacle of what our leaders consider a necessary amnesia that launched me in summer 2021 into a series of hypergraphic explorations connecting a deluge of new COVID data to what seem at first only tangential topics.

Three of the pieces are republished here in this second of what may well be by the end of the pandemic nineteen COVID essay collections. "A Spray of Split Seconds" weaves in police murders of children, Israeli apartheid, Minnesota nice, Daniel Defoe, and the Navajo Blessingway. The split second of an infection is no more an "innocent" social exchange than a cop's killing shot or a commodity purchase trailing back down long distances points South. "Vic Berger's American Public Health" seems by its index more on topic, but in addressing the U.S.'s self-own of a pandemic response pings from Belgium to China to South Africa, Brazil, Los Angeles, Ghana, the medieval English shore, Hungarian and Italian philosophers, and singer Phoebe Bridgers. "Don't Look Up . . . COVID's Infectious Period" uses the highly infectious Omicron COVID variant as a social radioisotope with which to trace the political animas that lead rightists and liberals alike into bending science to capitalist realism. It is in this sense that I called presidential chief medical adviser Anthony Fauci the Lysenko on the Potomac.

Why such expansive pictures, painting off the canvas of respectable commentary and onto the walls and windows of my Patreon garret and out into the proverbial street? Because the crux of the present pandemic—from its origins to its now years-long wend—has almost nothing to do with data or hypothesis testing or the difficulties of turning epidemiological understanding into policy. The meat of the matter isn't even about palace intrigue or parliamentary cretinism at the heart of the political class's present power.

The system's refusal to place everyday people's COVID well-being front and center is found in the mirror of the sense of manifest destiny, which I noted in my first pandemic piece in January 2020 helped bring about the virus itself.[7] And such self-reflecting presumptions are found far beyond even our favorite daily summaries of the pandemic online or in a newspaper. They're all the way out into our food, feelings, freeways, phones, and favorite films, reinforcing each other into a moral physiognomy without which we couldn't recognize ourselves. It's a mirror, like all mirrors, in which left and right are reflected back right and left, and, with the numbers infected piling up, the down direction of the dominant mode of civilization underlying all things ecological still looking grimly down.

The mechanics of public health policy matter, of course. With a defeat of the Build Back Better agenda, one of his own making, U.S. President Joe Biden announced that any agenda leaning politically left was over.[8] His administration now tacked to the right to save its political skin in what will likely be a bruising midterm election. Even before the pivot, the Biden on display presided over—save for a single week in November 2021—at least a thousand U.S. COVID deaths a day from August on, even with a working vaccine, months before the arrival of the Omicron variant, and long after Omicron's peak. It's like something other than virus or vaccination campaign is to blame.

In a classic case of externalizing domestic failure, everything bad was now to be hung upon Russia and China, even before the Ukraine invasion and Speaker Nancy Pelosi's junket to Taiwan.[9] One needn't be fans of the other powers to understand Biden was putting on his best Nicholas II, the tsar who fought Japan to ward off revolution at home. In a jaw-dropping op-ed, Biden COVID-19 Advisory Board members bioethicist Ezekiel Emanuel and epidemiologist Michael Osterholm argued that China's then-successful Zero COVID program represented a danger to the world.[10] Psychologists describe such an inability to admit a grave loss, spinning failure onto others instead, as *grandiose narcissism*.[11]

By that diagnosis, the whole of the U.S. political class is Trumpist now. A month later, the U.S. Centers for Disease Control and Prevention would abandon public health under the veneer that Omicron—and therefore COVID—was over. With what were previously "high" levels of community transmission (as high as 200 cases per 100,000 over the previous seven days) reset as "low," the very bases of public health intervention were just coded out of existence.[12] The CDC's own data also refuted resetting its recommendations for quarantine from ten days to five.[13] Think Trump's Malthusian neglect with a proper tone and better vocabulary.

Biden officials turned to acting surprised that their arguments that all is well—with at the time nearly 2,000 Americans still dying a day—convinced Congress to strip funding for anti-COVID programs from a larger appropriations bill.[14] So no new money for testing, treating, and vaccinating the uninsured, who are now on the hook for $195 tests.[15] No more free access to monoclonal antibodies. No additional oral antiviral treatments and scaled-back purchases of preventative treatments for the immunocompromised. Less funding for next-generation COVID vaccines. Even less of a push for vaccinating the rest of the world. Each of these an additional step down from an earlier abandonment of broader public health programs such as eviction moratoriums, stimulus payments, monthly child benefits, and the Paycheck Protection Program—despite infections on the increase in slowly heating hotspots nationwide and popping up inside the White House itself as if still serving as Trump accommodations.[16]

Even if funding is found—filling in a loss minimalist global vaccination campaigns also suffered—expectations that such biomedical "tools" pre- and post-pandemic emergence are enough champion systemic suppositions over results. "There is no possible downstream management of either nuclear conflict or mass-fatal zoonotic or other pandemic," public health ecologists Rodrick Wallace and Deborah Wallace encapsulated the matter:

> Elaborate, but basically medicalized, tactics of "early emergent pathogen detection and early vaccine development". . . do not constitute a viable public health strategy. Rather, such incessant medicalization indexes an underlying strategy aimed at

protecting existing neoliberal land use models and agribusiness structures, and, most centrally, the power relations behind
them.[17]

Characteristically, then, Osterholm, who was upbraided by Biden
officials for suggesting the United States needed to enter a four-to
six-week lockdown in late 2020, now helped argue that any lockdown
pursued by Chinese jurisdictions is not only useless but dangerous:

> Yes, China has weathered the pandemic well so far. Even with
> about four times the population of the United States, China has
> had fewer than 140,000 confirmed Covid cases and fewer than
> 6,000 deaths since January 2020, according to the World Health
> Organization. A vast majority of factories continued to operate.
> Early in the pandemic, China added thousands of hospital beds
> to its health care system in days.
>
> All of this seems like an enormous success when compared
> with the messy and often chaotic response to the virus in the
> United States, where more than 860,000 people have died and
> some 2,000 more die each day. Many hospitals are under siege.
> The economy has been disrupted.
>
> But this may very well be the future China is facing. Its pur-
> suit of zero Covid will prove to be a huge mistake. The policy has
> left it wholly unprepared for what will become endemic Covid.[18]

Our failures here in the States, Emanuel and Osterholm argued,
prepare us for an endemic COVID that has yet to arrive: "The coronavirus is not going to disappear—the world will have to live with
it." In other words, here's one shot of four rapid tests per household,
three masks, and a wad of Malthusian public health. Served up—as I
profiled Emanuel and Osterholm early on in November 2020 in the
first essay in this collection—by America's favorite eugenicist and an
Oprah-feted doom champion who backs down upon the slightest
political nudge.[19]

The op-ed isn't just about China or the Shanghai lockdown that for better and for worse China was forced to adjust in the face of Omicron.[20] It's about attacking Zero COVID, so that we do not enact it—or anything like it—in the United States. That's a classic feint. Attack Biden critics before they point out he helped match Trump in putting another half-million Americans in the ground. Anyone who now proposes a multipronged program is to be smeared as a China ally at the start of a reheated Cold War. The Sino-American cooperation propagandized just a couple years ago in *The Martian*, the Matt Damon vehicle, is opportunistically shelved.

The op-ed followed a *New York Times* front-page article that both stole from and tamed critical epidemiologist Justin Feldman's caustic roundup of the administration's first COVID year into a Biden win.[21] For a while there, *Times* commentator David Leonhardt was writing nearly weekly about the putative damage that efforts to control COVID impose, citing polling data to the effect that concern about COVID is at best a "very liberal" obsession.[22] In this version of the world, leftists don't exist.

In the *Times*'s business section, tech specialist Li Yuan has written a series of articles in the Biden vein that Zero COVID threatened the global economy and the Chinese people, comparing the campaign to the Holocaust and public health workers there to Nazis.[23] Yuan also compared Zero COVID to Mao's "zero sparrow" campaign, which, Yuan wrote, led to insect infestations and the Great Famine.[24]

Why such gutter snark? It's a signifier of a desperate moment in U.S. statecraft and the sociospatial limits of capital.[25] As historian Adam Tooze explains, both China's identity as much of the world's supplier of last resort and its initial successes in COVID control also made it conservative in pandemic economic policy.[26] China wasn't beholden to anxious multinationals bottled up all along their suddenly brittle supply lines.[27] And there is less chance of capital engaging in a spatial fix—pivoting to other suppliers elsewhere and circumventing congenital devaluation, unabsorbed overaccumulation, supply-chain finance obligations, and underconsumption—during a global shutdown. What is the point of the great labor arbitrage China represents, U.S. corporations and their media reps complained, if its government won't just sacrifice its workforce-populace during a pandemic for the greater (commodity) good?

Geographer David Harvey described the structural sources of such a crisis of faith:

> At times of savage devaluation, interregional rivalries typically degenerate into struggles over who is to bear the burden of devaluation. The export of unemployment, of inflation, of idle productive capacity become the stakes in the game. Trade wars, dumping, interest rate wars, restrictions of capital flow and foreign exchange, immigration policies, colonial conquest, the subjugation and domination of tributary economies, the forced reorganization of the division of labour within economic empires, and, finally, the physical destruction and forced devaluation of a rival's capital through war are some of the methods at hand.
>
> Each entails the aggressive manipulation of some aspect of economic, financial or state power. The politics of imperialism, the sense that the contradictions of capitalism can be cured through world domination by some omnipotent power, surges to the forefront. The ills of capitalism cannot be so easily contained. Yet the degeneration of economic into political struggles plays its part in the long-run stabilization of capitalism, provided enough capital is destroyed *en route*. Patriotism and nationalism have many functions in the contemporary world and may arise for diverse reasons; but they frequently provide a most convenient cover for the devaluation of both capital and labour.[28]

The United States's brightest bulbs pitching China a nationalist rebuke for refusing its tributary status can't grasp that the wealthiest of their own sponsors—cashing out on domestic commons—have already signed off on the end of empire stateside. The upside down is so internalized that the worst of failures are presented as great successes.

Reporter Apoorva Mandavilli, for one, wrote a *Times* series of "news analyses" declaring it's the nature of good scientific and public health practice that led the United States to its COVID trap.[29] In January 2021, Mandavilli described the CDC's "methodical" and "meticulous" approach as the cause for delays in public health response that are now being replaced by faster, if also less supported, decision-making. By August 2022, the CDC, rearranging the deck chairs, agreed such meticulousness the source of its failures.[30]

In actuality, the failure to get a handle on the outbreak is neither a matter of the provisional nature of science, nor, in the other direction, the need for speed, but rather the concerted refusal to engage in the kind of public health campaigns many poorer countries successfully undertook around the world even before the vaccine.[31] That is, approaches that Emanuel and Osterholm, U.S. leaders in the science of COVID, had now blacklisted off the board.

Indeed, the inter-imperial and domestic clashes around COVID that plaster this volume are markers of what Harvey identified as no mere anomalies but constitutive moments in the dynamics of accumulation.[32] There's an inner dialectic to be found at the point of eco-epidemiological collapse when the crises are pinned upon previous partners to mutual relief. Refusing to rescue Matt Damon off Mars or leaving fifteen million to their COVID deaths is a necessary part of global capitalism's reconstitution, even at this precarious conjuncture, when the land and labor from which capital needs to smash-and-grab a reset is found beginning to run out.

ONE BEGINS TO GRASP that we can't understand the nature of COVID solely with a microscope or mathematical model or Beltway commentary. All those may help, of course. They may also hinder.

By April 2022, the Biden administration had helped strip the U.S. capacity to keep track of COVID-19.[33] The Department of Health and Human Services ended the requirement hospitals report daily COVID deaths, overflow and ventilated COVID patients, and critical staffing shortages. Some U.S. states outright ended reporting COVID metrics, hospital bed usage and availability, and ventilator use. Some states scaled back COVID-19 reporting to as delayed a basis as weekly or simply ended such reports. Some hospitals followed NIH's lead changing definitions of COVID cases, including to only those patients that receive remdesivir or dexamethasone.

Some public health departments switched to replacing state PCR testing with at-home rapid antigen testing or ending such testing programs entirely. Unlike other countries, such at-home testing, provided by the state or bought at the store, is accompanied by no requirements to report results to public health departments.

The Biden administration helped enact a system-wide rollback that Trump, to much ridicule in May 2020, tried to talk us into:

> Could be that testing is, frankly, overrated. Maybe it is overrated. But whenever they start yelling we want more, we want more. Then we do more and they say we want more. When you test, you have a case. When you test, you find something is wrong with people. If we didn't do any testing we would have very few cases.[34]

By May 2022, with Omicron beginning to bounce back by way of new subvariants BA.4, BA.5, and New York City-grown BA.2.12.1, a calm to the point of comatose Biden administration entered conceptual meltdown. The White House, the CDC, and the COVID-19 Advisory Board all took different positions:

> The warnings from [CDC Director Rochelle] Walensky and other federal health officials seemed somewhat at odds with President Joe Biden's own stance. The attitude in the West Wing more closely mirrors that of most Americans, who have eagerly moved away from mask-wearing and other strategies to prevent infection . . .
>
> At the White House briefing, Dr. Ashish Jha, the new White House coordinator of the pandemic response, warned that if Congress fails to grant the administration's request for $22 billion in new COVID funding, Americans will suffer come autumn . . .

Dr. Ezekiel Emanuel . . . who led an effort to draft a new pandemic strategy called "The Next Normal," was more blunt in calling for the White House to improve its COVID communications strategy: "They need to step up their game."[35]

To stir up resolve, Walensky referred to the darkening maps of community transmission the CDC had abandoned in favor of the more optimistic measure of community levels.[36] The next day, the director went back to referring to the sunnier maps of community levels.[37] But Walensky's—and the White House's—discombobulation isn't just a matter of a trip of the lips. All these versions of "normal" that ask nearly no adjustment, including from the same Emanuel who objected to China having a strategy at all, are suffering from more than merely their communication.

For all these possible paths forward proposed—maybe also all those books shown together on the dedication page, the book now in your hands included—matter little with our leaders arriving upon the same willfully wrong choices time and again, as if such were always-already the answer to begin with. As if the same awful decisions—by Trump, Biden's once-COVID czar Jeff Zients, the soft eugenicist Walensky, and their equivalents in many governments worldwide—are every one the final click unlocking some ecstatic punishment. The historical threads are stitched down into these true believers' most base survival instincts until, if they are allowed to continue, everyone else is dead.

No masks, no vaccination, no sheltering-in-place, no eviction moratoriums all the way down to no nothin'. Some Americans apparently objected to such a prime directive. Columnist German Lopez reported:

Polling suggests that COVID—not the chaotic U.S. withdrawal from Afghanistan—jump-started Mr. Biden's political problems. His approval rating began to drop in July, weeks before the withdrawal.

That timing coincides with the rise of the Delta variant and reports that vaccine protection against infection was not holding up. Both came after Biden suggested for months that an "Independence Day" from Covid was near, setting up Americans for disappointment as it became clear that his administration would not fulfill arguably its biggest promise.[38]

Timothy Lenton's research group—as others before them—found it wasn't wealth that marked a country's success in controlling COVID.[39] Alongside the adaptive nature of governmental response, a matter we explore here in this volume in "Governance Is Key," the social trust people shared with each other and with their governments set COVID outcomes at the population level:

> Trust within society is positively correlated with country-level resilience to COVID-19, as is the adaptive increase in stringency of government interventions when epidemic waves occur. By contrast, countries where governments maintain greater background stringency tend to have lower trust within society and tend to be less resilient.[40]

The United States ran away from all of that. As public health dean Sandro Galea writes, the social divisions the United States is suffering as a matter of both historical principle and political expediency lead to public health sequelae—COVID included—that exacerbate the divisions.[41] A vicious cycle. Indeed, if some Americans lost faith in the administration's COVID policy, others embraced a libertarian sociopathy as a kind of reaction formation to governmental abandonment—embracing the suck—transmogrifying the resulting social vacuum into a virtue.[42]

What to do about such a mind fuck in the face of a collapse in social trust? Even if the refusal were spun as a form of rural autonomy from the state-supported productivism Angela Mitripoulos wrote of, the pain of a phantom limb of lost community requires mirror therapy.[43] Shattered communities need to be given the resources that will allow them to see themselves in more regenerative counterparts, if not in D.C. or in state capitals, then in the communities one county over that kept their wits and took care of each other during a pandemic.[44] We must find where representation and material realities meet.[45]

While the ongoing death drive is imposed on the exploited, some critics seem more taken by the story the rich tell of themselves. Philosopher Byung-Chul Han argues that capital individualizes (and monetizes) health as a form of death denial for its in-group.[46] He skirts around alternate possibilities. Health needn't be the commodity Mitripoulos described. That isn't the only option. By an array of ecosocialisms, anarcho-communisms, living Indigenous mythologies, and even the Rooseveltian interventions Biden promised but failed to deliver, health can also emerge as an epiphenomenon of people's well-being and sense of belonging far beyond the numerical fetish of statist population statistics. Scaling out these substitutes, as we describe throughout the book, requires of us sea changes in what counts as mutual recognition—with one another and other species.[47]

Without those destinations, however, Han ends up reflecting the very nihilistic individualization to which he objects. "Why revolution is impossible today," he titles one essay.[48] Han locates death as much in the "Botox zombie's" loss of identity as in physical decay, but he offers no path to generative meaning while the rest of us are still here alive.[49] One can subsume the facts of death (and defeat) without worshiping at their altar. Indigenous groups and various days of the dead appear to have a much better handle on the nature of these paths. We can learn to assimilate those insights without appropriating whole cultures, or, against science historian René Dubos, conflating objections to colonial genocide and a nostalgia for a lost Golden Age that never was.[50]

FROM MY ST PAUL, Minnesota, apartment, I try to *act* in favor of alternate futures every day, working with scientists and civilians alike in five different organizations dedicated to matching some of our terrible realities with sociohistorical corrections that the participants involved are together trying to work out along the way. We are trying to walk the talk and do so with other people, many with whom we share disagreements, including on exactly what to do about COVID.

I know not everyone can dedicate that kind of time and effort. There is more to life than the beautiful struggle. Bills have to be paid. Every metal and moral beam we recognize in civilization as worth saving requires many millions of hands to hold in place. But, as argued in this collection both directly and as an unspoken assumption, we must attempt a stab at acting beyond these constraints, as an affirmation that humanity is worth it all despite this hideous moment. These struggles are a means of discovering the ways in which all that we read and write—all those books in the collage—might meet up with the acts needed to turn wishful thinking into a better world. There is, then, a leap of faith in a science for the people. Doing, novelist Sheila Heti writes in another context, "causes the knowledge of it."[51] The *it* of such a science is a difficult and deeply humbling path. We will routinely stagger on it.

Act we must, however, as the microscopic and the geological—pandemics and climate change—are revving up faster than the capacity of this stumble of a system for a historical response. Act we must, as if our better selves are worth the seven generations Native cosmology imagines for us. If there's more to life than the beautiful struggle, can there be life without it?

In contrast, a Biden administration elected to volte-face Trump on COVID turned its position 360 degrees back to Trump positions. The "discombobulation" is deliberate. Its details and our disrespectful front cover here are necessary to help even "very liberals" make their own way out beyond the confines of party politics—Democrats vs. Republicans, Labour vs. Tories—that camouflage the more intrinsic damage.

In the face of an adaptive and ongoing pandemic that is producing millions of new infections a week worldwide and Omicron subvariants evolving out from under vaccine coverage, the administration, for instance, decided to declare victory on COVID-19. NBC News reported that in February, Impact Research, the administration's polling firm, recommended moving beyond merely dropping mask mandates and by default toward *discouraging* mask use.[52] Molly Murphy and Brian Stryker of Impact suggested that the administration make a play for November's midterm elections and "declare the crisis phase of COVID over and push for feeling and acting more normal." In what seem talking points from the Urgency of Normal campaign that encouraged moving students back into schools without adjunct interventions, Murphy and Stryker cited learning loss at school and COVID's effect on the economy as reasons to exit COVID as a reality.

Both problems arose out of decisions the Trump and Biden administrations made in refusing to provide adequate support for communities and households alike during a national crisis. At the same time, the Impact memo continued, aiming to eliminate COVID isn't the answer. In effect, with language reminiscent of Trump's chief of staff, Mark Meadows, the memo admits that COVID will remain the reality, which Murphy and Stryker also suggest the Biden administration ignore.[53] The CDC, other administration officials, and outside epidemiologists would follow up the memo by warning the American people of upcoming COVID spikes, including next fall and winter when Americans go to those very polls.[54]

Such realities are socially structured. In early July, Anna Peele interviewed the slated-to-retire Fauci for the *Washington Post* magazine, under a headline, "The Pandemic Is Waning":

> I am also aware that it would be a moral crime to transmit the coronavirus to Fauci. So when I got COVID two weeks before our interview, I obsessively parsed the guidelines from the Centers for Disease Control and Prevention: As long as I waited 10 days after my first positive test, I could still meet Fauci in person, right? No, I was informed by Fauci, via a member of his communications team. I would need to test negative three days in a row and wear a mask, even outdoors.[55]

So, no five-day quarantine for Fauci's circle along the lines a CDC under employer pressure recommended for Americans. And Fauci treats the possibility of infection after ten days as real. Exactly the kinds of precautions the People's CDC I helped found this year has recommended for the rest of the country.[56]

When Biden finally contracted COVID in July 2022, showing up to work maskless while infected, CDC Director Walensky took to the airwaves that, yes, the President would be treated with precautions above and beyond what the CDC recommended for the American people. After all, the Americans the administration abandoned are the labor force that *chooses* to go to work sick or alongside sick coworkers and the CDC is just accommodating them:

> Yeah, I think we can all agree that the president's protocols likely go above and beyond and have the resources to go above and beyond what every American is able and has the capacity to do.
>
> As we put forward our CDC guidance, we have to do so that they are relevant, feasible, followable by Americans, and that is Americans that live in urban jurisdictions and rural jurisdictions, that have resources and less resources, that have, you know, work constraints and many other things. So, when we put forward our guidance, we do so that they reflect such that every American is able to follow them.[57]

A growing class divide, which mainstream public health accommodates in the folksiest of fatalism, is treated as more sacrosanct than the obligations to control and prevent an infectious pandemic. The resulting damage is unlikely of any American's choosing. "For the period from June 29 to July 11 [2022]," the *Wall Street Journal* reported, "3.9 million Americans said they didn't work because they were sick with Covid-19 or were caring for someone with it, according to Census Bureau data. In the comparable period last year, 1.8 million people missed work for those reasons."[58]

Meanwhile, Walensky's office worked remotely throughout the pandemic.[59]

BY AUGUST 2022, CDC had dropped recommendations for quarantining at home and testing people without symptoms.[60] People who do still test positive should stay home for five days, the CDC continued, although people without symptoms now wouldn't know to. The contact tracing the administration promised but never really followed up with is now over, save in hospitals and nursing homes.[61] By autumn, the administration planned on ending funding for the very "tools" it long claimed lets the United States send everyone back to work in a pandemic.[62] No more federal support for vaccines, testing, and treatment.

The liberal establishment threw in entirely with the Biden administration's "return to normal": the Harvard School of Public Health, Randi Weingarten and the American Federation of Teachers, and— inviting arch-COVID minimizer Leana Wen to speak at its annual conference—the American Public Health Association:

> "What the CDC is, in my opinion, trying to do, they are trying to still be relevant, and maybe when they say something, people will listen to them instead of being completely 180 degrees away from what behavior is anyway," [Peter] Chin-Hong [an infectious disease specialist at UCSF] said.
>
> Bill Hanage, an epidemiologist at the Harvard T.H. Chan School of Public Health, agrees that the new guidance shows that the CDC is trying to meet people where they are.
>
> "I think that this is a point where you actually have to sort of get real and start giving people tools they can use to do something or not. Because otherwise, people will just not take you seriously," Hanage said.

As if the practice of public health was merely a popularity contest. And the refusal to pay people to stay home, never to be disputed, clearly now makes COVID a matter of personal choice.

Mike Osterholm, who the *Times* failed to identify as part of the administration's COVID Advisory Board, converged on this courageous line: "I think [the CDC] are attempting to meet up with the reality that everyone in the public is pretty much done with this pandemic."[63] A reality the administration worked hard to help manufacture by deft incompetence.

The administration knows full well the damage to come. It announced only a week earlier that it would be establishing a new Department of Health and Human Services office dedicated to addressing the debilitating Long COVID that as many as 23 million Americans have suffered beyond their initial acute infections.[64] An associated National Research Action Plan on Long COVID is to be pursued alongside the administration's efforts to "act more normal" and strip out programs in COVID prevention.

In other words, the supply of extremely difficult-to-treat Long COVID cases the administration now said it sought to mitigate will continue apace to accommodate an employer-led economy. Encephalopathy, dementia, cognitive problems, sleep disorders, pulmonary fibrosis, acute pharyngitis, pulmonary embolism, abnormal heartbeat, anemia, diabetes, and malaise and fatigue for all![65]

Given the bipartisan push to end COVID as an idea if not as an empirical fact, science writer Ed Yong's sense of defeat may be more an acknowledgment that a different public health is possible.[66] And that it's already underway. To passing references to the People's CDC and its radical public health practitioners and everyday people, Yong adds:

In 2018, while reporting on pandemic preparedness in the Democratic Republic of Congo, I heard many people joking about the fictional 15th article of the country's constitution: Débrouillez-vous, or 'Figure it out yourself.' It was a droll and weary acknowledgment that the government won't save you, and you must make do with the resources you've got. The United States is now firmly in the débrouillez-vous era of the COVID-19 pandemic. . . .

I have interviewed dozens of other local officials, community organizers, and grassroots groups who are also swimming furiously against the tide of governmental apathy to push *some* pandemic response forward, even if incrementally. This is an endeavor that all of American society would benefit from; it is currently concentrated among a network of exhausted individuals who are trying to figure out this pandemic, while living up to public health's central tenet: Protect the health of all people, and the most vulnerable especially. The late Paul Farmer, who devoted his life to providing health care to the world's poorest people, understood that when doing such work, victories would be hard-won, if ever won at all. Referencing a line from *The Lord of the Rings*, he once said, "I have fought the long defeat." In the third year of the COVID pandemic, that fight will determine how America fares against the variants and viruses still to come.[67]

What Yong misses in his respectable summary is that the resulting patchwork isn't just a reminder of what we have lost or what we might gain upon a reformation of a pivot, but perhaps a new world born out of the husk of the old. Are the People's CDC and other efforts a protest, a palliative, practice in parallel governance, or entrée to a revolutionary alternative? Or all these things together during what appears a punctuation of an historical moment?

In that spirit—of a history yet unwritten or alternate histories long discarded recovered to rationalize new futures entirely—let me thank Pandemic Research for the People, the People's CDC, Midwest Healthy Ag, the Southwest Mapping Project, and the Agroecology and Rural Economics Research Corps for their daily lessons in shared struggle and understanding the world.

I thank my co-authors in this volume, who are at one and the same time sincere and delightful: Alex Liebman, Allison Henry, David Bond, Fernando Ramirez, Ivette Perfecto, John Gulick, Julie Velasquez Runk, Kaitlin Enouchs, Katrina Anderson, Kenichi Okamoto, Kim Williams-Guillén, Lisa Kelley, Luis Fernando Chaves, Luke Bergmann, Meleiza Figueroa, Miguel Tinsay, Nicole Gottdenker, Philip Seufert, Rodrick Wallace, Sophia Kruger, Tammi Jonas, and Tanya Kerssen. I thank the editors at *Truthout* for the improvements they made to several of the pieces in this volume upon reprinting and my CUNY brother Kazembe Balagun for his kind help publishing the Rosa Luxemburg Stiftung commentary.

My sincerest appreciation for the hard work the Monthly Review Press team—Michael Yates, Martin Paddio, Rebecca Manski, and Susie Day—put in getting this book out shipshape and in short order. To Erin Clarmont for copy editing. And to John Bellamy Foster and the Press committee for their continual editorial support over the years. The essays were updated as close as we could to the publication deadline and edited for better reading. My deepest gratitude to John Gulick and Sophia Kruger for helping put an end to the endless endnotes and to Peter Cury for realizing yet another outrage of a cover design. And finally, to my Patreon supporters, whose kind contributions helped free some time to work on this book. The second of perhaps nineteen.

—AUGUST 2022

Biden's COVID Plan Isn't Enough

It is not inequalities that kill people. It is the people who produce and reproduce inequalities through their public and private interventions that kill people. In most cases, we have the specific names of those responsible for those inequalities and, therefore, for those deaths.

—Vicenç Navarro (2011)

JOE BIDEN'S CAMPAIGN PROMISED to "build back better." *Better than what?* one might ask. The Trump administration? That low bar hardly matches the expectations of the millions of voters who earlier this month risked health and welfare to make a change in our national trajectory.

Presuming Donald Trump's electoral defeat will lead to little more than some revenge firings, a parade of pardons for any Trump fixers still standing, and a practice run at the mechanics of a rightist coup for next time, what does a Biden administration promise us come January 2021?

Biden's transition team has released its program for the presumptive administration. Its economic plan continues the campaign's careful efforts to circumvent any whiff of economic populism in the face of 65 million unemployment claims filed since March 2020, much less the more foundational matter of a bourgeoisie selling off the infrastructure of empire at the end of the American cycle of capitalist accumulation.[68]

Biden's White House homecoming, New York Times columnist Charles M. Blow writes, is a restoration and not a revolution: "He is not so much a change agent as a reversion agent."[69] With U.S. inequality as measured by the Gini index the highest in the Global North outside Turkey, such a reversal may mark a revanche far more dramatic than merely, for some, a comforting return to Obama policy.[70]

A Biden administration that acts upon the wishes of its largest donors risks reconstituting the preconditions that led to the emergence of Trump in the first place. Could the so-called moderates of the extreme center that turned a sure thing of an election into a nail-biter possibly miss the perils of resetting the political pins for a fascist of even a modicum of competence greater than Trump?

Well, yes, they could, and willingly so, if the short-term demands of the billionaire class serve as impetus enough.

That kind of cultivated myopia is already programmatic. The transition team's plan to address the COVID pandemic dovetails with just such a regression. The plan's objectives, and the adjacent task force selected to see it through, telegraph a campaign aimed at rolling back COVID without changing the system that brought about the outbreak and all the other deadly pathogens in the epidemiological queue.

Plan Points, Good and Bad

To begin, the Biden COVID plan sports some good starting points, even under the loosened constraints that anything proposed, in all likelihood, would exceed what a murderously negligent Trump administration never bothered to offer.[71] "We're not going to control the pandemic," White House Chief of Staff Mark Meadows told CNN.[72]

The Biden plan declares the new administration will "always" listen to science and public health professionals and err on the side of transparency and accountability. It is time, Biden himself announced, "to end the politicization of basic, responsible public health steps."[73]

The plan calls for more testing—free and reliable—run by a Rooseveltian Pandemic Testing Board. Contact tracing would be run through a Public Health Jobs Corps. The Defense Production Act would finally be deployed to ramp up American-made personal protective equipment (PPE). Biden's plan calls for a national mask mandate that, reading between the lines, appears more suggestive than legally enforced. But such a notice on high would clearly offer a better model than the maskless pieholes currently flapping loose in a COVID-blitzed West Wing.

Although missing from the Biden COVID plan, presumably the incoming administration would be amenable to restoring an April U.S. Postal Service proposal, quashed by Trump, to ship masks to every U.S. household.[74]

The Biden plan calls for the kind of federal funding for state and local governments running low from COVID outlays or tax short-falls that the Trump administration out-and-out refused to provide in spiteful tightfistedness.[75]

The plan places vaccine rollout in the hands of scientists and federal staff, who will oversee safety, upload testing data for all to see, and testify to Congress uncensored about the campaign's logistics. It calls for $25 billion for vaccine manufacturing and distribution, free vaccines for all, and a handwave of a declaration opposing price gouging for any other new therapies. Enforcement will be key, as hospitals and insurance companies continue to charge patients for federally subsidized COVID tests.[76]

The plan also calls for establishing another task force, one to offer recommendations around racial disparities in COVID and other diseases.

It calls for creating a pandemic dashboard tracking local transmission at the zip code level. Publicly available COVID data are presently available at no finer level than U.S. county, although New York City just began to offer such zip code level reporting.[77]

Swerving past the entirely expected bump in the road that no plan survives its implementation, much is also missing from the very start here. And it isn't merely a matter of operational planning. With good will, funding, and the right people, that's fixable. What's carefully omitted from the plan is more emblematic of the U.S. political class's ideological presumptions—in this case, imprinted upon a major public health crisis.

Right up front, we get a sense of what the administration views as its America. The Biden COVID plan speaks of families, small businesses, and first responders, but not communities. The gap embodies a classical liberalism, the *dramatis personae* cited representing, respectively, the means of reproducing workers, petite capital, and the state's capacity for biopolitical intervention. Pathogens spreading far and wide rarely respect such utilitarian demographics.

Other "essential" heroes are similarly positioned. Threaded through the plan is a respect for science's place in helping infer the realities of an outbreak, something Trump abandoned. We also see science's long-standing role in upholding governance of a particular class character.

Indeed, a particular brand of science underlies the plan, setting the needs of the donor class ahead of stopping the COVID outbreak in any rapid order. The plan, for one, calls for hiring 100,000 Americans as part of a Public Health Job Corps to aid in contact tracing. That certainly sounds like a lot, but it isn't nearly enough by an order of magnitude.

The U.S. outbreak is presently off the charts at 11.4 million accumulative cases. COVID incidence clocked in as high as 193,000-plus daily cases this past week, with more than two million infected and over 15,000 dead since the start of the month, just as we are entering the winter wave of infections.[78] Texas alone has accumulated a million cases since March. California just joined that club. South Dakota is testing anywhere from 17 to 58 percent positive for COVID— depending on the measure, a staggering infection load.[79]

Hospital capacity is maxing out across 18 states, with overflow patients getting shuttled to other hospitals or released early.[80] Exposed health care workers are being forced to shorten their quarantine periods to return to understaffed wards.[81]

The Fitzhugh Mullan Institute for Health Workforce Equity at

George Washington University offers a county-level U.S. map of estimates of the number of contact-trace workers needed based on population size, tracer workforce, and the present outbreak load.[82] Even under heroic assumptions as to what contact tracers can accomplish daily, the projected personnel needed exceeds the Biden plan's capacity. For example, the metropolitan regions of Minneapolis and St Paul alone would need 6,000 of those 100,000 tracers the Biden transition team proposes, hardly anywhere near what is necessary to control the outbreak, even combined with the measly efforts by the states so far.

Of course, contact tracing depends on a lot more than infections and workforce. As *ProPublica* describes, counties with meatpacking-driven outbreaks are having great difficulty tracking cases among immigrants, many of whom speak other languages, don't have phones, or don't want contact with state officials for reasons of immigration status under Trump's Immigration and Customs Enforcement.[83]

So why the numbers gap between infections and Biden's contact tracers? The political class here simply can't afford the possibility that U.S. governance in late empire, focused on corporations and the stock market first, suddenly would be centered on hiring the American people to help the American people. FDR bunting is being placed on an austerity parade float.

The plan's numbers at best represent only a gesture toward the kind of public health responses which countries as different as Vietnam, New Zealand, and Iceland have demonstrated are necessary to get the outbreak under control in two months' time without a vaccine available.

What does it mean if the Biden administration, knowing full well the scale of response other countries have engaged to stop their outbreaks, begins budget negotiations with a Republican Senate for contact-tracing hires using numbers far from adequate for solving the problem?

There is an "anti-state-state" in the business of closing out interventions for everyday people in favor of interventions in favor of the powerful—even, or especially, for a pandemic encroaching upon both. Contrast, as historian Robert Brenner showed for the CARES Act, the open spigot with which entire industrial sectors were funded and the lousy one-time $1,200 for everyone else.[84]

Any righteous effort to control the outbreak would pay everyone to stay home for as long as a year, even should the two leading vaccine candidates prove efficacious. For a virulently capitalist state, however, such a reserve army of labor is allowed to fallow only so far as it disciplines those millions who are forced to work to survive, including during a dangerous outbreak.

In this context, lockdowns are suddenly turned into a front in a class war of neoliberal public health's own making. For the more affluent, able to electronically commute, "winning" racial capitalism never felt so redemptive.

From the very start of the city's outbreak, New York's subways were filled with Black and Brown workers on their way to work servicing the stay-at-home professional managerial class. Out in rural America, the Trump administration forced immigrant meatpackers back into COVID-splattered plants to help agribusiness supply the Chinese market.[85] No governor in the Midwest or the South, Republican or Democrat, will lift a finger to roll back such labor discipline. And now that Trump's done the dirty work, neither will Biden.

Objectives Domestic and International

A Biden COVID campaign that outstrips Trumpist neglect to mainstream applause can still represent a white flag waved at the virus. Controlling COVID isn't the primary objective. As for the Trump administration, opening the economy back up is. The agreement was most certainly the substance of the phone call Trump and Biden shared in April.[86] What differentiates the Biden effort is its conclusion that controlling enough COVID is necessary to make opening back up work.

The tension in balancing those two expectations is palpable, verging on nigh unintelligible strategy. In his first policy speech post-election to a room of business and union leaders, Biden said, "We all agreed that we want to get the economy back on track, we need our workers to be back on the job by getting the virus under control," adding that the United States is "going into a very dark winter" and "things are going to get much tougher before they get easier."[87]

The Biden plan accepts the premise that social distancing must be calibrated with keeping the economy going. "Social distancing," the plan claims,

> is not a light switch. It is a dial. President-elect Biden will direct the [Centers for Disease Control and Prevention] to provide specific evidence-based guidance for how to turn the dial up or down relative to the level of risk and degree of viral spread in a community, including when to open or close certain businesses, bars, restaurants, and other spaces; when to open or close schools, and what steps they need to take to make classrooms and facilities safe; appropriate restrictions on size of gatherings; when to issue stay-at-home restrictions.[88]

Flexible decision-making is always at a premium as outbreak circumstances shift, but the expectation we can so finely dial efforts in and out in time and space appears already a lost cause with an infection that spreads before symptoms appear.

Successful efforts controlling COVID abroad didn't operate under the premises the transition plan imposes upon the United States. The Biden plan locks an "evidence-based" CDC into the assumptions of a notorious model an Imperial College team presented early in the outbreak. Rather than the kind of all-out disease suppression China and other countries have successfully demonstrated, the Imperial model suggested the United States and the UK could toggle in and out of community quarantine as triggered by a set level of critical care beds filled.

Why err on the side of the kind of reopening that other models indicate routinely leads back to the pathogen rebound that keeps the country a COVID sink?[89] The primary objective is to keep the economy running, giving the little people of the country the money they need to survive only if they help someone else make profit.

Other plan points are organized around analogous predicates. The Biden plan issues a general call that patients suffering long-term COVID infections shouldn't be subjected to higher premiums or denied coverage for "this new preexisting condition." The plan accepts the concept of preexisting conditions, an insurance company contrivance denying all of us a right to a life history, and that insurance—even with a public option—should be anything but free to all.[90] Under the plan, drug prices aren't to be capped. Pharma executives are only to be shamed for a marketplace that Washington helped build.

In short, the "evidence" behind these interventions is tied directly to the prime directives of the society into which the Biden administration is to intervene. As my colleagues and I described the matter in March, "Models such as the Imperial study explicitly limit the scope of analysis to narrowly tailored questions framed within the dominant social order. By design, they fail to capture the broader market forces driving outbreaks and the political decisions underlying interventions."[91]

The same ideological finger trap is found in plan objectives directed internationally. The transition team uses disease as a new cold war cudgel, perhaps unsurprisingly, as even without reference to "Chinese virus" or "Kung flu," Biden ran to the right of Trump on China.[92]

The plan calls for reestablishing the White House biosecurity directorate Trump dismantled. It calls for relaunching PREDICT, the USAID program that sent U.S. scientists abroad to investigate early signs of potential pandemic strains. It calls for reestablishing the CDC's Beijing office.

All these efforts are organized around the notion that infectious diseases originate offshore, "including those coming from China." The insistence on externalizing disease is a time-honored practice but offers very little in terms of preventing the pandemics almost certainly to follow.[93]

The focus on specific GPS coordinates where deforestation or bushmeat might lead to a novel pathogen spilling over into locals misses what's driving emerging diseases. A more relational geography tags places such as New York City, London, and Hong Kong—key centers of the financing backing the deforestation and development that drive new infections—as the worst hotspots. U.S. investment firm Goldman Sachs owns farms in China's Hunan and Fujian provinces, but foreign direct investment pings so far and wide across the globe that the bourgeoisie across countries emerge as one big (albeit fractious) family.[94]

If not by Trump's death cult incompetence, the best and brightest of the Democratic Party are as constrained from acting upon this understanding by the prime directives of an imperial political economy. Biden himself took great pride in spearheading the Obama effort on Ebola in West Africa, but the administration's public health record was, at best, checkered with well-run failures.

It was under the Obama administration that swine flu H1N1, Ebola Makona, H5N2 (and other H5Nx), Zika, a cholera of UN sourcing in Haiti, the vaccine gap for yellow fever, H7N9, Ebola Reston, MERS in industrialized camels, the opioid crisis, and a surge in antibiotic resistance emerged.[95]

Such public health problems are no "natural" phenomena. We could have learned more, but it was Obama's National Science Foundation and National Institutes of Health that failed to fund scientific efforts to explore the roles agribusiness, deforestation, structural adjustment, and global circuits of capital played in these outbreaks.

Obama's wars contributed to global morbidity and mortality, including the 1.3 million deaths since 9/11 in Afghanistan, Pakistan, and Iraq alone. It was his bombing campaigns and proxy wars that helped spread cutaneous leishmaniasis across Syria, Eastern Libya, Yemen, and Iraq.[96] It was the CIA's operation against Osama bin Laden that helped destroy Pakistan's polio campaign.[97]

It was the Obama administration's refusal to bail out homeowners that allowed mosquitoes to incubate in the pools of abandoned California homes, leading to an outbreak of West Nile Virus.[98] It was that administration's refusal to seriously address consolidation in the food sector that allowed foodborne outbreaks to increase in deadliness and geographic extent.[99] It was Obama's CDC that only a couple years before the measles outbreak at Disneyland tagged

Disney as blameless for outbreaks (a carte blanche it refused to extend to the Hajj).[100]

It was the Obama CDC that built in anonymity for U.S. mega-farms that prove sources of avian or swine influenzas that infect even humans.[101] The strain typing and pathogen genetic sequencing conducted by the National Animal Health Laboratory Network, including at several federally funded public universities, were to remain confidential and for the livestock industry's eyes only.

All these failures were organized, identifiable even then, around serving capital and U.S. might first. The failures hit close to home, including a public health system that, over forty years of neoliberal management, was both neglected and monetized.

Indeed, the United States itself was a source of a pandemic. Contrary to the Biden plan's view of disease "out there," U.S. hogs were identified as the source for multiple genomic segments that contributed to the swine H1N1 strain that emerged outside Mexico City in 2009.[102] The meat dumping that permitted American companies to break into the Mexican market served as due cause why our group called the pandemic strain "the NAFTA flu."[103]

Successive administrations across party, including now Biden, have refused to acknowledge or act on U.S. responsibility in helping drive new infections.

Biden's COVID Advisory Board Is a Mixed Bag

The Biden COVID plan, then, offers a few good objectives bordering on obvious common sense. Several others are tellingly bad, permitting COVID the structural elbow room that no country placing public health first would allow. A model published earlier in the year offered that under the most pessimistic circumstances, we might be stuck with COVID-19 through 2024.[104] The conclusion seemed impossible to believe then.

The people invited to serve on Biden's COVID advisory board are similarly a mixed bag, embodying a mash of interests and ethoses already baked into the plan.

Marcella Nunez-Smith is one of the advisory board's three co-chairs. She is the associate dean of health equity at the Yale School of Medicine. Taking Kamala Harris's cue, the Biden team is jumping on the racial disparities COVID represents. The numbers are staggering: Black and Latinx COVID mortality rates are nearly twice that of the white population. Nunez-Smith appears an inspired choice to turn such stats into remediation, not just for COVID, but, as the Biden plan promises, public health beyond.

The approach may suffer an epochal drag, however. From Bill Clinton to *Hamilton*, the centrist wing of the Democratic Party has used such disparities as part of a bootstraps narrative. Four hundred years of racial capitalism and counting represent a perpetual Act One toward individualist redemption. A talented tenth can serve as an adequate placeholder in the political class running what historians Walter Johnson and Monica Gisolfi and geographer Ruth Wilson Gilmore describe as a modern plantation of a country.[105] On the other hand, as Keeanga-Yamahtta Taylor has written, such symbolic appointments aim to corral the votes of Black people, Indigenous people, and people of color for another generation.[106]

Sociologist Sonia Bettez found that in the late stage of the Clinton administration, such "disparities" discourse served as a deflection from the structural origins of public health damage:

> "Health disparities" emphasized race and ethnicity, individual responsibility, and medical care. This narrow focus omitted and diverted attention from root causes such as growing structural inequality, thus exculpating government of responsibility and forestalling socio-economic change. My analysis suggests that, because of their elite positions and qualifications, individuals who contributed to the discourse in government participated in transforming health inequities into "health disparities."[107]

Sociologist Elizabeth Wrigley-Field turned the classic disparities analysis the Biden administration appears ready to re-embark on in the other direction. She used COVID to show the structural inequities embedded in the country.[108] It would take 400,000 COVID deaths among white Americans to bring up their mortality rate to the lowest mortality rate Black Americans have *ever* suffered in all the years records have been kept. Everyday racial inequality is already as deadly as a pandemic.

Michael Osterholm, an infectious disease expert at the University of Minnesota and another advisory panel member, has a reputation for speaking frankly on matters of pandemic danger. He's appeared on *Oprah* to talk tough on swine flu H1N1. In the face of deep antipathy, he recently called for another four- to six-week lockdown for which workers should be paid to stay home, a position Biden steered clear of.[109] Osterholm is exactly right here, and such an intervention should be extended longer if necessary.

But Osterholm's tell-it-like-it-is is tempered by taking money from the poultry industry and a loyalty that has placed the imperium before scientific judgment.[110] Osterholm recently spoke on the likelihood that the next deadly influenza would emerge from poultry and hogs, but he long carried water for those industries. In 2010, he argued that "the best and safest poultry production in the world right now is occurring in ... very large facilities, where biosecurity is actually very high."[111] He asserted a single agribusiness company producing 70 percent of all poultry in India represented the best in production, with high standards of biosecurity and an excellent safety record. All H5N1 strains across Asia, even low-pathogenic serotypes, have been limited to "backyard range production." The same held true in the United States, with migratory waterfowl the source of infection: "[We] see very, very, very little influenza virus activity in our poultry production, where we have high biosecurity [as] required in large facilities."

Setting aside Osterholm's false dichotomy between backyard and intensive production, H7N9 in China, H5N2 in the Midwest (including across the industrial barns of his Hormel benefactors), and all the other H5Nx found in industrial poultry in Europe, disproved Osterholm's blanket assertions about industrial biosecurity down to bone and gristle.[112]

Upon COVID-19's emergence, Osterholm joined a coterie of U.S. epidemiologists who attacked China. Ma Xiaowei, the head of China's National Health Commission, announced in January that SARS-CoV-2, the virus that causes COVID-19, could be transmitted before symptoms appeared. "I seriously doubt that the Chinese public officials have any data supporting this statement," Osterholm told CNN. "I know of no evidence in seventeen years of working with coronaviruses—SARS and MERS—where anyone has been found to be infectious during their incubation period."[113]

It's remarkable that an epidemiologist of such experience would presume an RNA virus, even one that doesn't mutate at the rate of other such viruses, couldn't possibly evolve into a novel life history.

Ezekiel Emanuel, brother to the former Chicago mayor and Obama chief of staff Rahm Emanuel, represents a more odious addition to Biden's COVID advisory panel. In 2014, Emanuel argued against the worth and meaning of elderly life. He waxed against the tyranny of rising life expectancies and elongating morbidity.[114] While Emanuel initially set his position in terms of his own life (and death) choices and opposed assisted suicide, he painted his premises as matters of universal application. Along the way he omitted the class basis of his good health and family fortune and conflated productivity and well-being.

This isn't a misreading of his argument, as Emanuel later claimed. Five years later, Emanuel recapitulated his position to *MIT Technology Review* in stronger terms.[115] It's not just the dissolution of old age we need to avoid:

> These people who live a vigorous life to 70, 80, 90 years of age—when I look at what those people "do," almost all of it is what I classify as play. It's not meaningful work. They're riding motorcycles; they're hiking. Which can all have value—don't get me wrong. But if it's the main thing in your life? Ummm, that's not probably a meaningful life.[116]

Emanuel's argument serves more broadly as a neoliberal medical ethics, offering a rationale for rationing health care at a time when diseases of despair began to ravage rural areas that were turned into agribusiness sacrifice zones. Rural decline underpinned unprecedented decreases in American life expectancy, especially among poor and working-class whites in the Midwest and South, with the counties suffering the worst health declines undertaking the greatest switches from voting Obama 2012 to Trump 2016.[117]

Such an ethics, accepting the zero-sum of health care for profit at face value, folds in with the rightist necropolitics that emerged around COVID this year: save the economy, let the old die.[118] We must ask what Emanuel's appointment to the COVID advisory board will mean for Biden's interventions in nursing homes and hospital triage.[119] The appointment was not made without due vetting.

Match COVID Scale for Scale

None of us need pass our own understanding of COVID and its solutions through Joe Biden and his advisory board. We can pursue another program beyond Trump and Biden both.

• *Apply proven interventions.* Take notes and apply lessons already learned for beating COVID in countries the world over. China built a COVID-dedicated hospital in 10 days and flooded Hubei, the center of the initial outbreak, with 40,000 health workers. New Zealand implemented travel restrictions, placed incoming travelers into quarantine for 14 days and tested them regularly.[120] That country canceled public events, restricted gatherings, closed workplaces, deployed stay-at-home orders, restricted internal movements, restricted public transport to essential workers, closed schools, tested all symptomatic patients, tested selected asymptomatic people, provided income support replacing 50 percent and more of lost income, and coordinated public information. Two very different countries, their national campaigns in disease suppression without a vaccine, resulted in people being able to walk free outside without masks in four months' time. Should we feel four months is too long? We're already in month nine here stateside and worse off than in March.

- *Go for knockout.* Aim for COVID suppression. Gear up a national response to meet COVID scale for scale. Set a provisional deadline for the suppression campaign to give people an end date to which to look forward. Such a deadline will put impetus on the governments across jurisdiction to follow through with the task.
- *Scale up community health for the pandemic we have (not the one we wish we had).* Nationalize hospitals out from the onus of profits (and from the logic of firing medical staff during a pandemic).[121] Scale up hospital capacities, both urban and rural. Enforce health-based protocols and time off among health care workers to reduce staff decay. Socialize pharmaceuticals, not just testing. Supercharge all testing to within hours to permit contact tracing to work. Hire and deploy a million contact tracers. Hire and deploy a million community health workers to check up on people who need assistance in their homes—not just for their physical health, but for their emotional well-being. Win trust for a working vaccine with a full safety check.
- *Suspend capitalism.* That trust won't be won by denying people the means by which to survive the cure as much as the illness. Direct deposit monthly checks to all U.S. households. Enforce rent, mortgage, and debt abeyance. Municipalize restaurants and grocery stores to serve local neighborhoods free food. Retrofit and deploy hundreds of thousands of food trucks to cook meals house-to-house. Municipalize neighborhood brigades and other forms of mutual aid for compulsory stints of several days for able-bodied residents followed by quarantine.
- *Celebrate pandemic's end.* Upon the end of this outbreak, continue mailing support checks and insisting on debt abeyance to cover our return to day-to-day community life and a national celebration.
- *Reintroduce agriculture and nature.* To keep other such pathogens from emerging again, we must end global agribusiness, logging, and mining as we know them. We must preserve forest (and wetland) complexity, maintaining ecological buffers across bats, geese,

other natural disease reservoirs, our food animals, and our communities. We must reintroduce agrobiodiversity into livestock
and poultry to serve as an immunological firewall against deadly
pathogens both on farms and across landscapes. We must return
to letting livestock reproduce on-site so that herds and flocks can
protect themselves against pathogens by tracking immunity in real
time.

- *Return rural sovereignty.* Such interventions require unplug-
ging rural communities as agribusiness sacrifice zones in favor of
returning their locus of control. We must turn to the kind of state
planning that centers farmer autonomy, community socioeconomic
resilience, circular economies, integrated cooperative supply networks, food justice, community land trusts, and reparations. We
must undo deeply historical race, class, and gender trauma at the
center of land grabbing and environmental alienation.

- *Imagine humanity beyond the market.* On the world stage, we must
end the unequal ecological exchange between the Global North and
South. Healing the metabolic rift between ecology and economy
that drives pathogen emergence at the heart of modern agriculture demands we plant a different political philosophy that treats
agriculture as part of the ecosystemic functions—clean water, rich
soils, probiotic ecologies—upon which humanity depends. We
must shift our mode of social reproduction toward a regimen of
degrowth, decolonization, developmental convergence, debt can-
cellation, and disalienation of land and labor.

Such an ambitious program of interventions is required beyond
the COVID-19 virus, which is still evolving new variants in humans
and other animals. Other coronaviruses, avian and swine influenzas,
African swine fever, and a veritable zoo of other potential pandemic
strains circulate unscathed across agribusiness-damaged landscapes.
Without a fundamental shift, under the Biden administration, these
pathogens will be left to meander into a series of pandemic escapes,
one after another.

Many of these alternate interventions are already underway elsewhere. Despite the global nature of pandemics (and climate change), some countries are converging on foundational shifts in social ecology in response. The United States can join them, but only upon freeing itself of a system that by dint of its structurally enforced power dynamics treats the public commons as a plaything for the wealthy.

—*TRUTHOUT,* NOVEMBER 22, 2020

Bidenfreude

The Memory Police have done their work here, much as they did in my father's study, leaving it little more than a ruin. Nothing at all remains to remind a visitor that it had once been a place to observe wild birds. The researchers, too, have scattered.

—YOKO OGAWA (1994)

A JOKESTER ONCE CHARACTERIZED the Ivy League as a hedge fund with a campus attached to it. One might say something similar of the country in which the schools are based.[122]

The United States is abandoning what recently deceased political scientist Leo Panitch described as its responsibilities in managing global capitalism for the bourgeoisie worldwide.[123] With public health and other earmarks of the modern state abandoned within even its own borders, the United States seems now more a stock market with a country attached.

It's true, on the other hand, that the magical thinking of never-ending economic growth has long-anchored the American political ethos in settler expansionism.[124] *Nothing* is more important than perpetual growth. Everything else—even our shared humanity and life on Earth itself—is to be subsumed under that prime directive.[125]

But this year's COVID-19 outbreak alerted the world of a nation's identity turned inside-out like a smelly sock.[126] Rome wasn't built in a day, but the United States' nearly as fast a fall, however part of a *longue durée* decline from its peak as a center of capital, should flabbergast even the sharpest of radical observers.[127] For even a Biden administration may prove no prophylaxis for the COVID-19 outbreak and American decline overall.

Graphic Content

The potion of economic growth did *not* save the day during the pandemic. Those countries that kept their economies opened at the expense of their population's morbidity and mortality—the United States, Mexico, Chile, Belgium, among others—suffered worse COVID-19 outbreaks *and* greater economic losses.[128]

Wealth, on the other hand, remained protected, growing in record draughts and in ever greater concentration. Over the pandemic, March to December 2020, the collective wealth of America's 651 billionaires grew by more than one trillion U.S. dollars.[129] That's nearly four times the $267 billion in one-shot stimulus checks sent to 159 million Americans earlier in the year.

One can't help but be outraged. Toward the end of the year, a graph circulated on the online left showing a direct relationship between daily S&P Index closings for the top 500 companies' stock prices listed on the exchange and accumulative COVID-19 deaths in the United States.[130]

On its face, such a vulgarity of "dying for the market" seems a spurious correlation. Accumulative cases are always going to rise. So, we might better plot the S&P and COVID-19 hospitalizations for the days the market was open, in this case, March 17–December 18. Hospitalizations pinged up and down upon each COVID wave, marking the immediate state of the outbreak better than cumulative caseload.

We can see here stock prices split through the first two U.S. COVID-19 waves, with different closings in the index—high and low—at the same level of hospitalizations. Upon the start of each COVID-19 wave stock prices fell, bouncing back only on the wave's decline. Research

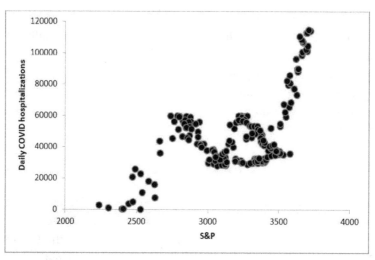

Daily U.S. COVID hospitalizations and S&P 500 closing index, March 17–December 18, 2020.

earlier in the outbreak showed just such a negative bias in stock closings, depressing the index more upon bad COVID-19 news than the
amount it bounced back upon good.[131]

So, the market *does* react to news in the real world, even as financialization—investing in debt and currency—is increasingly divorced
from the real economy (and the vast majority of people's everyday
lives). Or, in the more updated interpretation, as financialization
increasingly *drives* the real economy regardless of the various perverse outcomes.[132]

Geographer Albina Gibadullina recently plotted financialization
by industrial sector across countries.[133] She found that betting on the
debt backing the economy increasingly supersedes outright investment in real commodities. Sudden disasters don't roll our high-end
gamblers back to reality, however. Not even back to the capitalist reality of the kinds of use-value that might seem necessary to protect a
system in crisis.

Sociologists John Bellamy Foster, Jamil Jonna, and Brett Clark
describe financialization picking up in pace during the worst of
damage brought about by the present pandemic.[134] The resulting

impacts aren't felt just in stock portfolios or bond derivatives. With less revenue from elective surgery and other blows to projected profits, U.S. hospitals, for instance, are firing nurses during the worst outbreak in a hundred years, inside a broader trend in which hospitals are increasingly treated as portfolio assets first.[135]

Our S&P graph suggests that at the other end of the outbreak, even as hospitalizations are exploding in record number, with the vaccines rolling out and a Biden administration rolling in, things, from the vantage of capital, may be looking up.[136] Capital will survive—even prosper—through half-a-million U.S. deaths that its professional-managerial class largely dodged by staying at home.

So we may have here a positive bias later in the outbreak. Terrible news on the daily *doesn't* depress stocks now that the bourgeoisie appears in the clear.

Here, then, we find ourselves back at the vulgar interpretation we thought we'd circumvent in favor of nuance. Because the rest of the country is in *terrible* shape. Three to four times more of the population is hungry than an already unconscionable baseline.[137] Millions have filed for inadequate unemployment insurance.[138] Shoplifting of staples like food and diapers is at record levels.[139] Tens of thousands of COVID deaths, more than that of many countries combined, have been attributed to housing evictions alone.[140]

The overall trend apparent even in our rough graph from March to December—up, up, up—supersedes the dynamics of the stock market's blips here and there. The resulting massacre—COVID and otherwise—is teaching Americans an abject lesson, at least for those in a position to assimilate it.

The Extreme Center's Gambit

The lesson can be so easily lost. The tumult of a political class at odds with itself forces the country to choose sides that are not of its own making.

The hard part is not letting January's Trumpist putsch and the second impeachment that followed confuse matters. Certainly these histories count and defeating the fascist creep is always a front-and-center task. The roiling itself speaks to the bourgeoisie's struggles with administering an empire in decline home and abroad.

But we need to keep in mind that politicians of both major parties—Democratic and Republican—spent this past year organizing themselves around simultaneously bailing out billionaires, now far richer than ever in only a few short months, and minimizing paying the poorest of Americans trying to survive a deadly pandemic.[141]

Congress passed a lousy $1,200 of assistance per American earlier in 2020. It then dragged its ass for months at the end of the year before finally agreeing on another $600. A push to up the second payout to $2,000 was turned aside in the name of fiscal responsibility. The debate was cut off with a vote in favor of a military budget greater than the world's next ten largest military budgets combined.[142] Biden's latest offer to fold in another $1,400 nowhere near approaches what smaller countries have been offering their citizens monthly from the pandemic's start.[143]

The lesson couldn't be clearer. Under this system, Americans are to be given money to reproduce themselves *only* in the course of helping capital accumulate. Not even a pandemic is enough to interrupt imposing social identities tied largely to company productivity. People will just have to die if their living disrupts the very expropriation that brought about the pandemic.[144]

In short, the present U.S. system is a death cult. And it isn't administered just by Trump administrators propounding herd immunity into late summer, but by an incoming administration ready to get people back to work with vaccines that appear unlikely to stop transmission.[145]

The irony is that a system which for decades neglected public health as a commons, and so upon COVID-19 was unable to administer non-pharmaceutical interventions, may now display a remarkable incapacity to distribute a pharmaceutical one it took such pride in producing.[146]

In refusing to pay and protect the populace in its time of sacrifice, the political class may have lost the public's trust.[147] And the contacts and networks needed to connect people mind and body to public health as a shared fate were long destroyed for an S&P that the Biden administration aims to protect.[148]

Even months before inauguration, Biden and his COVID-19 response embodied as much of the epoch's exhausted spirit as Trump.[149] Whereas Trump represents the system's id, Biden campaigned as its science-touting superego, only now, once elected, he's back to acting its trap of a structurally imposed ego.[150]

Capitalist realism, as far down as its alienated bedrock of climate collapse and dehumanizing labor markets, is at this point as delusional as the flat-Earthism it looks down upon and the ecomodernism—thinking technology enough to reverse climate change—to which it gravitates.[151]

If the extreme center cannot hold, it is because in its ideological policing, blocking any alternative to the present shitshow, it appears, on the one hand, on track to accelerating civilization's environmental crash.[152] On the other hand, its celebrated failures of imagination open the way to the rise of more competent fascists.

Every step along the way the center champions "building back better" for the settler billionaires first and foremost. Even during COVID-19, the wealthy's successes continue to destitute much of the world, Global North and South.[153] And yet former president Barack Obama spent 2020 campaigning against even a whiff of socialist or liberationist amelioration—intervening against the Bernie Sanders campaign, Black Lives Matter, the NBA wildcat strike, and the Squad of democratic socialist representatives in Congress.[154]

Obama's purring negation emerged out of the same insipid source as Biden's decision to rehire agribusiness lobbyist Tom Vilsack for Secretary of Agriculture.[155] With whole swaths of rural countryside enraged enough by the damage of neoliberal agriculture to flirt with fascism.[156] Now that is some inspired thinking there! Let's return the country back to the conditions that brought about Trump in the first place.

Bidenfreude—relief in Trump's defeat but little joy—offers no exit out of the existential trap that the men from Hope spring upon the American electorate every four years.[157]

The only egress is disconnecting out of the neoliberal imaginarium. There are thousands of years of alternate paradigms—Indigenous, smallholder, working class—at fundamental odds with the present political class's tottering brinkmanship. It's time to start parsing through these alternatives, experimenting with them anew, whatever the lengths to which the Ivy-educated and other "best and brightest" scold us.[158]

—ROSA LUXEMBURG STIFTUNG, JANUARY 2021

A Spray of Split Seconds

But it seems the Government had a true Account of it, and several Counsels were held about the Ways to prevent it coming over; but all was kept very private. Hence it was, that this Rumour died off again, and People began to forget it, as a thing we were very little concern'd in, and that we hoped was not true; til the latter End of November, or the Beginning of December 1664, when two Men, said to be French-men, died of the Plague in Long Acre, or rather at the upper End of Drury Lane.

— DANIEL DEFOE (1722)

Those of us who survived the pandemic, and all the rest, passed through so many different worlds. Like time travellers. Some of us lived in the past. Some in the present, some in an unknowable future. If you lived in the past, you disbelieved the conflagration reflected in the eyes of those already looking back at you. You mistook the pity and anger, how they despised you. How, rightly, they despised you.

— JEFF VANDERMEER (2021)

I WATCHED THE VIDEO of young Adam Toledo's murder at the hands of a Chicago cop in March 2021.

I've had a rough relationship with such clips. In 2014, I took them on as a part of bearing witness to the cruel reenactment of the slave patrol upon which the United States still draws its daily political sustenance.[159]

I've held back since, watching only the first minutes of George Floyd's murder on a corner I routinely travel in Minneapolis, in part because of growing objections to the pornification of Black death. By Walter Scott's murder, shot eight times in the back by a Charleston cop, I couldn't stomach them any longer. I got the message. It's held since. I think about these murders—and the broader apartheid they represent—nearly every day.

But I have a thirteen-year-old. And for my own child's sake, I needed to see how we arrived at a cop killing a seventh-grader of the same age in an alleyway. I also took this one for the team. My son's mom refused to watch it but requested a sketch, with minimal detail, should we need to talk to him about it.

It took me a half-hour to report back. Because what I saw the first day the video was released didn't in any way, shape, or form line up with what the Chicago machine—from mayor to police to newspapers—described as its content.[160] No, Toledo did not draw a gun on the cop. Much as Floyd did not suffer a "medical emergency," as offered in early reports.[161] Nor was Winston Smith—not the protagonist of George Orwell's 1984, but another Black man gunned down in Minneapolis in June—a "murder suspect."[162]

Did Chicago think lying for two weeks would buy it time? Is that how low it thinks of the population it ostensibly governs? Was there an expectation that politicos could continue to play all sides into numb inaction?

"Behind every cop who murders a 13-year-old child," tweeted civil rights lawyer Alec Karakatsanis,

> there is a city lawyer working to keep the video secret, a prosecutor lying about it in court, a mayor giving cops more money and weapons, and a professor with a consulting firm deciding which "reform" will make the most money.[163]

Chicago had invested in ShotSpotter tech that triangulates gunshots only in the West and South Side neighborhoods.[164] An ABC-7 team investigation found Chicago police rushed to 37,763 ShotSpotter alerts but reported no crime 86 percent of the time.

A police unit with Officer Eric Stillman at the wheel on March 29 arrived within minutes of such a report—and two 911 calls—in the predominantly Latino Little Village neighborhood. The video shows Stillman exiting the car, running down an alley, and tackling twenty-one-year-old Rubin Roman, who was later shown to have shot the gun. Roman apparently handed the gun off to Toledo upon police arrival.

Stillman catches up to Toledo from behind. Stillman flashes his strobe light on Toledo the way the police line in Minnesota hit protesters outside the Brooklyn Center station where Officer Kim Porter, Daunte Wright's killer, served.[165]

The strobe aims to confuse and disorient. A confused and disoriented Toledo is given a split second to "drop his weapon," which he has already left behind the gap in a fence where Stillman finds him. Toledo puts up both hands before Stillman fires.

My initial thought was that Toledo didn't have a chance to process any of it. But he does get his hands up. It's Stillman who can't match the description in his head of a report of an armed man with the reality of the unarmed boy before him.

THE INSTINCT WAS NEVER Stillman's alone. It's programmed in. And not just in Chicago. A 1967 Supreme Court ruling awarded qualified immunity, which

> protects state and local officials, including police officers, from personal liability unless they are determined to have violated what the court defines as an individual's "clearly established statutory or constitutional rights."[166]

A 1989 follow-up, the *New York Times*'s David Kirkpatrick writes, set a precedent that protects police who violate even that loose standard:

"The calculus of reasonableness must embody allowance for the fact that police officers are often forced to make split second judgments—in circumstances that are tense, uncertain and rapidly evolving—about the amount of force that is necessary in a particular situation," Chief Justice William H. Rehnquist wrote in the majority opinion. . .

[The case] became "the lodestar" and "created this impression that almost nothing is out of bounds," said Barry Friedman, a law professor at New York University and the director of its Policing Project. . . .

The same standard also became embedded in the training and practices of American police—"part of law enforcement DNA, often unnoticed as it works in the background to determine our actions," a magazine for police officers declared in a 2014 article about the ruling.[167]

In other words, as in the case of twelve-year-old Tamir Rice, killed within seconds of Cleveland Officer Timothy Loehmann's arrival, better to show up shooting first.[168] The split seconds harbor police, "fearing for their lives," from all consequence.

As Hannah Fry describes in her review of the dangers of such standards, by Goodhart's law, "once a useful number becomes a measure of success, it ceases to be a useful number."[169] In this case, police start to game the split second buffer in the service of the kind of BulletProof Warrior protocol in which Jeronimo Yanez, Philando Castile's police shooter, was trained.[170] Better to shoot first and survive.

The context of any situation police arrive upon is thereby jettisoned entirely. Columbus, Ohio, police arrived upon a flaying brawl to shoot sixteen-year-old Ma'Khia Bryant four times in the head.[171] She had called the police for help.

"Many critics," writes Kirkpatrick,

say the [Supreme Court] standard's narrow focus on the moment an officer pulls the trigger obscures questions about the many choices that led up to the confrontation, noted Rachel Harmon, an authority of police law at the University of Virginia. For example, she said, did the officer rush recklessly into danger or take steps to defuse the situation?[172]

The split second can extend in duration. Upon an hour-and-a-half negotiation with nineteen-year-old Christian Hall on an Interstate 80 overpass last December, Pennsylvania State Police gunned down a pellet gun–armed Hall who, when shot, was holding up his hands.[173]

"There's no requirement that a member of law enforcement wait for a weapon to be pointed directly at him or her before deadly force can be used," Monroe County First Assistant District Attorney Michael Mancusco said of Hall's murder.[174] Imminent danger isn't a criterion.

Contrary to prosecutorial insistence that such circumstances are algorithmic in their action, police do not have to follow through with what Mancusco insisted was a classic suicide by cop.[175]

The rest of the Chicago video records Toledo's agonized (and agonizing) death from a sucking chest wound. Toledo's mouth is a vomit of blood. He gargles an inhuman sound.

His body is small. He's five feet tall and ninety pounds.[176] He has a start of preadolescent gangliness, but nothing near the growth spurt that anyone would mistake for what right-wing commentator Sean Hannity called "a thirteen-year-old man."[177] Of course, the size of men—a panicky Scott shot in the back or weeping Floyd calling for his dead mother—does not embody the rationale for a sanctioned and trained short-circuit in judgment.

Police aren't the only occupation with the cultivated prejudice of an angel of death.

One of my students this semester remarked that Floyd's murder reminded her of the repeated studies that show U.S. doctors think Black people feel less pain.[178] The doctors, I'll add, insist, like their brethren in blue, on conflating such anti-empirical caricatures and the behaviors individual patients—no angels they—partook upon their own untimely demise.

Even Black doctors can't protect themselves. Susan Moore, as knowledgeable as any patient could possibly be, was gaslighted by her attending physician that, no, she was neither short of breath, nor in pain.[179] Sent home early, Moore, who filmed her maltreatment for Facebook, died of COVID-19 two weeks later:

> "This is how Black people get killed, when you send them home and they don't know how to fight for themselves," Dr. Moore told her camera.[180]

WHAT POLITICS AND CULTURAL baggage are smuggled into a diagnosis may extend still further out.

Late-night talk show host Stephen Colbert has been commenting on the cruel truth of the police murders. If I've checked in on the show recently, however, it's because Colbert is engaged in a contrary polemic on the pandemic. Post-Trump, and as early as February, Colbert repeatedly boostered the Biden administration's pandemic efforts as Happy Days Are Here Again, and that this summer he'd be able to enjoy a drink at a local club to hear band leader Jon Batiste's first gig back.

Trump was a liar. And nearly everyone knew it, even his supporters.[181] If the Biden administration lies, it's as much in deference to the structural demands of an empire in decline that I described previously as a scramble to stay ahead of American disappointment.[182] The result? Mind-boggling incoherence. Nearly within a week of Federal Reserve Board Chairman Jerome Powell announcing the United States as near "full reopening," CDC director Rochelle Walensky, fighting back tears, went off script at a press conference, pleading with Americans to continue to follow COVID safety protocols.[183]

U.S. daily cases have since declined, but some states are still in full-spectrum crisis. The Biden administration demanded Gretchen Whitmer of Michigan, one of the most progressive governors in the country, to lock down her state during a rager of a resurgence instead of sending her a surge of vaccines.[184] The governor had been targeted in a kidnapping plot in part for a previous lockdown.[185] Spinning off responsibility upon the states—especially blue states—is exactly what

Democrats had condemned of Trump.[186] And represents a political tin ear about the difficult spot that a member of their own party found herself.

The widening gyre recapitulated the American exceptionalism that allowed the virus wide entree to begin with earlier last year.

The Institute for Health Metrics and Evaluation at the University of Washington projected U.S. COVID deaths are wildly underestimated. In May, the Institute estimated 905,000 Americans had died of the disease, 58 percent more than on record.[187] Even that number was likely an underestimation.[188]

As other sources of mortality have declined during the outbreak in some states, COVID deaths likely make a *larger* proportion of the deviation from the average mortality rate. Other infectious deaths—for instance, from influenza, respiratory syncytial virus, and measles—declined. With the elderly especially hard hit by COVID since the start of the pandemic, age-associated mortality from ischemic heart disease and other end-of-life morbidities also declined.

It's a strategy in calculation that Restoration author Daniel Defoe took to the London plague of 1665:

The Second Week in *June,* the Parish of *St Giles's,* where still the Weight of the Infection lay, buried 120, whereof though the Bills said but 68 of the Plague; every body said there had been 100 at least, calculating it from the usual Number of Funerals in that Parish as above.[189]

On the other hand, as described by social epidemiologist Sandro Galea in a talk at the National Institutes of Health, other U.S. co-mortalities have *increased* during the COVID period, including cerebrovascular diseases, Alzheimer's and dementia, diabetes, and hypertension.[190] The feds more recently reported that the United States saw remarkable *increases* in heart disease, diabetes, and other common sources of mortality during the pandemic.[191] Many people may have failed to go to the hospital upon dangerous symptoms, fearing catching COVID or being blocked from access.

Doctor and medical sociologist Howard Waitzkin objected to IHME's stat readjustment on two other grounds. He noted on the Spirit of 1848 listserv that public health data worldwide, including the United States, are insufficient at best. Waitzkin's student was unable to follow up on infant mortality for migrant farmworkers:

> In brief, there was no way reliably to link a birth certificate in one state with a death certificate in another state (assuming a death certificate was produced) so even the mediocre reported infant mortality rates in the USA at the national, state, and county levels were underestimates. Mortality reporting from U.S. nursing homes, prisons, police departments, military institutions, and many other settings show similar deficiencies, often based on incomplete or inaccurate diagnoses recorded in death certificates.[192]

Waitzkin and others targeted more acute objections to IHME and its director Chris Murray around methodology, including a failure of transparency, lack of access to primary data, and problematic statistical modeling. The WHO's World Health Report 2000 that Murray co-chaired was subjected to similar criticisms, says Waitzkin.[193]

The Institute, Waitzkin continues, is funded in a major way by the Gates Foundation to the tune of *$600 million* and subjected to its undue influence.[194] This past year, as Tim Schwab writes in *The Nation*, IHME

> projected a far less severe outbreak than other models, which drew the attention of Donald Trump, who was eager to downplay the danger. At a March 31 [2020] press briefing, the White House's coronavirus response coordinator, Debbie Birx, with the president at her side, used IHME charts to show that the pandemic was rapidly winding down.[195]

The projection laid cover for opening up the states early on, a ruse that epidemiologists at Stanford University paid by the airline sector also attempted underestimating COVID mortality.[196]

Still other work pushed back in the other direction again, that we were getting pummeled worse than presumed. COVID's typically quoted case fatality rate of 1.5 percent missed the damage to so-called long-haulers, infecteds who suffer symptoms long after the initial infection.[197] Alexis Dinno and Jarvis Chen of Harvard worked out a back-of-the-envelope calculation on the Spirit of 1848 public health listserv:

- 28-day case fatality rate: 1.5 percent
- 20 percent hospitalization means that with 1.5 percent dead, 18.5 percent survived hospitalization
- Deaths rates of those 18.5 percent for six months post-hospitalization is one out of eight or 12.3 percent
- 29.4 percent of those who left hospital are rehospitalized
- So 1.5 percent original CFR + (18.5 percent x 29.4 percent x 12.3 percent) produces a new case fatality rate of 2.2 percent

With the politics swirling around all these numbers, policy decisions drawing upon them—some over others—appear baked in.

But unlike doctors and university researchers, U.S. public health officials have long had free range beyond the technicist thunderdome to conduct social experiments on whole populations by commission or omission without being subjected to malpractice, Institutional Review Board supervision, Freedom of Information requests, or, given Fauci adoration, public shame.[198]

THE WIDELY CIRCULATED CONTENTION that U.S. police require less training than a cosmetologist may not pass muster on a technicality.[199] But police stateside, killing many more civilians per capita than in other countries, receive much less training than their counterparts abroad.[200]

Setting aside the validity of another set of numbers—IQ tests speak more to what police departments believe matters—dumber cops are at a premium. A New London, Connecticut, police cadet's lawsuit appealing his application's rejection was itself rejected by a federal court:

> [Robert] Jordan, a 49-year-old college graduate, took the [police] exam in 1996 and scored 33 points, the equivalent of an IQ of 125. But New London police interviewed only candidates who scored 20 to 27, on the theory that those who scored too high could get bored with police work and leave soon after undergoing costly training.[201]

Critical judgment appears to be thought a liability.

Whereas one cop—or CDC administrator—is trained to jump to conclusions to protect themselves first and foremost, and in doing so also delivers the political class's cruelest messages about whose lives are worth what, others cultivate a myopia that renders them unable to see the worst of crimes. I'm not just talking privatized surplus value or wage theft, by far the worst property crime in raw numbers alone.[202] We have to limit our expectations of what qualifies as even permissible conversation in American company.

The brutal long-hauler mortality and the racial disparities in COVID deaths, both hidden out in the open, got me thinking of John Balcerzak, the president of the Milwaukee Police Association from 2005 to 2009.[203]

Balcerzak was originally fired in 1991, later reinstated, when as a patrol officer he returned a drugged-up fourteen-year-old Konerak Sinthasomphone, of Adam Toledo proportions and bleeding from his rectum, back to cannibalistic serial killer Jeffrey Dahmer in spite of Black bystander protests that the kid's life was in danger. Without essentializing matters too badly, one can't help but think the two white men shared a near-automated mutual understanding.

Much of what has been written to explain Dahmer can be found in part in the mirror of the representatives of the state that *refused* to capture him, despite the smell of another body, which Balcerzak and his fellow officers whiffed on visiting Dahmer's apartment. Plentiful data aren't enough.

What critic Jenny Diski writes of biographer Brian Masters's Dahmer[204] could as easily be applied to Balcerzak and the CDC:

> It's important, says Masters, that Dahmer is not a moral idiot. He knows right from wrong. But that is no proof against possession. The Devil only triumphs over a man capable of putting up a fight against him. Corruption must have a decent medium in which its bacilli [or viremia] can multiply. Dahmer was finally taken over, but there were periods when he tried for normality.[205]

From Dahmer to Balcerzak to a Weeping Mary of a Walensky—what an outrage of a 4-6-3 Braves double play! A slimy false equivalence, some will dismiss. But one can't help but hear in Diski's summary an exhaustion in the industry of death our three infielders share:

> The strongest and most awful image of both Dahmer and [serial killer Dennis] Nilsen is that of housekeeping in hell. Both come to a point where the bodies pile up around them—Dahmer taking a shower with two corpses in the tub—the smells are intolerable, the logistics of disposal impossible, and they are condemned to a seemingly unending task of dismembering, eviscerating, dissolving, and scrubbing away at the disorder and putrefaction they have created.
>
> All the classic images of hell are present in each of those flats, inhabited by the ghost of Hieronymus Bosch and the two increasingly bewildered, dull-minded men, who finally long to be caught so that their nightmares can stop.[206]

Look, reasonable professionals asked, with hundreds of COVID bodies still stored in refrigerated trucks on New York City wharves a year later, why not just call the pandemic off?[207]

THE FOG OF PANDEMIC, a class of epidemiological modeling pulled by contradictory interests, and just sheer exhaustion of a self-own of a public health response complicate our understanding of what COVID is doing and what to do about it.

The failure to act isn't necessarily merely a matter of not knowing the details or the unknown unknowns to reference the recently passed Donald Rumsfeld. Knowing full enough the order of mortality in play, the Trump administration's favorite intervention appeared malicious neglect.

If such Rumsfeldian horror differs from Walensky's anguish, since dabbed away by the Biden White House, it is in its "inability to reflect," as Errol Morris put it.[208] In ethnocentric terms that speak to Morris's upbringing, Rumsfeld, untouched by history, is

> the least Jewish person I'd ever met: no guilt, no self-loathing, no remorse, no self-doubt, no nothing. Just a kind of glib self-satisfaction—which I see with Trump, by the way. A glib kind of narcissistic self-love, almost like he's masturbating in public. And it's kind of gross.[209]

Other estimates projected 40 percent of U.S. COVID deaths could have been avoided.[210] As Sandro Galea described figure after figure in his talk, COVID's damage isn't just the roulette of chance encounter and immunogenetics. It's structured by race, class, and their interaction.[211]

Demographers Theresa Andrasfay and Noreen Goldman reported that the United States suffered yet another year of decline in life expectancy.[212] COVID helped shave off another 1.13 years from the American population. Black and Latino populations were estimated to be hit with four times greater a reduction than whites.

A March Familes USA report summarized research showing a third of COVID deaths were tied to the lack of health insurance.[213] The effect was multiplicative: "Each 10% increase in the proportion of a county's residents who lacked health insurance was associated with a 70% increase in COVID-19 cases and a 48% increase in COVID-19 deaths."

Controlling for stay-at-home orders, school closures, and mask mandates, another study, published in November, estimated that lifting eviction moratoriums state-to-state resulted in between 365,200 and 502,200 excess coronavirus cases and between 8,900 and 12,500 excess deaths.[214] Other research showed the impact to be cyclical. Renters in New York City COVID hotspots faced four times the likelihood of eviction (and back to greater exposure to COVID).[215]

What role are scientists to play in such a thatch of causes? A NIH staffer who helped moderate Galea's talk summed it up this way:

> We live in a society that is a capitalist society, that by its very nature generates inequality. But it is the only economic system that really generates enough wealth to make progress. So our role often is to manage those inequalities and try to mitigate them as we move forward and make progress across the country.[216]

Shades of a call by China's leader Xi Jinping's that the *New York Times* looked down its nose at six months later: "Science has no borders, but scientists have a motherland."[217]

The necropolitics extend far beyond such celebrated negligence and taking one for the economy. One op-ed placed our severe loss as a worthy warning to China that the United States was ready to sacrifice American lives.

The cruel flippancy isn't all 2020. At the beginning of 2021, environmental health scientist Jeffrey Shaman's group at Columbia University estimated 105 million Americans infected to that point, projecting 29 million more would be infected if even the inadequate nonpharmaceutical interventions in place were rolled back starting February.[218]

President Biden begged Americans to hold on to July 4, but by early April, the Texas Rangers allowed full-capacity attendance at opening day of the baseball season at Globe Life Field, with the state rolling back all mask mandates as it sits toward the bottom in vaccine inoculations.[219] The Atlanta Braves, in another state far behind in vaccination, started allowing full-capacity May 7.[220] Masks will still be required when fans aren't eating and drinking, a requirement so far largely unenforced to this point of the season.

University of Southern Mississippi's Justin Kurland and colleagues reported a link between NFL games with large numbers of fans attending and subsequent COVID infections in locales near the stadium.[221] A more recent WHO study found the same following European Championship soccer matches.[222] This "final" reopening followed exactly in line with the earlier reopenings or no closings at all that many U.S. states pursued through the entire outbreak.[223] But post-Trump flippancy isn't just a Southern thang.

Andrew Cuomo, the governor of New York who earned undue praise as the can-do anti-Trump during the early pandemic, continued his rivalry with New York City Mayor Bill de Blasio by demanding the city open up faster than the mayor first planned.[224] The rush proved an appropriate bookend to what began as a fiasco:

> New York Governor Andrew Cuomo, however, reacted to de Blasio's idea for closing down New York City [in March 2020] with derision. It was dangerous, he said, and served only to scare people. Language mattered, Cuomo said, and "shelter-in-place" sounded like it was a response to a nuclear apocalypse.[225]

The week delay and subsequent errors in public health protocol—improper patient transfers, insufficient isolation, procurement gaps—amplified New York deaths into what was then the world's primary epicenter.[226] All compounded, as health ecologist Deborah Wallace wrote for Pandemic Research for the People, by the long austerity program Cuomo pursued, including helping shed hospital beds in the thousands over his tenure.[227]

Hero Cuomo later was found to have covered up thousands of the COVID deaths that followed in statewide nursing homes.[228] As part of a month-long campaign, his aides excised 9,000 deaths from a state report on the matter, part of a campaign of repeatedly overruling state public health officials.[229] State scientific reports were buried. The release of the administration's own audit of the numbers was delayed. Health Department letters informing state legislators of the matter were never sent.

Cuomo's administration had dismissed criticism that forcing hospitalized nursing home patients who recovered from COVID back to their nursing homes helped spread the virus, contributing to 15,000 resident and home aide deaths. The administration also undercounted nursing home cases by the thousands and, eliciting an FBI investigation, underreported them to the Justice Department. Cuomo copped to the tactic, declaring he did so to rob Trump of political ammunition and a possible federal investigation.

Cuomo signed legislation that included language his staff stuck into a budget bill shielding health care executives from the threat of COVID lawsuits.[230] Two years previous, the Greater New York Hospital Association padded Cuomo's campaign coffers with $1.25 million to the Cuomo-controlled New York State Democratic committee. The rider would not provide the governor personal indemnity. Cuomo hired a personal attorney to defend him and his staff against any criminal charges for the nursing home deaths.[231] He would need lawyers on other matters. Cuomo aides, with family ties to lobbyists, spearheaded efforts to slime co-workers who accused the governor of on-the-job sexual harassment:

> Cuomo's powerful secretary, Melissa DeRosa, is married to Matthew Wing, his former press secretary who now serves as a top communications exec for Uber. Her father, Giorgio DeRosa, is a partner and chief Albany lobbyist for the influential Bolton St. Johns firm. Brother Joseph and sister Jessica also work at the firm.
>
> Chief of staff Jill DesRosiers, meanwhile, is life partner of Harry Giannoulis, president and co-founder of the Parkside Group—another Empire State lobbying behemoth. . . .
>
> Bolton St. Johns similarly cleaned up while repping some of America's most powerful corporations in Albany. The Durst Organization paid $60,000; United Airlines $30,000, and Pfizer $33,000 to lobby Cuomo's office.[232]

The efforts to cover for COVID and Cuomo's harassment got tied together. Larry Schwartz, a former Cuomo aide and now the state's vaccination czar, lobbied state Democratic leaders to support Cuomo during his political crisis:

> In one case, a county executive, who spoke on the condition of anonymity for fear of retaliation, said that after Mr. Schwartz had discussed the governor's political situation, he then pivoted directly to a conversation about vaccine distribution.
>
> In another example, a second county executive said Mr. Schwartz called immediately after a different Cuomo administration official had called about vaccine distribution.
>
> The second executive's legal counsel filed a preliminary complaint on Friday with the state attorney general's office's public integrity bureau about a possible ethics violation by the governor's office, according to an official with direct knowledge of the complaint.[233]

The complaints implied a Trumpian trade of county vaccines in return for support for Cuomo that Schwartz denied:

> Local officials in recent months have quietly raised worries that the Cuomo administration may have viewed its control over vaccine as a means to reward or punish local officials.[234]

Less connected staff similarly bore the political brunt of just trying to do their jobs.

Cuomo made staff work for free helping him write a book about his COVID prowess for which he received $4 million. His handling of the pandemic, including dismissing expertise in Trumpist terms, drove out nine top state health experts, including the state's deputy commissioner for public health, the director of the bureau of communicable diseases, and the state epidemiologist, who were asked to match their health guidelines to the policies Cuomo introduced without input at those press conferences for which he was so praised.[235]

De Blasio, now teaching pandemic leadership at the Harvard School of Public Health, tried to outcompete the governor in incompetence. Alongside driving out his health commissioner, he handed over the city's COVID contact tracing to an inexperienced crony who led the city's hospitals system and believed sheltering-in-place would not help curb the outbreak.[236]

City Comptroller Scott Stringer sued de Blasio for failing to turn over documents relating to the city's response to the outbreak, including how it failed to process $1.4 billion in medical supplies purchased in the early weeks of the pandemic.[237] The city lost track of ventilators and protective gear. It spent millions on masks that proved to be non-surgical.

In February this year, Cuomo let restaurants open up to an unenforceable 25 percent capacity, long before the vaccination campaign was even really begun. By April the CDC had joined Cuomo's New York—not just Texas—reversing course on nonpharmaceutical interventions and waving through reopening the country with the vaccine campaign at the time only a third complete.

But certainly the threats of poor planning and lessons left unlearned, including the nearly 2,000 New Yorkers found dead in their apartments the week ending early April 2020, can be put aside, officials argued. By June, New York City had what health officials took to labeling "functional immunity," a neologism that, with 76 percent of its 5 million target vaccinated at the time, presumably means that the city is comfortable with opening up.[238]

AS PHILOSOPHER SLAVOJ ŽIŽEK described, it's by these unknown knowns that commissars of various stripes pretend ignorance in the service of imperial expediency.[239]

I like "Those Nerdy Girls" over at @dear_pandemic. They're a group of epidemiologists who are middle-of-the-road on the science of the pandemic, but solidly so. Alongside a variety of sources, they keep me abreast of some of the fast-accumulating COVID research. "Middle-of-the-road" and only "some" data, as we noted with Officer Balcerzak, aren't enough. The questions asked and premises assumed are critical.

In May I took issue with their presentation of the CDC's new mask recommendations, which declared that those vaccinated could take off their masks in most situations. I objected if only because one data-backed result can greenlight a whole bunch of others that are not. That's the difference between epidemiology and public health:

> @dear_pandemic You present three propositions that while appearing logically interlocking, and cemented together by an implicit appeal to governmental authority, may not be justified as a deductive progression. 1/11
>
> You say, 1) CDC says masks off in most situations for those vaccinated. 2) Some places may still require people wear masks. And 3) we still haven't hit necessary benchmarks to drive the virus below its Allee threshold, under which the virus burns out on its own. 2/11
>
> You present the two last propositions as caveats: the second as a matter of level of jurisdiction (some places may still insist on masks) and the third as a second-order necessity that you spin off here as the responsibility of the unvaccinated. 3/11
>
> But the second two propositions aren't mere caveats. Their states depend on the first proposition that the U.S. has green-lighted dropping masks. 4/11
>
> Setting aside that reduced risk of transmission under vaccination is neither zero, nor captures its statistical dispersion, greenlighting taking off masks increases the likelihood circulation continues above the replacement you caution. We have only 1/3 of the population vaccinated. Multiple variants of documented vaccine resistance of a variety of orders are in increasing circulation. We know little of the relationship between breakthrough infections and superspreader events, as the New York Yankee cluster suggests. And we still offer nearly none of the contact tracing or targeted isolation pursued in other countries.[240] 5/11
>
> As you write, some businesses may still require masks for entry, but others, taking CDC's lead but not its rationale, will not. Is everyone at our neighborhood bars vaccinated? Many of

the establishments don't care. Biden has given them their plausible deniability. 6/11

It may be that the administration tried to leapfrog state efforts to roll back mask mandates entirely by pushing, but not requiring, no masks if and only if you're vaccinated. The administration appears to have willfully confused public health for individual choice under an honor system millions of Americans long violated by dint of necessity or because follow the leader or as a matter of vice signaling. It's a buffering that can be tolerated epidemiologically only at a herd immunity the U.S. has given up on. 7/11

In other words, the underlying data—from the state of population vaccine coverage to the still fully populated exposure matrices across host type to the mix of evolving variants already within U.S. borders against which American public health is unwilling to actively intervene—do not support the timing of the recommendations. And we were getting so close. 8/11

If anything, at the very least, shouldn't we make this a matter of the precautionary principle?[241] Or lessons learned? Pretending away China yesterday led to the deaths of 500,000 to 900,000 Americans. What will ignoring India or Indiana do today? Has Biden reversed Trump's dismissal of COVID as a blue state problem to one of an unvaccinated red state problem now that the professional-managerial class is protected? 9/11

As public trust is an epidemiological variable, the insistence of the CDC and Fauci to engineer such ill-supported policy may cater to an American exhaustion that could have been avoided if we had intervened as other countries did from the start, but it also only acts to further degrade public health as both discipline and practice. 10/11

I know it's only an Instagram post here, but one can't help but read between its lines a refusal to take on these issues openly. In the face of the kind of anti-science superstition you are fighting, we can err on the side of presenting science as something other than still socially bounded. 11/11

Those Nerdy Girls didn't reply to the comments. A subsequent post on science communication included the advice to ignore trolls.

IT WASN'T JUST INCORRIGIBLES like me. More august public health scholars objected to the CDC's new recommendations:

> Dr. Leana Wen, an emergency physician and public health professor at George Washington University, called the change "stunning" in a Friday interview with NPR. "CDC seems to have gone from one extreme of overcaution to another of basically throwing caution out the window."[242]

David Holtgrave and Eli Rosenberg, Dean of Public Health and Professor of Epidemiology at SUNY Albany, respectively, assured anyone disturbed by the CDC decision that they weren't alone:

> Unfortunately, we are still not across the finish line in the U.S. pandemic. There is still a COVID-19 death about every 2.5 minutes in the nation, and serious racial and ethnic disparities exist (e.g., in disproportionate access to vaccination services). There are six major concerns about the decision to roll back some key safety measures when in fact we need all of the tools we have in the COVID-19 prevention toolbox for perhaps just a short time longer.[243]

The first of the six concerns is that the CDC did not inform the vaccinated what risks they still faced. The vaccines aren't perfect. And the surveillance system isn't up to capturing all the breakthrough infections. Second, the CDC threw the vaccinated who wished to support public health by continuing to wear masks under the social bus. Mask use in some circles would be stigmatized, Holtgrave and Rosenberg predicted. It has been.[244]

Third, the CDC offered no follow-up in getting the unvaccinated vaccinated, an omission to which we will return. Fourth, as touched on above, there's no means by which most businesses or other institutions can verify any unmasked is vaccinated. They shouldn't. Under the previous recommendation, they didn't have to as a matter of public health course. Fifth, the policy would have been better tied to a specific milestone to aim for, such as only fifty to a hundred U.S. daily COVID deaths. Finally, we need all tools—biomedical and non-pharmaceutical—to get us to a true pandemic finish line (rather than a passing interruption in some quarters).

Infectious disease reporter Ed Yong elaborated on what long-documented public health strategy comprised:

> The U.S. also largely ignored other measures that could have protected entire communities, such as better ventilation, high-filtration masks for essential workers, free accommodation for people who needed to isolate themselves, and sick-pay policies. As the country focused single-mindedly on a vaccine endgame, and Operation Warp Speed sped ahead, collective protections were left in the dust. And as vaccines were developed, the primary measure of their success was whether they prevented symptomatic disease in individuals. . . .
>
> Ian Mackay, a virologist at the University of Queensland, famously imagined pandemic defenses as layers of Swiss cheese. Each layer has holes, but when combined, they can block a virus. In Mackay's model, vaccines were the last layer of many. But the U.S. has prematurely stripped the others away, including many of the most effective ones. A virus can evolve around a vaccine, but it cannot evolve to teleport across open spaces or punch its way through a mask.
>
> And yet, the country is going all in on vaccines, even though 48 percent of Americans still haven't had their first dose, and despite the possibility that it might fall short of herd immunity. Instead of asking, "How do we end the pandemic?" it seems to be asking, "What level of risk can we tolerate?" Or perhaps, "Who gets to tolerate that risk?"[245]

The CDC position wasn't just a violation of ideas. National Nurses

United, representing thousands of nurses, left to garbage-bag gowns
early in the pandemic, demolished CDC talking points:[246]

- **A continued high number of Covid cases in the United States,**
  with more than 35,000 new detected infections reported each
  day, and more than 600 people dying from Covid each day.
  Yesterday, 780 people died from Covid-19.
- **Circulation of Covid variants of concern** that are more transmissible, deadlier, and may already be or may become vaccine
  resistant.
- **Unanswered questions about vaccines.** Nurses emphasize that
  it's unclear how well vaccines prevent asymptomatic and mild
  Covid infections, how well vaccines prevent transmission of the
  virus, and how long protection from vaccines will last.
- **The CDC announced they would no longer be tracking
  infections among fully vaccinated people unless they result
  in hospitalization or death.** This means that the CDC is no
  longer tracking data necessary to understand whether vaccines prevent asymptomatic/mild infections, how long vaccine
  protection may last, and to understand how variants impact
  vaccine protection.
- **The CDC "recognized" scientific evidence on aerosol transmission but refused to update guidance based on science.**
  Nurses say the CDC needs to fully recognize aerosol transmission and update its Covid guidance accordingly to prioritize
  measures that prevent and reduce aerosol transmission (ventilation, respiratory protection, testing to identify asymptomatic
  cases). "If the CDC had fully recognized the science on how this
  deadly virus is transmitted, this new guidance would never have
  been issued," said NNU President Jean Ross, RN.
- **Preventing and reducing transmission of Covid requires multiple layers of protective measures.** Nurses say this includes
  masks, distancing, and avoiding crowds and large gatherings—
  in addition to vaccines. Importantly, it also includes protecting
  nurses and other frontline workers from workplace exposure

to the virus. Vaccines are only one important component of a robust, public health infection control program. "All of our protective measures should remain in place, in addition to vaccines. This pandemic is not over," said NNU President Deborah Burger, RN. "Nurses follow the precautionary principle, which means that until we know for sure something is safe, we use the highest level of protections, not the lowest. The CDC is putting lives at risk with this latest guidance."

- **The recent guidelines are unjust and will disproportionately harm Black, Indigenous, and people of color.** "There has been so much inequity in the vaccine rollout and racial inequity in who is a frontline worker put most at risk by this guidance. The impact of the CDC's guidance update will be felt disproportionately by workers of color and their families and communities," said NNU President Zenei Triunfo-Cortez, RN.

- **National Nurses United said the new CDC guidance underlines the importance of OSHA issuing a long overdue OSHA emergency temporary standard (ETS) on infectious diseases without delay.** "If OSHA does not issue a Covid ETS immediately, we will undoubtedly see more unnecessary, preventable infections and deaths, as well as long Covid cases among nurses and other frontline workers," said Triunfo-Cortez.[247]

Fifteen months late, OSHA finally got around to instituting, rather than merely recommending, the emergency occupational standards for the health sector.[248] Employers are now expected to keep infected workers off-site, notify workers of COVID exposure, and report worker deaths and hospitalizations.

Most other sectors remain exempted,[249] including the food industries through which COVID raged, from farm to processing to grocery store and restaurant:

The new standard "represents a broken promise to the millions of American workers in grocery stores and meatpacking plants who have gotten sick and died on the frontlines of this pandemic," Marc Peronne, president of the United Food and Commercial Workers Union, which represents 1.3 million workers, said in a statement.

Debbie Berkowitz, a former OSHA official who now works at the National Employment Law Project, said the new rules fail to protect many low-wage workers, such as slaughterhouse employees who work shoulder-to-shoulder on production lines.[250]

Pushing off pestilence upon the "essential" workers is one of modernity's ancestral features. "It must be confest," Daniel Defoe copped,

> that tho' the Plague was chiefly among the Poor; yet, were the Poor the most Venturous and Fearless of it, and went about their Employment, with a Sort of brutal Courage; I must call it so, for it was founded neither on Religion or Prudence; scarse did they use any Caution, but run into any Business, which they could get Employment in, tho' it was the most hazardous; such was that of tending the Sick, watching Houses shut up, carrying infected Persons to the Pest-House; and which was still worse, carrying the Dead away to their Graves.[251]

THE IMPACTS OF REPEALING the mask mandate ripped through the body politic. Despite the pushback from our essential workers, Heroes of the Front Line, the American people followed the leaders. Freedom rang! People—vaccinated or not—hit the bars and restaurants, documented superspreader sites, to toast repudiating the latex-fisted rule of the scientists.[252]

My son's school reopened with only five weeks left in the semester. Despite making physical attendance optional, Minnesota governor Tim Walz refused to wait until the fall when all students would likely be vaccinated. Within a week, new cases were detected among those who went back to the kid's school.

Back east, de Blasio—who closed schools a week later than his public health staff advised, contributing to an estimated 22,000 excess deaths in New York City—preemptively *banned* online school for the next year.[253]

By the Thursday before the Memorial Day 2021 weekend, "As Pandemic Ebbs" *St Paul Pioneer Press* headlined the AP report, 1.8 million Americans traveled by air, with airports such as Orlando reaching 90 percent capacity.[254] Despite the open skies—feel free to move about the country, to use a post-9/11 line—flight crews were being subjected to record assaults largely due to expectations that masks be worn in airports and in the air, as if passengers got the impression somewhere that wearing masks was over.[255]

The Republican states long had left the public health orbit, but Democrats since have joined them. The political landscape beyond fractures. There's the usual. Leftists and liberals opposed Trump together. Now many liberals rally around Biden, while many leftists object to neoliberal restoration.[256]

At the same time, Biden is making a gesture of a Keynesian spending program that Republicans, making appeals to "the working man," are trying to kill while Biden also abandons rolling back student debt and berates unemployment beneficiaries for refusing to return to work.

Some liberals are objecting to CDC falling back on mask recommendations, while there are leftists who object to any lockdown as a matter of emotional well-being or economic survival in a capitalism little of their choosing.

As the nurses noted, the CDC announced it would no longer tabulate mild COVID cases for the vaccinated.[257] We're back at Trump's suggestion that if we stopped counting cases, we wouldn't have so much COVID. Does Biden differ from Trump more by degree (and tone) than kind?[258]

It's a question for much of American public health as well. Before the year was out, Leanna Wen, who we quoted expressing shock at the CDC's new mask mandate, would take a full turn and berate administration officials for not opening up fast enough.[259] By August 2022, the American Public Health Association had invited Wen to speak at its annual conference. Harvard School of Public Health profs and Randi

Weingarten of the American Federation of Teachers supported even further loosening of COVID recommendations for quarantining at home and ending testing people without symptoms.[260]

IT'S WORTH QUOTING YONG at length on the structural ethnography in play, both acted out and led by Biden's CDC:

> Framing one's health as a matter of personal choice "is fundamentally against the very notion of public health," Aparna Nair, a historian and an anthropologist of public health at the University of Oklahoma, told me. "For that to come from one of the most powerful voices in public health today . . . I was taken aback." (The CDC did not respond to a request for comment.)
>
> It was especially surprising coming from a new administration. Donald Trump was a manifestation of America's id—an unempathetic narcissist who talked about dominating the virus through personal strength while leaving states and citizens to fend for themselves. Joe Biden, by contrast, took COVID-19 seriously from the off, committed to ensuring an equitable pandemic response, and promised to invest $7.4 billion in strengthening America's chronically underfunded public-health workforce. And yet, the same peal of individualism that rang in his predecessor's words still echoes in his. "The rule is very simple: Get vaccinated or wear a mask until you do," Biden said after the CDC announced its new guidance. "The choice is yours."
>
> From its founding, the United States has cultivated a national mythos around the capacity of individuals to pull themselves up by their bootstraps, ostensibly by their own merits. This particular strain of individualism, which valorizes independence and prizes personal freedom, transcends administrations. It has also repeatedly hamstrung America's pandemic response. It explains why the U.S. focused so intensely on preserving its hospital capacity instead of on measures that would have saved people from even needing a hospital. It explains why so many

Americans refused to act for the collective good, whether by masking up or isolating themselves. And it explains why the CDC, despite being the nation's top public-health agency, issued guidelines that focused on the freedoms that vaccinated people might enjoy.

The move signaled to people with the newfound privilege of immunity that they were liberated from the pandemic's collective problem. It also hinted to those who were still vulnerable that their challenges are now theirs alone and, worse still, that their lingering risk was somehow their fault. ("If you're not vaccinated, that, again, is taking your responsibility for your own health into your own hands," [CDC Director Rochelle] Walensky said.)

Neither is true. About half of Americans have yet to receive a single vaccine dose; for many of them, lack of access, not hesitancy, is the problem. The pandemic, meanwhile, is still just that—a pandemic, which is raging furiously around much of the world, and which still threatens large swaths of highly vaccinated countries, including some of their most vulnerable citizens. It is still a collective problem, whether or not Americans are willing to treat it as such.

Individualism can be costly in a pandemic. It represents one end of a cultural spectrum with collectivism at the other—independence versus interdependence, "me first" versus "we first." These qualities can be measured by surveying attitudes in a particular community, or by assessing factors such as the proportion of people who live, work, or commute alone. Two studies found that more strongly individualistic countries tended to rack up more COVID-19 cases and deaths.

A third suggested that more individualistic people (from the U.S., U.K, and other nations) were less likely to practice social distancing. A fourth showed that mask wearing was more common in more collectivist countries, U.S. states, and U.S. counties—a trend that held after accounting for factors including political affiliation, wealth, and the pandemic's severity. These correlative studies all have limitations, but across them, a consistent pattern emerges—one supported by a closer look at the U.S. response.[261]

The domain violation—applying individualist interventions to structural problems—is *de rigueur* at this point and extends far beyond pols washing their hands, if you'll excuse the bon mots.

"I'm watching a press conference about that Miami building ollapse," observed *Organizing Work*'s Marianne Garneau,

> and I can't believe how through-the-looking-glass we are with hypersubjective, individualistic discourse. The elected officials are praising what heroes the first responders are, and not giving any factual update about death count or the search. When it comes to whether the twin building in the same development risks collapsing, they're saying that *if* residents *feel* unsafe, resources will be made available to them to relocate. No comment on the actual structural integrity.
>
> The reporters are talking about how family members of collapse victims are feeling frustrated with authorities, but chalking this up to trauma and grief. We can't even describe reality anymore except in terms of individual perception and feeling. Obviously that goes hand-in-glove with a lack of institutional accountability, as in this case.
>
> Also, the left is completely on this subjectivizing bandwagon, if not driving it.[262]

To Yong's Durkheim we might add a Marx who asks in what ways the imperial moment waves through such pathological behavior even, or *especially,* among our public health elite.[263] Elsewhere we've written on how upon neoliberalism's rise, public health was neglected or monetized on the far side of the U.S. cycle of accumulation.[264] As independent scholar Nick Jackson underscores, American (and other metropole) public health practitioners embody the "hidden agency" by which such annihilation is rationalized (and enforced) as a Kantian duty.[265]

As pathetic as American public health has been for decades, the CDC's decision—albeit subjected to still ongoing and widespread condemnation—effectively destroyed what little was left of public health as a concept here.

One sees in the U.S. vaccine-abetted reopening all the failures of engineering and empire the wonder of the *Titanic* represented. Author Joseph Conrad presented the sunk unsinkable as a trope of sociotechnicist fantasy and the diseconomies of scale and inequality:

> You build a 45,000 tons hotel of thin steel plates to secure the patronage of, say, a couple of thousand rich peoples (for if it had been for the emigrant trade alone, there would have been no such exaggeration of mere size), you decorate it in the style of the Pharaohs or in the Louis Quinze style—I don't know which—and to please the aforesaid fatuous handful of individuals, who have more money than they know what to do with, and to the applause of two continents you launch that mass with 2,000 people on board at 21 knots across the sea—a perfect exhibition of the modern blind trust in mere material and appliances.[266]

The kind of idealist empiricism philosopher Ludwig Wittgenstein warned about.[267]

One immediately recalls the hog hotels being built in China, a thousand head per floor patrolled by robots, whole campuses at this point, unsunkable sinks for African Swine Fever and swine influenzas still clunking through their irresistible evolutionary ratchets.[268]

THE DISCORDANCE SPILLS OVER abroad.

The *New York Times* ran an amazing photo.[269] By its terse caption, the *Times* had no idea how amazing. In the car on the passenger's side, the *Times* failed to identify Peter Daszak, the president of the EcoHealth Alliance and, strangely, also a member of the WHO team that investigated the origins of the COVID-19 outbreak in and around Wuhan. The team posted its final report in March.[270]

I say "strangely" because Daszak is a central figure in the lab leak theory of the origins of the outbreak. The EcoHealth Alliance used NIH and likely Department of Defense funding to bring coronavirus gain-of-function studies from a post-moratorium United States to China, including the Wuhan Institute of Virology.[271] Whether the lab leak actually happened, the EHA connection is a matter of the scientific record, it isn't conspiratorial bunk.

It happens that I am a proponent of the field hypothesis of the COVID's origins.[272] I believe the genomics of the virus and the sheer numbers of SARS-like strains circulating over tens of thousands of bats, wild food animals, and livestock likely favor origins "out there" in a south-central China landscape of post-BRICS development.

But for the past decade, such marginal figures as Pulitzer Prize–winner Laurie Garrett, Princeton's Matt Keeling, Yale's Alison Galvani, and Harvard's Marc Lipsitch have sounded vociferous alarm about the increasing likelihood of lab leaks. More acutely here, the absurdity of having someone so integral to the lab leak possibility helping lead the investigation—its report declared the lab leak "extremely unlikely"—is a violation of any investigatory protocol. And this at the highest level of public health diplomacy. Or, maybe, *because* it's at the highest level of such diplomacy. The *Times* writes:

> One member of the team of experts, Peter Daszak, a British disease ecologist who runs EcoHealth Alliance, a New York-based pandemic prevention group, pushed back against the criticism of the team's work and of China's level of cooperation. He said the lab leak hypothesis was "political from the start."[273]

Elsewhere:

> The experts had said that officials at the Wuhan Institute of Virology, which houses a state-of-the-art laboratory known for its research on bat coronaviruses, assured them that they were not handling any viruses that appeared to be closely related to the coronavirus that caused the recent pandemic, according to

meeting notes included in the report. They also said that staff members had been trained in security protocols.[274]

The EHA-Wuhan team's own publications and the gray literature around the possible spillover event in a Yunnan cave in 2012, samples from which were brought to Wuhan, suggest otherwise.

I traced the EcoHealth Alliance's role in helping move the gain-of-function studies to China in *Dead Epidemiologists*.[275] I also weighed in on the two hypotheses.[276]

While I believe the field hypothesis is the right one, the WHO report, however interesting some of its data and details, has little to do with scientific integrity. And the WHO leadership agreed, remarkably abandoning its own team's report.[277]

SO, AGAINST DASZAK'S VERY political denial, all epidemiology is now politics. To some, an efficacious vaccine means continued caution is symbolic of a left giving the political right power to question the vaccine. If you wish to defeat the right, the argument goes, get a vaccine and hit the bars. Shop, America's Mayor Rudy Giuliani suggested post-9/11.

By June, India loomed over such hedonic power of the now, with reports its B.1.617 variant was powering through even some of the few vaccinated there. The South African B.1.351 demolishes the AstraZeneca vaccine. Brazil's P.1, now ours too, significantly reduces Pfizer protection, even as that vaccine protects against the British B.1.1.7 and the South African variant. The Moderna vaccine shows nearly five times decline in mean factor of neutralization titers against P.1 and, although good against the B.1.1.7, a twelve-fold decline against the B.1.351 strain.[278]

More recent work indicated that the Pfizer vaccine works against the B.1.617.2 variant, now known as the Delta variant, but with a reduced efficacy in producing neutralizing antibodies particularly after the first shot.[279] The result puts a damper on some governments' strategies around getting a single shot in as many people as possible first. The study looks like solid science—paid for by a list of pharmaceutical companies interested in showing the reality that we'll need booster shots here on out—in part because many governments chose to avoid suppressing outbreaks early on.

The younger demographics some suggested protected the Global South—as well as here in the United States—are starting to suffer more serious COVID damage (beyond merely that the elderly are getting vaccinated out of the mortality equation).[280] The open-air ventilation of the slums and possible low-dose exposures of previously circulating coronavirus may not be protecting the poor any more either, if they ever did.

It's like the virus evolves or something. On the demand side, as my father and mathematical epidemiologist Rodrick Wallace models, the failures of statecraft and institutional cognition set the course of the rebounds sloshing at increasing amplitudes across the planet for months at a time.[281] To be filtered out only at the borders of states that can pivot on the public health dime the United States, the richest country in the history of humanity, says it doesn't have.

As our team led by evolutionary biologist Kenichi Okamoto modeled in December, an outbreak is a dialectic.[282] Our public health responses can change viral life history, including, in some parts of the parameter space, out from underneath prophylaxes or quarantines. And, one would hope, vice-versa, that changing our interventions can change viral evolution in our favor.

Evolutionary geneticist Cock van Oosterhout and colleagues warned about the new variants:[283]

1) The faster the virus burns through a population of susceptibles with only partial natural immunity left behind, against the Biden moment, the *more* complete the vaccination campaign must be.

2) Transmission rates aren't just about infectiousness. A successful variant could lean on a change in its life history, including lengthening its transmission period. I'd say whether that would select for a less acute infection

is an open question. The relationship between virulence and infectivity is a multidimensional object we have no business pretending to predict.

It needn't end up that way, of course. Perhaps all these possible complications aren't enough to punch through vaccination's secular blanket that the United States, however reluctantly, appears—maybe—on its way to sharing with the world.

Yes, the vaccines work (against most variants presently circulating). In opposition to raw vaccine skepticism, data are now in that the vaccines do presently lower viral load and reduce subsequent transmission. To what level from person to person is always an open question, but the sterilizing immunity is at least partial.[284] If the vaccines have problems in blocking subsequent variants, a COVID infection alone doesn't do nearly the same damage. Any adverse effects from vaccines, even rarely death, don't anywhere nearly match the deaths from letting COVID run free.

If vaccine skepticism were the main standard, we'd be in the medals. But there's much more involved. Even without inducing herd immunity, vaccines can drive local outbreaks below their population of replacement. As China showed, the arduous contact tracing and rapid testing *we still refuse* to pursue in this country can root out the last of circulating virus by isolating those few still infected.

Life is in danger everyday anyway, a more louche argument goes. If we find ourselves back where we started, shrugging our shoulders at a new outbreak half a world away all over again, that doesn't mean we're in danger. It's been a horror of a plague year already. The damage in risking a type 2 error—preparing for an outbreak that proves a nothingburger—is too much to bear. Substitute back the type 1 error—failing to prepare for a nasty outbreak—that trapped us in the first place. It's a risk already built into the system, a mirror in which at the very least we can recognize ourselves, as Yong observed.

So, setting aside that last bit of caustic sarcasm, by all means enjoy a beer outdoors with friends. It neither marks a betrayal of global solidarity, nor—contra Colbert, who later copped to getting Long

COVID—does it celebrate the end of the pandemic. If the Kiwis can attend rugby matches in their unmasked thousands almost a whole year ago because their government extirpated their outbreak, we can poke our tan-lined faces up for a pint.

If only, one would hope, to blow off steam for our return to the task still at hand that we can't wave away as *Pandemic's* season finale. We are still obligated to fight for people across the Global South—from the South Side of Chicago to South America—still subjected to the worst of the pandemic.

FOR EVEN AS SARS-2 isn't as swift an evolver as other RNA viruses, as it typically "spell-checks" its genome upon replication, the millions of infected worldwide allows the coronavirus broad experimentation. The SARS-2 evolutionary tree looks like one of those Higgs boson figures—we see a spray of emerging variants.[285]

It appears this variation in part explains why a vaccine-led herd immunity presently may be dead in the water as a public health goal. It isn't just a matter of the failure of hitting some vaccination threshold—although that will likely also trip us—both within any one country and worldwide. Or even a slow decay in vaccine efficaciousness (something to which we alluded and to which we'll return). It's that herd immunity may not be what we think.

In reality, population immunity appears an ongoing negotiation in time and place.

Lewis Buss's group tested for COVID antibodies in blood samples from what was a largely uncontrolled outbreak in Manaus, the capital of Amazonas state in northern Brazil.[286] They found the population there 76 percent infected by October 2020 but had not achieved the vaunted herd immunity. Even with a young population and low death rates, the outbreak in Manaus continued to march on, including in the face of nonpharmaceutical interventions.

The team speculated the result may be due to overestimating the attack rate. The population hadn't been so infiltrated. Or maybe it's because immunity wanes and those infected are returned to the pool of susceptibles. It may be a matter of an antigenic shift that resets the immunity clock for the virus like a cache of video game health points picked up through the maze of the favelas. But if we are to take the results on their face value, the key lesson may be that populations may differ in what counts as herd immunity.[287] Indeed, *there may be no threshold at all.*

No worries, we can still defeat the virus. But as we touched on above, many countries, including the wealthiest, choose not to engage in the contact tracing and case isolation to drive the pathogen population below its rate of replacement. That's "big government," a pejorative, even if the military-industrial complex and police militarism are too.

Early in the pandemic, as we also noted, the Global South seemed somehow protected, with relatively few cases there. Hypotheses orbited around a variety of mutually inclusive possibilities: truncated surveillance, younger demographics, open-air (and therefore ventilated) slums, and prior exposures to SARS-like coronaviruses producing herd immunity before the fact.[288]

But Brazil and, by mid-May, India shelved much of those expedient hopes, with shades of Dahmer's bathtub:

Hundreds of corpses have been found floating in the river or buried in the sand of [the Ganges] banks. Those who live close to where they have washed up, in the northern state of Uttar Pradesh, fear they are Covid-19 victims.

India has been overwhelmed by a devastating second wave of the pandemic in recent weeks. It has recorded more than 25 million cases and 275,000 deaths, but experts say the real death toll is several times higher.

The bodies on the river banks, taken together with funeral pyres burning round-the-clock and cremation grounds running out of space, tell the story of a death toll unseen and unacknowledged in official data.[289]

Uruguay's 2020 success controlling the outbreak lost out to 2021 complacency, government concerns about the economy (leaving restaurants open), and getting squeezed between two major epicenters, Argentina and Brazil.[290] The country's model Tetris program—test, trace, and isolate—faltered in the face of the ensuing onslaught.

Journalist Sarah Jaffe summarized the Colbert ilk's toxic positivity:

"Why isn't everyone back to normal?" They'll complain, ignoring that the pandemic is still ravaging the world—in places where the goods we consume are produced, in neighborhoods where the service workers they depend on live.[291]

Marching essential workers into COVID's maw is a global sleight of hand.

The reductionist's favored answer appears to be to vaccinate the planet. But that still requires the very public health networks countries failed to build for the previous year's nonpharmaceutical responses. It's also a program that was attacked from the very start.

There are the structurally rigged roadblocks represented by, for instance, monetizing what is clearly a public good:

Three of the leading Covid vaccine manufacturers have paid out $26bn in dividends and stock buyouts to shareholders in the last year—enough to cover the cost of vaccinating the population of Africa, say campaigners.

The People's Vaccine Alliance argues that the profits made by the companies are inappropriate when most of the world cannot get the vaccines they need, which are expensive and in short supply. Campaigners want to see the companies waive their patents and help set up factories to make affordable versions of their vaccines around the world.

The alliance estimates that Pfizer has paid out $8.44bn in dividends, Johnson & Johnson $10.5bn in dividends and $3.2bn in share buybacks, and AstraZeneca $3.6bn in dividends.

The demand for vaccines, at a time when the global economy is at a standstill, is responsible for a new wave of billionaires, it says. Uğur Şahin, the founder of BioNTech, which partnered with Pfizer to produce the vaccine he and his wife invented, now has shares worth $5.9bn. Stéphane Bancel, the CEO of Moderna, which produced a vaccine with similar mRNA technology, is worth $5.2bn.

"This is a public health emergency, not a private profit opportunity," said Anna Marriott, a health policy adviser at Oxfam, which is part of the alliance. "We should not be letting corporations decide who lives and who dies while boosting their profits."[292]

The market doesn't just enrich publicly financed companies whose commodities work, it also enriches those whose products don't work.

The *New York Times* has been reporting on the problems of U.S.-based Emergent Biosolutions, a politically connected pharmaceutical company that won an early no-bid, high-cost, paid-up-front federal contract to produce Johnson & Johnson and AstraZeneca vaccines in the millions.[293] Emergent's long-criticized Baltimore factory, which never earned regulatory approval, mixed up inputs for the two vaccines and trafficked vaccine waste through its production unit. Emergent's two other plants were tagged by regulators as "obsolete" and suffering quality control problems.[294]

The foul-up cut off vaccines not only stateside but for countries across three continents.[295] Even as Emergent hadn't delivered a single usable vaccine dose under Operation Warp Speed and had been placed by the FDA under investigation, its board of directors awarded five executives millions in bonuses:

> Dr. Robert Kadlec, a former Trump administration official who oversaw the agency that awarded Covid-19 contracts, had previously worked as a consultant for Emergent. Dr. Kadlec has said that he did not negotiate the Emergent deal but did approve it.[296]

Trump administrators weren't the only politicos looped in:

> Since 2018, federal campaign records show, [Emergent founder

and CEO Fuad] El-Hibri and his wife, Nancy, have donated at least $150,000 to groups affiliated with the top Republican on the [House] panel [to which El-Hibri was to testify], Representative Steve Scalise of Louisiana, as well as Mr. Scalise's campaigns. At least two other members of the subcommittee received donations during the 2020 election cycle from the company's political action committee, which has given about $1.4 million over the past 10 years to members of both parties.[297]

Yet another Pharma Bro that Congress helped launch and who representatives can now performatively chastise to keep the shell game going.[298]

THEN THERE ARE THE more acutely targeted obstacles to riches.

We touched on the lowbrow campaign Andrew Cuomo launched upon his own public health programs. Very Mussolini and his late trains that transport administrators were bullied by the regime into failing to report. Perhaps only a little less fashy than Governor Rick DeSantis who sent state police, guns drawn, to raid a Department of Health epidemiologist's home. Rebekah Jones had blown the whistle on Florida's efforts to manipulate case data.[299]

Noises early in the pandemic out of WHO, NIH, NIAID, and the *Financial Times,* among other surprising outlets, suggested all pharmaceuticals, vaccines included, would make open medicine available to all at no cost. Sentiments were turned into action or, to start, a platform—the WHO COVID-19 Technology Access Pool, or C-TAP—to be made accessible to all private and public entities aiming to produce medicine.

Bill Gates, with overwhelming influence on public health up into UN executive offices, put a kibosh on the effort, getting the Covid-19 ACT-Accelerator launched under the WHO flag.[300]

The Gates-run Accelerator—like the Vaccine Alliance Gates launched in 1999—organized R&D and distribution under the old model of intellectual property. That included COVAX, the WHO effort to distribute the vaccine to nations that couldn't afford the mad dash for vaccine access among the richer countries. "[COVAX]," *New Republic*'s Alexander Zaitchik writes,

> aimed to provide vaccines for up to 20 percent of the population in low-to-middle-income countries. After that, governments would largely have to compete on the global market like everyone else. It was a partial demand-side solution to what the movement coalescing around a call for a "people's vaccine" warned would be a dual crisis of supply and access, with intellectual property at the center of both. . . .
>
> One year later, the ACT-Accelerator has failed to meet its goal of providing discounted vaccines to the "priority fifth" of low-income populations. The drug companies and rich nations that had so much praise for the initiative a year ago have retreated into bilateral deals that leave little for anybody else. "The low- and middle-income countries are pretty much on their own, and there's just not much out there," said Peter Hotez, dean of the National School of Tropical Medicine in Houston. . . .
>
> The timeline for supplying poor and middle-income countries with enough vaccines to achieve herd immunity, meanwhile, has been pushed into 2024. . . . The truth repeated so often throughout the pandemic—no one is safe until everyone is safe—remains in force.[301]

Gates and his ilk have again turned virtue hoarding into a front for genocide. As Zaitchik continues:

> It embodies Gates's philanthropic approach to widely anticipated problems posed by intellectual property–hoarding companies able to constrain global production by prioritizing rich countries and inhibiting licensing. Companies partnering with COVAX are allowed to set their own tiered prices. They are subject to almost no transparency requirements and to toothless contractual nods to "equitable access" that have never been enforced.

Crucially, the companies retain exclusive rights to their intellectual property. If they stray from the Gates Foundation line on exclusive rights, they are quickly brought to heel. When the director of Oxford's Jenner Institute had funny ideas about placing the rights to its COVAX-supported vaccine candidate in the public domain, Gates intervened.[302]

In short, Gates and the pharmaceutical giants his foundation represents are the bottleneck through which the Global South can't get its COVID vaccines. "The artificial shortage of vaccines," South Africa intervened at the WTO TRIPS Council in February, "is primarily caused by the inappropriate use of intellectual property rights."[303]

STATESIDE, FORMER DEMOCRATIC PARTY presidential candidate Howard Dean, a medical doctor and a lobbyist at the Dentons firm, has been helping lead the industry charge protecting intellectual property. In March, Dean wrote in *Barron's*:

IP protections aren't the cause of vaccination delays. . . . Every drug manufacturing facility on the planet that's capable of churning out Covid-19 shots is already doing so. But there are almost 8 billion people on Earth. Even if we max out production—and we are—it's going to take over a year to fully vaccinate the global population.[304]

Lee Fang at *The Intercept* has been writing a series of articles debunking these talking points:

Dean's claim that global vaccine manufacturing is already at capacity is patently false. Foreign firms have lined up to offer pharmaceutical plants to produce vaccines but have been forced to enter into lengthy negotiations under terms set by the intellectual property owners. The [WTO] waiver, however, would allow generic drug producers to begin copying the vaccine without delay.[305]

An army of a hundred lobbyists has been launched upon the Biden administration and U.S lawmakers to oppose unexpected signals that the administration would back efforts for a temporary WTO waiver:

> "The drug company lobbyists are saying the TRIPS waiver won't increase the supply of vaccines, but if that's true, why do they oppose it? Because they think it will in fact expand production," noted James Love, director of Knowledge Ecology International, a group that supports the waiver petition.[306]

The sausage-making behind lobbying Washington—distributing talking points and collecting congressional signatures—recapitulates Pharmaceutical Research and Manufacturers of America's successful efforts at blocking anti-HIV generics a generation ago.[307]

Hollywood is also supporting the bipartisan push against the WTO waiver, if only because it would represent an intolerable precedence.[308] Better a few million more dead from COVID than letting Bollywood produce a Modi Comics Universe or some kid sell some knockoff DVDs on the streets of Jakarta. Talking points are extending to publishing and that paragon of respecting artists' rights, the music industry:

> Neil Turkewitz, a former Recording Industry Association of America official, blasted the proposal on Twitter, claiming it will harm musicians, performers, and other cultural workers who are already struggling.
>
> "As COVID has undermined the livelihoods of creators around the [globe emoji], you want to further expand their precarity—in the name of justice?" Turkewitz wrote.[309]

Fang reminds us of the crackdown early on in the pandemic against a couple of cowboy hospitals that 3D-printed replacement parts for what were a limited supply of ventilators, as if the unauthorized parts and not an economy of scarcity and a legislated repair monopoly were the problem.[310]

China appears little constrained by such self-medication, as it were. It has its own problems, of course, but took full advantage of the historical moment to send out far more vaccines than the United States first appeared to be willing to supply.[311]

The United States has since upped its offer, as much a matter of pharmaceutical diplomacy competing with China as any gesture of global solidarity.[312]

At least this country now appears attuned to these dynamics. Earlier in the year, the U.S. ideological apparatus's self-regard spun a failure to help as offering exactly that. The *Star-Tribune* headlined this *Washington Post* dispatch, "U.S. Pledges to Help Devastated India."[313] The article's last paragraphs, on the other hand, read:

> Many countries have provided aid. Singapore sent oxygen containers to India on Saturday. Germany was airlifting 23 mobile oxygen-generation plants to the country.
>
> India worked with private companies to ship 80 metric tons of liquid oxygen from Saudi Arabia. China and Russia have offered help. And Pakistan [Pakistan!] is ready to give ventilators, digital X-ray machines, protective equipment and other supplies to India, Pakistani Foreign Minister Shah Mahmood Qureshi tweeted.
>
> "We believe in a policy of #HumanityFirst," Qureshi wrote in what appeared to be a thinly veiled jab at the United States.[314]

Forcing the pharm companies to serve humanity first may not be the loss leader it seems. The sector's objections, and the passing collapse in stock prices Alexandria Ocasio-Cortez among others celebrated, may be as much about conditioning the political class as about any sting to quarterly margins.[315] The long-range projections, Matt Stoller writes, are glowing:

> On an investor call last month, the CEO of Pfizer, Frank D'Amelio, discussed what would happen to revenue from his vaccine product as the Covid pandemic ends, what he called the "durability of the franchise." He told analysts not to worry.

People in rich countries will need annual booster shots, and that is where Pfizer will make real money. For these annual treatments, Pfizer will be able to charge much more than it does now. The current price for a Covid vaccine, D'Amelio noted, is $19.50 per dose. He told analysts of his hope Pfizer could get to a more normal price, "$150, $175 per dose," instead of what he called "pandemic pricing."[316]

What the variants win from a host system intent upon profitably denying itself herd immunity, the industry wins from the variants' proliferation.

MOST PEOPLE KILLED BY cops are adults. Cold comfort there and offering none to the families and communities of the Adam Toledos of the world.

A couple weeks ago, Sgt. Michael Davis killed seventeen-year-old Hunter Brittain during a traffic stop.[317] Lonoke County, Arkansas, fired Davis, in part for failing to engage his body camera during the stop. Brittain's passenger reported:

Davis pulled them over and Brittain's truck wouldn't shift into park. So Brittain got out with a blue oil jug to put behind his truck's tires and keep it from hitting the deputy's vehicle. That's when Davis fired.[318]

In April, four Knoxville, Tennessee, cops lost control of the situation in a high school bathroom and killed seventeen-year-old Anthony Thompson, shooting one of their fellow officers in the process.[319] The Knoxville DA refused to press charges against the officers.

COVID may offer an analogous wet blanket.

The U.S. caseload and hospitalizations *were* until recently in steep decline and that extends to pediatric cases.[320] New vaccinations are in decline too. So, infection hotspots, including among children, continue to percolate, particularly in the Midwest and the South.[321]

With older people increasingly vaccinated in the United States—
not so much elsewhere—the average age of patients hospitalized or
killed by the virus is in decline.[322] But it may be more than a matter of
a shift in protected demographics. The virus may also be adapting to
younger patients.

Reports from Minnesota to Brazil signal intermittent increases
in pediatric cases and deaths.[323] Like the police murders, pediatric
COVID isn't in the sphere of adult impact, but letting the kids loose
may cause damage beyond their role as a potential vector for parent
and teacher.

Vibhu Parcha and colleagues reported results of a retrospective
cross-sectional analysis of U.S. pediatric cases:

> Among 12,306 children with lab-confirmed COVID-19, 16.5%
> presented with respiratory symptoms (cough, dyspnea), 13.9%
> had gastrointestinal symptoms (nausea, vomiting, diarrhea,
> abdominal pain), 8.1% had dermatological symptoms (rash),
> 4.8 percent had neurological (headache), and 18.8% had other
> non-specific symptoms (fever, malaise, myalgia, arthralgia and
> disturbances of smell or taste). In the study cohort, the hospi-
> talization frequency was 5.3%, with 17.6% needing critical care
> services and 4.1% requiring mechanical ventilation.[324]

The relative risk of hospitalization was worse in Black (1.97 [95
percent confidence interval 1.49–2.61]) and Latino (1.31 [95 percent confidence interval 1.03–1.78]) children. The CDC reported
in September, before the winter spike, that 75 percent of pediatric
COVID deaths were BIPOC children.[325]

The typical asymptomatic infections kids host do not necessarily mean
an absence of serious morbidity. A University of Texas study reported
multisystem inflammatory syndrome (MIS-C) three to four weeks post-
infection in children.[326] The children—especially those that suffered
Kawasaki disease, depressed ejection fraction, and aneurysm—are in
effect life-haulers, requiring monitoring the rest of their lives.

UCSF's Monica Gandhi and Kyle Hunter dismiss these concerns as part of a "fear-based" response to the Delta variant now dominant in the United States:[327]

- Children are not high-risk for severe disease.
- Children are not vectors, although the source study they cite says "less likely."[328] A study of New York City schools found *less* COVID in students and school personnel than in the greater community.[329]
- The Delta variant isn't hospitalizing children any more than others, although an optimistic *Times* report shows (slight) increases in Britain.[330]
- By definition, the more people vaccinated, the more COVID cases detected will be registered in those vaccinated, if only as a percent of the declining caseload.

Against the Swiss cheese model of multiple interventions many epidemiologists support, Gandhi and Hunter oppose WHO[331] and Los Angeles's[332] insistence that masks are needed:

Messaging heightened anxiety and new masking guidelines around the delta variant also sends a confusing message about vaccines and their effectiveness. One reason the vaccines are modern miracles of science is that they "teach" our immune system to create lasting protection against variants by harnessing the power of our B cells and T cells.

If you are vaccinated with one of the three vaccines approved in the U.S., your memory B cells can adapt and produce antibodies for whatever variant it sees, while your T cells prevent severe disease, even when your immune system has not seen the delta variant before.[333]

The pharmaceutical companies that manufactured these "miracles" disagree, suddenly fast-tracking the plans for booster shots they previously projected further out:

Pfizer said Thursday it is seeing waning immunity from its coronavirus vaccine and says it is picking up its efforts to develop a booster dose that will protect people from variants.

It said it would seek emergency use authorization from the US Food and Drug Administration for a booster dose in August after releasing more data about how well a third booster dose of vaccine works.

"As seen in real world data released from the Israel Ministry of Health, vaccine efficacy in preventing both infection and symptomatic disease has declined six months post-vaccination, although efficacy in preventing serious illnesses remains high," the company said in a statement emailed to CNN . . .

Israel's health ministry said in a statement earlier this week that it had seen efficacy of Pfizer's vaccine drop from more than 90% to about 64% as the B.1.617.2 or Delta variant spread.[334]

The CDC and FDA disagreed: "Americans who have been fully vaccinated do not need a booster shot at this time."[335]

Why? Science writer Carl Zimmer explains how the effectiveness of a vaccine depends on the population tested out in the real world:

It's possible, for example, that people who choose not to get vaccinated may be more likely to put themselves in situations where they could get exposed to the virus. On the other hand, older people may be more likely to be vaccinated but also have a harder time fending off an aggressive variant. Or an outbreak may hit part of a country where most people are vaccinated, leaving under-vaccinated regions unharmed. . . .

Israel's numbers could also be different because of who is getting tested. Much of the country is vaccinated. During local bursts of new infections, the government requires testing for anyone—symptoms or not—who came into contact with a person diagnosed with Covid-19. In other countries, it's more common for people to get tested because they're already feeling sick. This could mean that Israel is spotting more asymptomatic cases in vaccinated people than other places are, bringing their reported effectiveness rate down.[336]

Perhaps the pharmaceutical companies are trying to veer away from their own success. Biotech specialist Brian Orelli told Keith Speights that the vaccines' extended protection—to which we will return—cuts into the companies' revenue stream:

It's really hard to make an argument for the valuations of Moderna and BioNTech right now if these vaccines are one and done over a couple of years. They really need to have ongoing sales until they can get growth from other drugs in their pipelines.[337]

CDC, veering on policy day-to-day, has now pivoted to talking with the companies about a third shot:

President Joe Biden's chief medical adviser acknowledged that "it is entirely conceivable, maybe likely" that booster shots will be needed.[338]

For their part, Gandhi and Hunter are aiming to get kids back to school in the fall come hell or high water.

THE CONCERN FOR KIDS and COVID far outpaces that for kids killed by cops.

That might be a matter of the scale of the children affected, although little but passing notes have been posed in the mainstream press over the Black and Brown kids the virus has killed or damaged. And killing a single teen in a high school bathroom broadcasts a message far beyond the other kid in the bathroom that day—screaming pleas at the cops to save his dying friend—or the greater student body. It can shake a city to its core.[339]

In just the past couple years, children stateside and abroad have been shoveled into the U.S.'s punitive maw.

In April, the Supreme Court ruled in favor of the option of jailing juveniles for life.[340] Justice Brett Kavanaugh, who demanded during his 2018 confirmation hearing that he shouldn't be held responsible for what he did as a kid, wrote the majority opinion.[341]

For years, the New York Police Department illegally collected a database of fingerprints of juveniles as young as eleven.[342] The NYPD also maintains a juvenile facial recognition database of thousands of children and teens caught in the system.[343] The collection, and previous efforts to collect juvenile DNA, moved public defenders to advise kids to avoid entering the new game truck[344] the NYPD is driving around town:

> A senior counsel for Brooklyn Defender Services, which represents around 35,000 people per year, professionally advises not to go anywhere near this thing. "As a criminal defense attorney, I would advise every young person to stay away from the Police Foundation's so-called game truck, a mobile surveillance arcade, for their safety and for the protection of their personal information," MK Kaishian wrote to *Gizmodo*, pointing to DNA harvesting. "If this venture was really about providing harmless activities for young people to engage in, there would be no need for police involvement."[345]

By a genetic fallacy, police elsewhere are targeting kids for the pre-crime of their demographics as part of a program in predictive policing. "[A Florida] county police department," Priyam Madhukar tells us—describing the next generation in school-to-jail pipeline—

> has created a secret list of kids it thinks could "fall into a life of crime." According to documents revealed by the *Tampa Bay Times*, students can be labeled as "at-risk youth who are destined to a life of crime" if they get a D in a class, have three absences in a quarter, get a single discipline referral, or have experienced childhood trauma.

If a list like this existed when I was a teacher in East Baltimore, the vast majority of my students would have been placed on it—not because they were likely to develop into "prolific offenders," as the Pasco County Sheriff Office's intelligence manual suggests, but because the combined forces of concentrated poverty, institutionalized racism, and decades-long disinvestment make hitting at least one of these indicators almost unavoidable.

The sheriff's office uses data from the school district, the state's Department of Children and Families, and its own records to categorize certain children as "at risk of becoming criminals." The school district has defended the policy, but privacy experts have challenged the legality of the practice, noting that federal law allows schools to share student data with police only under very specific circumstances. Additionally, misuse of sensitive data can put children at risk of being unfairly targeted or impact their long-term trajectory if the designation follows them through the school system. . . .

The police intelligence manual also suggests that having "low intelligence" or coming from "broken homes" are predictive factors in determining whether children will break the law.[346]

No indication if the scale by which "intelligence" is measured here is the same by which police are hired.

Much in the spirit of Chicago's ShotSpotter system, flooding the West and South Sides with police incursions:

Research has shown that increased contact between students and school resource officers can result in higher rates of arrests even for minor, non-criminal offenses. As the intelligence manual directs officers to leverage their relationships with students to find "seeds of criminal activity," it's also possible that children on the list will be questioned about or used to surveil the communities they come from.[347]

In 2018, El Paso, Texas, police went full Israeli Defense Forces on a bunch of unarmed neighborhood kids, pulling a gun on them, egging them on, threatening witnesses with extrajudicial reprisal, and arresting two teens who had nothing to do with the crime the police were called for:

> The incident started after police officers responded to a report of criminal trespassing at an apartment complex at 6719 Sambrano Ave., officials said.
>
> Julian Saucedo, 17, and Jacob Saucedo, 15, were arrested on suspicion of interfering with a police officer. Neither was arrested on trespassing charges.[348]

Along the same border, the Biden administration continues the previous administration's kiddie cages. In May, the Associated Press reported 21,000 unaccompanied migrant children—including toddlers—were being held across two hundred facilities in twenty-plus states.[349] Five facilities host a thousand children in overcrowded conditions. Many of the facilities are run by private contractors presently under investigation for physically and sexually abusing immigrant children. More than likely the prison bus Immigration and Customs Enforcement outfitted with child seats to transport detained children on field trips is still in operation.[350]

The hypocrisy of Vice President Kamala Harris's "do not come" speech in Guatemala was widely commented on.[351] It directly conflicted with her year of campaign speeches against Trump's detention centers, including defending the reasons why migrant children left for the United States in the first place.[352]

Extending out beyond the border, in June, the Supreme Court limited human rights suits against corporations, in this case around child slavery in Africa.[353] Six Mali citizens trafficked into slavery when children had sued Nestlé USA and Cargill:

> Justice Clarence Thomas, writing for an eight-member majority [joined in a concurring opinion by Justices Sonia Sotomayor, Stephen Breyer, and Elena Kagan], said the companies' activities in the United States were not sufficiently tied to the asserted abuses.

The companies, he wrote, drawing on the plaintiffs' suit, "did not own or operate farms in Ivory Coast. But they did buy cocoa from farms located there. They also provided those farms with technical and financial resources—such as training, fertilizer, tools and cash—in exchange for the exclusive right to purchase cocoa."[354]

What happens in Mali, stays in Mali:

The plaintiffs said the companies "knew or should have known" that the farms were using enslaved children but failed to use their economic power to stop the practice. (The companies have denied complicity in child labor.)

The flaw in the plaintiffs' case, Justice Thomas wrote, was its failure adequately to tie the companies' asserted conduct to their activities in the United States.[355]

If not the United States directly or U.S.-based companies, U.S. allies, backed with billions of dollars in foreign aid, engage in war crimes against children.

Forty percent of Gaza's population are kids.[356] Israel's "Operation Guardian of the Walls" this year was both targeted and indiscriminate. Yes, the occupants of the building in which the Associated Press and other media outlets were situated were forewarned before it was leveled. From Minneapolis to Gaza, media are targeted in an effort to control the information out.

But the strafing lines of bombs through a densely populated Gaza City are also reminiscent of footage of U.S. napalm dropped through Vietnamese jungle. Stochastic terror and collective punishment as a form of prevention. Even the loss of the AP building had its deadly impact on the neighborhood around it—from dust, loss of work, and destruction of roadways, gas lines, and water lines. All summing up to a message that *any* resistance to apartheid is to be paid for in dead kids.[357]

"Mowing the grass" is what Israeli forces call it.[358] It is, as reporter Arun Gupta observes, "the language of genocide."

Insisting kids return to schools even in the face of a likely next wave of COVID cases isn't necessarily predicated upon a national ethos organized around children's well-being.

I'M NOT THE ONLY one to notice the incoherence stitched through reactions to epidemiological realities. One Facebook friend noted earlier in the year before CDC's reversal on masks:

> IDK what's worse. To see covid news and headlines from the cdc saying brace for impact and impending doom while simultaneously watching people behave like the objective reality is the exact opposite and clapping at Coney Island re-openings, and other crap like that.

José Halloy, a physicist who studies sustainability and collective dynamics in natural and artificial systems and is part of the Paris group that helped force the WHO to backtrack from its Wuhan report rejecting a potential lab leak,[359] threw up his hands at France's own response in a Facebook post:

> I'm going to drop epidemiology. Obviously, the government has understood everything since they are not listening to anyone. The waste and the under-utilization or even the non-utilization of the scientific community is depressing. Their political choice is now clear: no extra effort, no change, no investment, nothing. They hope the storm passes while we vaccinate (too slowly). This strategy has not prevented closures of sacrificed economic sectors, and semi-lockdowns. This has already doubled the total number of deaths from January to April, not counting the sequelae and long COVID, collateral deaths as a result of hospital saturation, and it continues, and will continue. I wish them good luck with the management of variants.
>
> I am not a doctor or a leader. The sick and the dead are not my problem. I still look at the situation no longer for the company,

but simply to protect my family. We are privileged, at worst we can take refuge in different countries, one of which is among the least affected in the EU.

The presidential election is coming soon. I imagine a party that rubs its hands together without saying anything or doing so much will have everything in its favor. For me, and here, the "curvature of the waves" is over.

It isn't just those in power. Geographer Salvatore Engel-Di Mauro warned that the left in capital's core routinely followed its opposition's lead, and should expect

reorientation among most leftists in core countries, the sort that happened with nuclear weapons, imperialism, and anti-communism by the 1990s, reorienting away from those issues as if they were suddenly irrelevant.

There may be a danger that such wealthier bandwagonistic leftists will forget about the pandemic while it still rages elsewhere, like most leftists do regarding Ebola, constant war in places like eastern DRC, etc. Debates on whether China is socialist, for example, are incredibly blissful of the wider context and inter-relations. . . . There is zero internationalism subtending such leftist debates. While indirectly reaping the material benefits of many of those horrors.

Or maybe there is no such danger and even if such reorientation happens it is irrelevant in the larger scheme of things, given the level of influence the left has in general. As you reckon, the pretense (or possibility of such pretense) that the pandemic is over just because a small minority of the world population is mostly vaccinated is exactly why Pandemic Research for the People remains possibly even more important than before.[360]

That can't possibly be the case! And yet here's what Joshua Ginsberg, the president of the Cary Institute of Ecosystem Studies, admitted in a letter to the *New York Times:*

During a virtual conference with colleagues from around the globe, I used the past tense in referring to the Covid-19 pandemic, and was politely corrected. While life in the United States often feels post-pandemic (it is not), much of the rest of the world is experiencing the depressing, frightening and deadly acceleration of Covid-19 that overwhelmed America for much of the last 15 months. I have rarely felt so embarrassed by my own implicit smugness.[361]

Each complaint implies that losing context, much as the police's arrival upon a street scene, appears exactly the system's objective.

Our team described how the focus on the emergency of each new emergent disease threat, clearly a necessary task, also often serves as the very means by which to avoid addressing the disease's structural origins. Context implies that causality intersects responsibility.[362] That's total anathema to a system rationalizing its own power as always-already justified.

Public health is too much a commons to be anything other than neglected or sold off. The fallacy is also folded into promoting every suddenly commodified solution.

"Just because the roof doesn't send a bill every month doesn't mean that it doesn't need to be paid," Robert Norlund, turning back to the Miami condominium collapse, told the *New York Times*.[363]

Norland's company found condominium boards prioritized monthly maintenance costs while failing to set funds aside for major repairs. Objections to the suddenly steep repair bill were a topic of conversation around the Champlain Tower pool just days before the collapse, even as major cracks had been identified years previously.[364]

Filtering out shared threats as beyond the ken of identities organized around individualized economic units—the bedrock of liberalisms from classical to neoliberal—wasn't just a detachment that Florida officials continued to exhibit post-collapse, as we quoted Marianne Garneau earlier. It was a form of unintended suicidal ideation on the part of the residents themselves.

I'm not blaming the victims here. A corrupt city inspector didn't help.[365] But the traumatic bonding found in identifying with market failure is ironically a systemic matter, extending well beyond beach-front real estate and, in my field of interest, to the farmers presently buffered by the Midwest's ecological collapse: dying soil, polluted water, falling water tables, and particulate ammonium nitrate, ammonium sulfate, and hydrogen sulfide. Few changes on any single farm will be enough to roll back such destruction.

If only even such inadequate responses were pursued! For upon the end of many an emergency, or its presumed end regardless of the damage's actual state, returning to the normal that causes the crisis is a form of collective anterograde amnesia. The larger population of the Global North is taught to fail to form memories to protect the system that threatens their lives.

"Capitalism," artist Chiara Acu observed, "will try and fool us into thinking that [the pandemic] didn't even happen."[366]

PUBLIC HEALTH—PREVENTIVE MAINTENANCE for population health—works. Even based in a neoliberal context on the rawest economism or as a matter of power's self-preservation.

Defoe commented on the ways and means London's plague humbled the poor and kept their population under a Malthusian carrying capacity of rebellion.[367] By this point of the crisis, he claimed, charity wouldn't otherwise have been enough. Indeed, the rich's own poor planning saved them. For had they hoarded Stores of Provisions in their Houses at any scale, they would have been ransacked.

The dubious rewards of such an accelerationism isn't worth so many poor lives lost. There are better ways even under a political thumb we can still aim to break. Indeed, Defoe describes the many programs London's city lords pursued in an effort to control the plague: the previously alluded to charity, as well as stay-at-home orders, quick burials, epidemiological analysis, isolation wards, contact tracing, community health officers, occupational quarantines, public events cancelled, restaurants closed, and errand helpers. Little of which has been pursued in the United States during COVID.

Such public health support bears significant impact beyond emergencies. Ten years ago, health policy analysts Glen Mays and Sharla Smith found that U.S. mortality rates from preventable deaths—sources like infant mortality and cardiovascular disease, diabetes, and cancer—fell between 1.1 to 6.9 percent for every 10 percent increase in local public health spending.[368]

In 2018, Trust for America's Health put out a report on the effective decline of just such funding.[369] CDC's budget then was $7.15 billion, which, adjusting for inflation, was flat for the previous decade. Most of the CDC's budget goes to states and municipalities. There's also a CDC Prevention and Public Health Fund, from which about $625 million a year also goes directly to states and municipalities.

The report described the Public Health Emergency Preparedness (PHEP) Cooperative Agreement Program as the only federal program that supports state and local health departments to prepare for and respond to emergencies. Except for onetime bumps for the Ebola and Zika outbreaks, core emergency preparedness funding had been cut by more than one-third (from $940 million in 2002 to $667 million in 2017).

The report went on to identify precipitous declines in public health funding at the state level. Thirty-one states cut their public health budgets 2015–16, with spending lower that year than in 2008. The budget cuts out of the Great Recession were never restored.[370]

The impact was felt at the local level too. Local health departments cut 55,000 staff the decade following the Recession. By this system's logic, an acute emergency is also grounds for such cuts. Thousands of health staff were furloughed during the COVID outbreak from declines in more lucrative surgeries.[371]

The Trust for America report went on to describe the incoming disasters for which the United States appeared unprepared in 2018. They sound like headlines of the past month: weather disasters, flooding, wildfires, extreme drought, hurricanes, infectious disease outbreaks, deaths of despair, including out of racial disparities, opioids, and the regional disparities that both cost Hillary Clinton the 2016 election and continue to drive governmental distrust.

Trust for America's Health placed particular focus on pandemics and the need to fully fund the Pandemic and All-Hazards Preparedness Act, the Hospital Preparedness Program, the Project BioShield Act, and PHEP.

The organization finished up by suggesting increased funding for public health at all levels of jurisdiction—fed, state, and local. The report called for preserving the Prevention and Public Health Fund, funding for preparing for public health emergencies and pandemics, establishing a standing public health emergency response fund, and surge funding upon an emergency to avoid the delays that were apparent in the Ebola outbreak, the swine flu pandemic, Hurricane Sandy, and Zika.

It called for a national resilience strategy to combat diseases of despair, for preventing chronic disease, and for expanding high-impact interventions across communities.

The recommendations were wrapped in the worst of language and precepts. Trust for America's Health accepted the class character of the state. Public health is a means of cleaning up messes that capitalist production produces. Public health outcomes were pitched in terms of Returns on Investment.

All terrible. And yet in the present context, radical, if only in pushing back against the damage of an empire at the end of its cycle of accumulation, organized around helping billionaires squeezing what's left of the commons and turning capital back into bunker money.

The problem is twofold. Ed Yong's complaint of a lost competence in and cognition of the commons isn't just a COVID thing. It was decades in the making. The preponderance of the rich in the United States is committed to failing to recognize the resulting threat. Even, or especially, some of the philanthrocapitalists funding health interventions.

Congressional Democrats, for one, are slashing back a $30 billion infusion of pandemic preparedness funds presently slated in the $3.5 trillion infrastructure bill.[372] The money was to restock medical and mask stockpiles and proactively develop vaccines. A limited notion of public health, but something of a step forward nonetheless.

The poor, then, even should that funding be placed back in, are likely to ransack those Stores of Provisions. Paying for a fascist gambit blocking such raids is, like its predecessors, unlikely to end well.

CLEARLY THERE REMAINS OPPORTUNITY in such abject failure. American epidemiological myopia is so culturally bounded that our brightest minds celebrate the very damage they simultaneously condemn.

Jennifer Szalai's review of Michael Lewis's new book following five public health "renegades" who objected to the Trump administration's response to COVID-19 included these two paragraphs:

> [Lewis] describes a health care system whose for-profit operations are so entrenched that hospitals last spring couldn't even avail themselves of a nonprofit lab that was faster and free, because the hospital computers were incapable of coding for a $0 test. Staffers at the lab eagerly awaited a shipment of precious nasal swabs from the Strategic National Stockpile that turned out to be a bunch of Q-Tips. A venture capitalist offering to help alleviate the nasal swab shortage procured 5,000 eyelash brushes. . . .
>
> He ends with what's apparently intended as a heartwarming epilogue about [renegade Charity] Dean's decision, a year into the pandemic, to enter the private sector. She has named her venture the Public Health Company. "We're going to do private government operations, like Blackwater," she says. For some readers, her reference to a notorious mercenary force might sound ominous, but there's no skepticism and no pushback from Lewis, nothing to suggest that he might see it differently from how Dean does: as the brilliant idea of an honorable person whose only intention is to do the right thing.[373]

LEWIS'S BOOK IS A GOOD read and defends the public health rank and file upon who we depend, but who's left behind in the epilogue of such a gold rush? Earlier in the U.S. vaccination campaign, I posted @ ChiVaxBot maps showing the gap between COVID deaths and vaccination by Chicago zip code. Some of my connections reposted them. I read objections underneath those posts to the effect that, well, it's early on, as if transitory dynamics—y'know, our lives as they are happening—aren't also deeply political.

The latest maps, as of mid-July 2021, show the sociospatial disparity between COVID deaths and completed vaccinations still in place.[374]

It's such a classic result that it embodies a law in the public health literature long on the books. Tudor Hart's Inverse Care Law declares, "The availability of good medical care tends to vary inversely with the need for it in the population served."[375]

Social reformer Florence Kelly found the disparities in sanitary hygiene in the Chicago of the late 1800s:

It is needless to suggest that the sweat-shop districts as they have been described are the natural abodes of disease and the breeding places of infection and epidemics. While the system does not create these conditions, it penetrates the regions where they exist and thrives upon an atmosphere which a higher form of industry could not breathe. It is true the normal or ordinary death rate in the wards mentioned is not conspicuously greater than in others; possibly the vital statistics of certain localities within wards might show the actual and relative effects of bad sanitation more forcibly; at least, disease and all death-laden agencies pervade these communities, and if they have escaped pestilence in the past, they still may be ripening for plague in the future.[376]

A municipal geography that recapitulates its pattern across health crises from cholera, dysentery, scarlet fever, smallpox, and the aftermath of the Great Fire in the mid-1800s through 1918 and HIV and the heat wave of 1995 refutes Florence on the point the source isn't systemic.[377]

Chicago continues this long tradition in deciding that the South and West Sides are to be subjected to ShotSpotter surveillance but are apparently unworthy of the effort at distributing the latest in medical innovation during a pandemic.

And even those vaccines that made it to poorer neighborhoods earlier in the year still found themselves in white people's deltoids. White and wealthier showed up at vaccine clinics for poor people in cities and towns across the country: D.C., Dallas, New York, rural Florida, and North Minneapolis, among other places.[378] A June Chicago Department of Health report showed the life expectancy gap between Black and non-Black residents widened to nearly a decade, in part due to COVID exposure and the Tudor Hart effect.[379]

We see the priorities repeated time and again as if an epistemic bedrock. It's why Chicago Mayor Lori Lightfoot, another Democrat, spent $281.5 million earmarked for COVID on police instead.[380] The city's Department of Health received only $18 million, the Office of Emergency Management $8 million, the Department of Family and Support Services less than $200,000, and the Office for People with Disabilities $2,000. Another $68 million went unspent while tens of thousands of residents were denied rental relief.

Lightfoot wasn't alone:

Heat-seeking cameras that see you in the dark, sometimes even through walls. Firepower and vehicles for "dealing with crowd management security and potential civil disturbances." "Specialized crime scene mapping technology," encrypted radios, and data-collection software for "gathering intelligence and enhancing surveillance." Using federal funds earmarked for Covid-19 relief, these and hundreds of other requests to militarize police forces have been green-lit on the U.S. taxpayer's dime.

Using stimulus from the multi-trillion-dollar CARES Act, which passed in March 2020, the Department of Justice has awarded at least $845.8 million of emergency grants to state and local law enforcement officers across the U.S. and its colonized territories. The relief has gone to more than 1,800 of these agencies, ranging from $30,000 boosters for small-town cops to tens of millions of dollars for a single police department in states like Florida and Texas.[381]

Perhaps that money could have helped keep Adam Toledo home or at school in an enrichment program that Chicago, which in 2013 closed fifty schools in the poorest neighborhoods, should have been able to pay for.[382]

Cook County nurses went on a one-day strike protesting unfilled positions numbering in the hundreds during the pandemic even as the county where Chicago is located got a billion dollars in COVID money:

> Nurse Cathleen Armstrong said in her 23 years at Cook County Health, she's never seen staffing and morale as bad as they are now.
>
> "The staffing is so bad that patients can be here for several days without someone to wash their face," Armstrong said, noting that washing a patient's face is usually the job of certified nursing assistants, and nurses are not the only workers in short supply. "We're always short-staffed."[383]

Days ago, the Biden administration moved from turning a blind eye to surreptitiously defunding nurses and teachers to *urging* state and municipalities to spend their COVID funding on police.[384]

Focusing on vaccines alone at the expense of these extrapolating societal determinations of health—even as successful vaccination campaigns depend on the latter—evokes author Michael Chabon's description of the appeal of the adventures of Sherlock Holmes as "the bourgeois thirst for tidy adventure."[385]

I DIDN'T THINK I was going to get into an ongoing contretemps with Those Nerdy Girls, twenty-three epidemiologists fielding the public's pandemic-related questions. I had pushed back against one of their posts earlier.[386]

After all, the Girls' Instagram posts are a valiant effort at containing the veritable tidal wave of misinformation from the strange convergence of anti-vax yoga moms and Trumpists. This testimony before the Ohio legislature on the magnetizing properties of the COVID vaccine and its interface with 5G towers is as nutty as it gets.[387] Shannon Kroner on the vaccine's impact on miscarriages is another one.[388] And on and on.[389]

But it begs whether the Girls' effort is about sweeping together any and all objections to the present state of the pandemic response. The posts are beginning to take on the smell of Bill Nye's alliance with Monsanto.[390]

They recently posted this punchy post:

FACT OVER FALSEHOOD: A new occasional series.

The bad news: Setting the record straight on vaccine misinformation is a daunting job.

The better news: Evidence-based strategies are effective in beating back bad info, and we can all help! Today we launch a new occasional series that fights back against vaccine myths using an evidence-based "truth sandwich" approach . . .

VACCINES ARE OUR BEST BET IN THE RACE AGAINST NEW VARIANTS

Fact: COVID-19 vaccines are powerful weapons to fight all current strains of COVID-19

Falsehood: Bad actors are peddling a dangerous myth that COVID-19 vaccines seed new viral strains. This is FALSE and is a well-worn page out of the anti-vaxx playbook. Similar falsehoods have been used to sow doubt during previous global vaccination campaigns.

More facts: In the race against variants, vaccines are our best bet. As we vaccinate as many people as possible, as quickly as possible, we stop the virus from spreading. Slowing the spread means fewer opportunities for the virus to mutate, which will help prevent the emergence of new variants.[391]

They're referring to, among others, HIV discoverer Luc Montagnier's assertion that the vaccines may be driving new variants.[392] I don't think the vaccines are to this point responsible for the new variants, which were long evolving before the campaign began, but Those Nerdy Girls reject the possibility out of hand moving forward. Clearly the physical vaccine injected in our arms doesn't "seed" new variants that are transmitted on, but there may be more here than what the Girls neatly package.

Here was my response:

"Bad actors," you say? Do you not even hear yourselves? This is the language of prosecutors and the national security apparatus. The latter helped bring about the surge of emergent diseases post-1980 if only by knocking out governments that objected to handing over resources to American multinationals that are helping drive the deforestation and development behind spillover events. 1/13

We might agree on the obnoxious nature of anti-vax propaganda—clearly the vaccine injections themselves do not "seed" new variants. But trading one set of virulent oversimplifications for another only highlights the ugly underbelly of your brilliant posts. *Who* are these bad actors, for instance? 2/13

Because when you spray a room with bullets, someone you perhaps didn't intend to hit might fire back. Or maybe conflating targets is exactly the kind of bad faith association that the security apparatus whose language you're drawing on has long indulged. Patrice Lumumba is a communist—he wasn't—therefore he must be assassinated. As if he was mere reason enough to kill another country's elected leader. 3/13

"What is he talking about?" If you're unable to see the course of engagement you've chosen here, it may speak to the limits of the scientism with which you're steering your IG account of state here. 4/13

For one, vaccine efficaciousness and effectiveness, as you well know, are two different things entirely. Boston University

Dean of Public Health Sandro Galea spoke to NIH on exactly this point. The triumphs of biomedical science, he said, do not obviate the failures of public health at other levels of biocultural organization, including the agencies and industries you tacitly defend. 5/13

Our team went one step further and argued that under imperial capitalism, biomedical foci are used to run discussion of the structural causes of disease emergence off the road.[393] It is deployed as a form of Gramscian hegemony.[394] 6/13

In that way, stripping out public health and nonpharmaceutical interventions in favor of biomedical commodification allows pathogens the time they need to engage in the interdemic selection that leads to the emergence of new viral variants.[395] So by that causal pathway, yes, vaccines under a capitalist model *do* "seed" new variants at the level of the metapopulation.[396] 7/13

So if modes of intervention are forced into competition because the state has a class character and won't engage in social medicine because that might alert everyday people that their needs can be met beyond a market economy that expropriates them, then, yes, having to wait a year before the kind of vaccination campaign the political class favors begins did in fact have something to do with the deaths of half-a-million Americans. 8/13

Finally, vaccine escape—beyond mismatched coverage and as a matter of *positive selection* on the virus—is a stalwart of the molecular and clinical literatures. So any broadstroke dismissal that vaccines don't lead to new variants is as ill-informed as the anti-vaxx bull propagated elsewhere. 9/13

It seems, then, that vaccines are *not* the best bet in the race against new variants. Instead, it's keeping novel diseases from emerging in the first place. And keeping those that do emerge from spreading by organizing governance around public health and the public commons. Both interventions require replacing a mode of social reproduction organized around profit that sacrifices millions annually, including this year by COVID. 10/13

Yes, vaccination is critical, but you've positioned yourselves as speaking to empirical realities. Serving these "truth sandwiches" may just be the next generation of the PR science many practitioners have long complained about. 11/13

Recently deceased evolutionary geneticist Richard Lewontin spoke to the resulting fallacies: "Conscientious and wholly admirable popularizers of science like Carl Sagan use both rhetoric and expertise to form the mind of masses because they believe, like the Evangelist John, that the truth shall make you free. But they are wrong. It is not the truth that makes you free. It is your possession of the power to discover the truth. Our dilemma is that we do not know how to provide that power."[397] 12/13

Until you switch out of using science as a form of policing, you will repeatedly find yourself protecting the powerful who both helped bring on the outbreak and let it churn through the U.S. Who, indeed, are the "bad actors"? 13/13

Now, it didn't help matters that one "cryptosammyog" claimed three minutes before I posted these comments that the literal vials of vaccines did seed variants. "Its a fact," he declared without facts. What a mess all this is.

"The Apprehensions of the People," Defoe observed of 1665, "were likewise strangely encreas'd by the Error of the Times; in which, I think, the People, from what Principle I cannot imagine, were more addicted to Prophesies, and Astrological Conjurations, Dreams, and old Wives Tales, than ever they were before or since."[398]

The two stumbles here aren't disconnected. A failure of governance one side issues apologia for opens up the Conjurations of another.

POET SAEED JONES TWEETED that the vaccines might mean some of us are exiting out of the pandemic earlier than others.[399] Likely to grave resentment, as sci-fi author Jeff VanderMeer began us in the epigraph at the top.

The grand bifurcation that splits the country slops over into what stage of the epidemic we find ourselves. Those affluent enough to stay home while "essential workers" risked death to service them can now hit the restaurants and bars again unafraid. Like they're a different species. As Ayn Rand disciple Zack Snyder puts it: His Batman's superpower is being rich.[400]

The resulting personas of a variety of social standing incarnate the historical process.[401] They work only to the extent they match material realities or, for the more swaggering, their practitioners avoid buying into their own gimmick. For the pandemic, as we described, may roar back. This virus or the next.

Unbeknownst to me, I myself struck a persona the past year.[402] It served its public and private purposes. I am grateful it helped a lot of people make their way through the early months of COVID. But I found myself tapped out.

It dawned on me that the storyboard in which I only half-sensed I was participating wasn't up to a denouement worthy of the scale of the danger. Look around. Observe the celebratory refusal to learn from the calamity. There are irresistible momenta that return us to exactly what caused the disaster. Our best and brightest are on the case. Liberal and conservative. Democrat and Republican. Ideologue and technicist (an ideologue by another name).

I shaved my bonhomie mustache as much for my well-being as for the phail of a "resolution" the pandemic is converging on. My students this semester commented on the missing prop. I told them I had hung up the stache on the wall for now.

A day later, a reporter called to sketch out a story he had in development along the lines that COVID would likely go endemic among poor people and the Black and Brown. I agreed. I pointed out many a disease that went that way if on other temporal scales, including HIV and TB. I could sense the reporter's despair fishtailing his queries. Upon hanging up, I went for a long walk in the sun.

SUCH REGIME SHIFTS—bad-to-good health and back again—can be detected in near-real time.

A burst of new measures have been proposed for *projecting* ecological regime shifts into the future, as in climate change or eutrophication of a lake: greater population variability; greater autocorrelation; a slower rate of recovery after perturbation; changes in skewness in population distribution; and a change in spectral density ratio, indicating a shift from high to low frequency processes.[403]

Our team is investigating the possibilities of using these to detect such shifts for the better.

We might, for instance, aim to detect spatial signals preceding agricultural shifts (and associated health impacts) for localities defined by proximate agroecological processes tracked by county census data and more distal shifts in regional dynamics. We might be able to detect which U.S. counties are already shifting into a more regenerative regional food system. And where.

Which localities represent spatial thresholds across which regime shifts—say, from conventional to regenerative production along an agricultural index we've devised—originate and spread?[404] Does the spatial geometry and connectivity affect where and when such agricultural shifts occur? For instance, would the initial emergence of a regime shift be accompanied by an increase in regional spatial variance that, on the other end of an inverse-U curve, declines as the diffusion of the change propagates outward? Does the level of exposure to these changes weight local effective resilience?

Clearly the nature of the efforts to spread regenerative agriculture differs from the interventions dedicated to blocking disease emergence. On the other hand, we've proposed the former as exactly the way to the latter. Trying to control disease outbreaks after they've already emerged is too much shutting the barn door after the horse has bolted. Changing how livestock, poultry, and crops are grown in a landscape may keep such pathogens from emerging in the first place.

But maybe we're too late (although such a possibility never forswears the attempt). One could imagine COVID kicking us out into the next round of racial capitalism in time and space. The billionaires are already out in the lead, profiting enormously from the state murder the pandemic represents.[405]

Will the rest of the country be pulled into new vicious cycles rather than the virtuous ones our team proposes? With the United States on the wrong end of its cycle of accumulation, something more Latin American, without the latter's nod to social medicine, may be on its way. Police shooting down children in alleyways already has a certain favela bouquet. Although killing George Stinneys and Emmett Tills is also a long American tradition.

INDEED, SCIENCE APPEARS TO have signed on to such a trajectory.

Evolutionary biologists Heather Heying and Bret Weinstein resigned from Evergreen State College when students there tried to force them off-campus in a twist on the annual Day of Absence that highlighted the importance of minority students and faculty. Since then, the couple has landed on the Joe Rogan show, moderated the Sam Harris-Jordan Peterson debate, and scored Princeton University fellowships.

Although I have spoken seriously about the possibility COVID originated as a lab leak, I find it really strange that the two evolutionary biologists, as per their appearance on Bill Maher's show, wouldn't know the evolution of virulence modeling that's been around for four decades showing that a virus can evolve greater deadliness if presented with an effectively bottomless supply of susceptibles as humanity presently offers.[406] Or that a virus could evolve such virulence by interdemic selection.[407]

Nor are these two apparently aware of the evolutionary genomics that suggests SARS-2 was circulating among humans for *years* before Wuhan.[408]

Finally, Weinstein asserts that the polybasic furin cleavage sites open to host proteases snipping at the spike protein's S1/S2 juncture were found in SARS-2 and nowhere else and so are a sign of lab origins.

As I balked in August:

Such sites repeatedly arise in nature. They may not be present in the 2019 bat sample as initially proposed, but have been inferred in SARS-2 ancestors, alongside [SARS-like] strains expressing widespread spike conservation and recognizing both bat and human ACE2. The furin cleavage sites have been identified in MERS, so are not solely a function of putative genetic engineering or gain-of-function.[409]

People want to make a real argument in favor of the lab leak theory, okay, fair enough. But apparently making a dull one gets your Princeton fellowship renewed.

Five months later, Weinstein, no Richard Lewontin he, placed himself on the Derek Chauvin jury, judging the police officer and George Floyd's killer:

A textbook case of reasonable doubt. Not only are there reasons to question Chauvin's guilt, but it is hard to imagine how an impartial jury, following standard instructions, could have escaped that conclusion. Derek Chauvin may have caused George Floyd's death, but the established medical facts alone would seem to preclude certainty.[410]

For the real jury was influenced less by the typical free pass the Supreme Court and the state-supported blue wall issue officers, but by the demonstrations in the streets:

Today, if the mob is convinced and motivated enough, their cause becomes the righteous one. Whether jurors accede to this out of fear for their own safety, or out of fear of the damage that may be done to innocent people if their verdict reignites violence, or because they are convinced by the mob that there is some higher principle whose value exceeds their duty to the accused, it must not stand. The will of the mob has no place in court. Likewise, no conviction that emerges from a mob-influenced court can be legitimate.[411]

Clearly Weinstein identifies with Chauvin. The jury were those kids at Evergreen.

NOW IN THE OTHER direction, evolutionary geneticist Kristian Andersen badly presents the case in favor of the field hypothesis of the virus's origins, on which I still place most of my purse of prior probabilities.

In a *New York Times* interview, Andersen, who in recent weeks has gotten flak for an early 2020 email to Anthony Fauci raising the possibility of an engineered virus, continues to conflate a designed virus and a lab leak.[412] They're not the same. A field sample could sneak its way out of a lab's back door without first being manipulated or even allowed space to evolve through serial passage.

Without evidence, he dismisses the lab leak possibility as without evidence. It's the kind of appeal to both incredulity and authority that the *Times* tried to leave him room to reverse out of.

Instead, Andersen, no Lewontin either, declares no regrets. That's been the case for some time. His sweeping declarations about the origins of the virus in his March 2020 *Nature Medicine* paper were unsupported even then.[413]

He finishes by claiming his work apolitical, even as modern science's origins, and continued practice, are intertwined with capitalism's beginnings and the state's imperial character. Why, we might ask, did Andersen send his initial concerns to Fauci to begin with?

With these two sides of the origins argument, one grasps the speed at which U.S. institutional cognition is rotting away.

THE ROT GOES BOTH ways: political class to science and back again.

Computational geneticist Yaniv Erlich and immunologist Daniel Douek have suggested applying gene drive technology to stopping coronavirus outbreaks by making horseshoe bats immune.[414]

With CRISPR genomic engineering technology, scientists can precisely edit DNA and introduce selfish genetic elements that spread through a population faster than by Mendelian inheritance.[415] Scientists have introduced rapid sterilization in mosquito populations with the aim of eliminating the pests, which critics claim only allows other mosquitoes to immigrate and replace their predecessors.[416]

The application here appears more hubris and ideology than science. Or just science as raw ideology.

The molecular and ecological follies are numerous:

Developmental geneticist Kim Cooper and her team at the University of California, San Diego, engineered a gene drive that spread a genetic variant through 72% of mouse offspring in her lab. That isn't efficient enough to quickly spread the desired trait in the wild.

What's more, creating a gene drive in bats would be much harder than it is in mice, because bat researchers lack the genetic tools available in mice, said Paul Thomas, a developmental geneticist at the University of Adelaide in Australia, who is trying to engineer mouse gene drives.

And unlike mice, which can breed at 6 to 8 weeks of age, bats take two years to reach sexual maturity, so it would take much longer for a trait to spread throughout wild bat populations than in lab mouse populations.[417]

As with almost all such proposals, the ecology is missing:

Biologists also say that Erlich's proposal is unlikely to work in the wild—even if researchers get bat gene drives to work in a lab—because bats are incredibly diverse.

There are 1,432 bat species, including multiple horseshoe bat species that carry coronaviruses and pass them among each other. . . .

Engineering one gene drive in just one bat species would not solve the problem, biologists say.[418]

Then there are the bats themselves:

"We don't know the implications of wiping out coronaviruses in bat populations, because we don't know how bats have evolved to coexist with these viruses," said virologist Arinjay Banerjee of the Vaccine and Infectious Disease Organization at the University of Saskatchewan in Saskatoon, Canada.[419]

While well on point, these criticisms also miss a bigger picture.

As agroecologists have argued, the line between nature in the broadest sense and agriculture *should* be fuzzy.[420] But not in the direction proposed here. Erlich and Douek aim to turn the stochastic abundance of the forest into just another megafarm.

Under the cover of respectability, the proposed intervention plunks due cause for a disaster of its moneybags' own making upon nonhuman species minding their own business engaged in the ecological metabolism upon which, it so happens in passing, humanity depends.[421]

The solution proposed here represents a click forward in the ratchet of capitalist realism's hyperrational irrationality. We must further doom ourselves, it is argued, to save the system that along the way rewards researchers.

Erlich is also chief scientific officer of MyHeritage, a genetic genealogy company, and founder of Eleven Therapeutics, which perhaps, if lucky, will one day become the Blackwater of biotech startups.

THE POLICE MURDERS OF George Floyd and Breonna Taylor go hand-in-hand with the assassinations of Berta Cáceres and other peasant activists attempting to stop deforestation around the world.[422]

All such murders back hideous political economies of racist terror and expropriation that, along with the pain and punishment they embody on their own, also drive so much of Earth's ecological damage, pandemic included.

Cáceres and her colleagues are by far more efficient virologists than the Erlichs and Doueks of the world.[423]

No ecohealth that fails to assimilate this underlying oppression is worth its weight in vaccines saved. As already long pursued outside the North American context, efforts must be made to explicitly integrate these fundamental clashes into agroecological research.[424]

Our team at the Agroecology and Rural Economics Research Corps made one such humble effort here, tracing the continuum of structural violence imposed upon peasants (and an array of strategies that could be deployed in response).[425]

THE STATE OF KENTUCKY pursues such violence. It charged a single cop solely for the bullets that *missed* Breonna Taylor while she slept.[426]

A paramedic, Taylor saved many a Louisville life. In turn, the State sacrificed her in body and good name so that it could reserve the right to kill more Black people in such an arbitrary way. The State aims not only to preserve a monopoly on violence, but on murder without due cause.

More acutely, the Place-Based Investigations squad that killed Taylor was being deployed to clean out Elliot Avenue for Vision Russell gentrification.[427] Taylor's death is folded into the kind of serial forced displacement, as social psychologist Mindy Fullilove writes, that characterizes the histories of nearly every Black community in America (or Indigenous group on Latin America's commodity frontier).[428]

Using data collected by the nonprofit Fatal Encounters, the Decolonial Atlas mapped the fatalities of police violence in various U.S. cities over the past decade, including both race/ethnicity of the victims and the racial demographics of the neighborhood.[429] We see Eric Garner, Freddie Grey, and Mike Brown were only individual examples of a larger trend in their neighborhoods relating police murders, demographics, and place.

It's not just community groups, there's a whole subfield that's emerged in peer-reviewed public health around statistically testing and describing the social exposures police brutality and shootings represent. According to Cody Ross's 2015 analysis, Hennepin County, where George Floyd was killed, clocks in at nearly twice the relative risk of Black people being shot by police while *unarmed* to whites being shot when *armed*.[430]

Hennepin represents the second greatest of such gaps in
Minnesota. The first? Ramsey County, where Philando Castile was
killed. Other counties with comparable disparities? Glynn County in
Georgia where Ahmaud Arbery was murdered and Jefferson County
in Kentucky where Taylor was shot dead.

Taylor's double murder isn't a bug in the system. It's a feature. This
is America. This is as much *your* America as the cops who killed. And
we don't get to walk away from that kind of damage. The shopping
malls and bike lanes and brunch cafes lining many a former Elliot
Avenue, some burned down in the riots that are starting to follow
each new police murder, are directly implicated in the settler colonialist cause-and-effect.

The vicious cycle is perhaps best crystallized for me by Patience
Zalanga's photos of the looted Target across the street from
Minneapolis's Third Precinct, Derek Chauvin's precinct, burned out
in the riots.[431] In a context of low breastfeeding rates among Black
women and the cost of its commodity replacement, Zalanga observed
how many of the shelves for baby formula were looted.

The sole officer Kentucky charged in the Taylor raid was later acquit-
ted.[432] The Ohio officer who killed Ma'Khia Bryant went uncharged.[433]
Arkansas gave the deputy who killed Hunter Brittain at that traffic
stop a whole year of jail he's expected to exit early on good behavior. Hennepin County refused to charge Minneapolis Officer Mark
Hanneman for killing twenty-two-year-old Amir Locke on another
botched no-knock.[434] Cook County refused to charge Eric Stillman,
the Chicago cop who killed Adam Toledo in that alley.[435]

Illinois's state attorney for Cook County, Kim Foxx, explained the
Stillman decision: "The case law that we rely on recognizes that police
officers are often forced to make split second decisions and judgments
in circumstances that are tense, uncertain and rapidly evolving."

THERE ARE ALTERNATIVES TO such deeply cultivated cultural
instincts.

We know in health that the rare adverse effects of vaccination—

producing morbidities and mortalities many multiple orders below letting disease run free—are far outweighed by the benefits of induced herd immunity.

One can object to the pharmaceutical sector—demanding tighter regulation and appropriate subsidies that undercut profit epidemiology—and still embrace vaccination as a principle. Indeed, the two together are ideal, ensuring widespread coverage. As City College of New York alum Jonas Salk put it, giving his polio vaccine to the world for free, "There is no patent. Can you patent the sun?"[436]

Sandra Roush and Trudy Murphy review basic vaccination's historical benefits.[437] The numbers of lives saved across diseases are *astounding*.

We're talking a 92 percent decline in cases of diphtheria, mumps, pertussis, and tetanus and a 99 percent decline in deaths. We're talking 80 percent-plus declines in deaths from hepatitis A, acute hepatitis B, Hib, and varicella. We're talking the (near) end of endemic transmission of poliovirus, measles, and rubella here in the United States and smallpox's eradication worldwide.

The absence of measles that U.S. skeptics cite as due cause for forgoing the MMR vaccine is due to the vaccine! And as a measles outbreak of 20,000 cases in France 2008–2011 makes clear, any such victory is conditional on continuing vaccination. More than 80 percent of France's cases occurred in unvaccinated people.[438]

Much as presently over 99 percent of U.S. COVID deaths are happening in the unvaccinated.[439] While that difference declined in the months to follow, it remained largely categorical.[440]

CLEARLY VACCINES ARE A foundational public health intervention. So, it's an outrage that Tennessee is moving to banning outreach for teens not just for COVID, but *all* vaccines![441]

But, as I described to Those Nerdy Girls, vaccines are also oft not enough. Indeed, the modeling literature is full of perverse outcomes along the lines we discussed around Cock van Oosterhout's work that speak to the complex parameter spaces that pathogen populations and their interventions share.

Three more come to mind. In the first, vaccines can turn chickens into ducks. The allusion is to a potential problem in China's campaign of regularly vaccinating its entire population of chickens against H5N1, the infamous bird flu.[442] While unprotected chickens are killed in short order by the virus, leading outbreaks to burning out, the kind of damage Boris Johnson was prepared to impose upon the British people, vaccines may turn many chickens into a reservoir of the virus from which new variants can emerge.[443] Much in the way ducks appear to act for many avian influenzas.

In some sense, this is a reiteration of the debate in late 2020 over whether the COVID vaccines offered only *disease immunity*, by which the vaccinated were protected from getting sick but in some cases could still transmit the virus, or full *sterilizing immunity*, by which infections could not be passed on to susceptibles.[444]

Evidence eventually rolled in to the effect that sterilizing immunity was the norm, but the University of Minnesota's Mike Osterholm, who serves on Biden's COVID advisory committee, declared five of those six studies may have showed nothing of the sort. Some local outbreaks of the Delta variant since proved greatest in the vaccinated. Seventy-four percent of new July COVID infections in Provincetown, Massachusetts, were identified in fully vaccinated patients.[445] That might be a marker of how successful the Massachusetts vaccine campaign has been, but also that the vaccines, while protective from the worst of disease, are not sterilizing.

The second caveat is that in some circumstances, vaccines may help select for increased virulence.[446] A strong immune response is more than likely to keep the pathogen from getting a foothold to begin with. It might also help clear a viremia that does get such a hold. But another option is that viral inoculates that can replicate against the stronger (if also incomplete) tide of a vaccine-charged response might survive enough to reach a transmission threshold.

Indeed, bats' strong immune systems appear to explain the coronavirus infection's deadliness to start.[447] Upon infecting someone who isn't vaccinated, the Nietzsche pathogen—what didn't kill it made it stronger—might cause that much more damage.

Disease ecologist Luis Chaves, one of my co-authors, pointed out a paper promising a vaccine that could wipe the betacoronaviruses off the map as a human danger.[448] Certainly not the durable franchise Pfizer promised its investors. But also a possible source of an unexpected outcome if successful. A moonshot that explodes the moon.

A general vaccine may lock out less virulent variants that produced a more "natural" vaccination, clearing the field for even more virulent strains.

The trap has been documented in industrial poultry, if out of different control mechanisms. Microbiologist Andreas Bäumler placed virulent salmonella's emergence on the eradication of two related strains that helped occupy the disease niche.[449] Once those strains were removed upon culling infected birds, Bäumler claims, immunity to salmonella that produced enteritidis declined.

ANALOGOUS COMPLICATIONS SPILL INTO notions of nature. A commenter on editor Michael Yates's Facebook page made a good-faith, Earth Day effort at pinning this kind of alienation between humanity and the environment to our species' origins.

I proposed the following adjustment:

Many nonhuman species engage in niche construction—manipulating the environment to their own needs.[450] Think on the humble beaver. Ecological succession is categorical.

Alienation didn't emerge upon our own speciation either. Even as we engaged in local extirpation of our own food sources, various megafauna among them, our metabolism was still embedded in the landscape upon which we depended. Yes, the growing civilizations that followed routinely destroyed regional watersheds and soils. But still within the bounds of humanity's relationships with nonhumans. Those bad decisions were punished by local collapses.

Capitalism is something else entirely. It projects humanity out beyond its ecological fabric as a *prime directive* rather than as a

side effect. Our rush to strip Earth of its regenerative power for
some minuscule cabal's offshore profits makes mass extinction
the only outcome. Should we continue that path.

In short, a secular trend punctuated by a sudden objectification,
abstract in conception and all too real in impact, what our group in
our Mike Davis chapter describes as projecting us off the planet's surface and out of the ecological matrix upon which we depend.[451]
Artist Eric Nord replied:

And the question of CAN we humans learn to live within the
"bounds" set by nonhuman needs seems at least partially confirmed by indigenous communities who proactively developed
sustainable land stewardship practices. My takeaway from this
is that we're not hardwired for either blissful symbiosis or earth
rape.

Earlier in 2017, I combined Nord's two points this way:

We are bound to our environmental context, including the vast
webs of energy and information exchange, pathogens among
them, that are at best tangential to civilization's command and
control. . . .
   We can embrace humanity's ingenuity without pretending we
need to extract our identities—as if iron and oil—out of the ecosystemic matrix.
   Making that conditionality work, properly situating our
Feuerbachian *Vergegenständlichung,* our citified projections,
within the web of life on which we depend, well, that's where the
real science of the 21st century now lies.[452]

INDEED, SUCH AMALGAMS ARE more than just good ideas. They
exist in the real world.
   I've taken to the morbid joke that Elon Musk, the American bil-

lionaire and son of South African apartheid now building rockets, is indeed taking us to Mars. He and his class aren't taking us by spaceship. They're turning Earth into a dust bowl. We're going to Mars without leaving Earth. Like Jeffrey Dahmer (or the city of New York) with a larger tub.

Cognitive dissonance isn't merely a matter of spin or a source of despair, however. It could also represent the path out.

Earlier this month a friend and colleague from Australia showed our meeting the sunrise in her farm window. It was the same sun marking my incipient daily trip for an afternoon coffee. It was the same sun from only a slightly different angle of a mere 9,400 miles not only later in the day and three-quarters a day behind but during a different season.

I gave the opening talk at a conference Down Under earlier in the month. Someone took a photo of me on the auditorium screen in Sydney. There was a bigger hall in Melbourne and a large contingent online from Brisbane to which the Sydney talk was also streamed.

It was a lively crowd, young, many Trots, who upon the Q&A integrated what I shared about industrial agriculture and new infectious diseases in scathing attacks upon capitalism. There was no pussyfooting around the c-word.

If I tried to direct traffic a bit in my responses, it was only along the lines that the "working class" wasn't enough of a solution. While we needed the spirit of the *Communist Manifesto* that many people brought to the mic, we also needed the strategy (and cast of thousands) embodied in the *Eighteenth Brumaire*.[453] How, for instance, to engage smallholders across the urban-rural metabolic rift? Or in the Global South?

Such a path might also weigh on the side of antihistoricist Alain Badiou to the effect that politics is really found in events and on the street rather than in opinions or even facts.[454] The logic of capital (and its alternatives) and the logic of struggle are incommensurate save in the acts of a communist proletariat. Including out of all the forms such a tactical communism might now take. The intervention, declares Bruno Bosteels introducing Badiou, authorizes itself.[455]

132 THE FAULT IN OUR SARS

If you can detect surprise in my face in the photo the organiz-ers posted of the Oz event—and that might be just an artifact of a moment caught by a pic—I was indeed initially stunned. Rooms full of people together, about half not wearing masks. I mean, that's the United States during a full-bore outbreak. Restaurants and bars filled up whatever the state of a county's outbreak. The Texas Rangers open-ing up the new baseball season at full stadium capacity. Stupid shit is our game plan.

But here, Australians were gathering because they could. The coun-try then had taken care of the outbreak without a vaccine. None, or very little SARS-2 presently circulates. They don't have to wear masks. Astonishing to anyone stateside who has been beaten down into pre-suming a failed nation-state is the natural order.

No wonder there are American flat-Earthers who believe Australia doesn't actually exist.[456] There is no alternative, goes the land of the free.

OUR EARTH STATESIDE IS indeed a different geometry. Solutions, as in a Lysistrata Gambit this time, emerge out of social manifold of a far different curvature from even that of an Oz I virtually visited and that is ruled by its own rightist man behind the curtain.

Although hitting the bars and dating sites have gotten some American men laid during COVID, forgoing the vaccine—and an albeit tenuous exit out of the pandemic—may revoke that passport: "What do women want? For men to get Covid vaccines."[457]

At least in some circles. Given how contentious even the notion of shared fate has become in the face of accumulating global crises, a sex strike or a finely plucked raised eyebrow may not be enough. Hedonic nihilism across any and all genders is one reaction to catastrophe. There may be plenty of fish of your stripe.

Along with presenting the first cogent hypothesis about the origins of the sex bias in COVID deaths, our little book *Dead Epidemiologists* had something to say about getting men to cooperate with public health campaigns.[458] It appears somebody read it, even some of the passages we left only in passing between topics more of our interest.

I was watching the local news in April. The broadcast interviewed Leah Witus, a Macalester College prof here in the Twin Cities, on her research showing commercials aimed at getting men to get the vaccine were more successful with a male voiceover than a female one.[459] The researcher expressed the necessary irony of the result in exactly the terms we described the race driver Denny Hamlin PSA we proposed in our book, including returning to the fight against gender inequality on the other side of saving us all.

I don't think I've now earned tenure at Macalester, but the book, as Nick Cave has said of some of his songs recorded years ago, still offers surprises.

SUCH CELEBRATIONS ARE COMPLEX things. The verdict against Derek Chauvinist was welcome, of course. The feelings, however, were mixed. Joy or relief tempered by the disgust for the depraved—and smug—indifference Chauvin, one man no PSA can save, displayed snuffing George Floyd on that Minneapolis corner.

The mix of working-class witnesses couldn't stop the murder. They tried.[460] Only a thorough thrashing would have interrupted those cops that day. A note for next time. As the witnesses testified, they will continue to be haunted by late-night visitations. George at the window. George at their bedside.

The justice served here isn't blind, of course. For decades Minnesota cops held carte blanche—the hideous pun intended—to kill Black and Brown people as they please. Or as they were directed. Minnesota Twins baseball star Rod Carew couldn't even jog in his own neighborhood.[461] Black man running is a crime in progress.

Now, in the other direction, it took burning down a part of the city to deliver the message such structurally prescribed extra-adjudication would no longer be swept aside by a boosterist curling broom. Indeed, to Bret Weinstein's point, well, yeah, Minneapolis knew it had to deliver a guilty verdict. Otherwise, the city would have been torched fo realz (and not just in the pages of the *New York Times*).[462] A jury decision that nullified the usual blue wall of silence that Weinstein embraces.

The lesson couldn't stick, however. Not even through the trial. Murdered motorist Daunte Wright—not ten miles from Minneapolis, but right up against North Minneapolis—was Philando Castile all over again. And Operation Safety Net, deploying three thousand National Guardsmen, was a revanchist collaboration, liberal to right-ist—from Governor Walz to the Boogaloo Bois—to dictate the demos runs nothing but the orders of the Itasca Project, the regional round-table of corporatists and NGOs that exercises power far beyond any elected body.[463]

A state that named lakes after summering slaveholders who bailed out a financially struggling University of Minnesota can't recognize itself except in the "good deeds" of Jantelagen apartheid.[464] The soci-opathy is considered exactly polite behavior.

The way out of that trap is backing the bravery of the families of Twin Cities police murder victims, who for decades have fought the oft-lonely battle against the blue line that runs from the Third Precinct through the State Capitol. The path ends in dismantling the power structure that is so in love with itself.

SUCH A SUCCESS MIGHT be ruinous in all the right ways, in part because of the inevitable *Bittereinder* reaction built in from the start.

As Alain Badiou on the Paris Commune persuasively argues, what happens out on the street is philosophy in practice.[465] Louis Althusser, for one, writes of a Lacanian interpellation when police hail some-one.[466] In recognizing the call, the civilian constitutes him or herself the subject of power.

Slavoj Žižek extends the subjectivization to prior to the encoun-ter, wherein even the innocent carry an abstract and indeterminate guilt.[467] Under most circumstances, when those stopped formally acknowledge their subjection, however unfair, the impasse is resolved.

But to many whites—individually and as a group, participants and observers—even that concession isn't enough. By a Fanonian soci-opathy mined from deep within the country's metaphysics—from its behavioral bedrock, down to slavery, lynchings, and Jim Crow—arbitrarily disconnecting the order of punishment from a subject's actions represents an important punctuation to white identity.[468]

To many whites, killing Black and Brown people for the *wrong* reasons is exactly an act of justice. As if hundreds of years of chillingly capricious precedence are jurisprudence enough. The murders—and the rationalizations that follow—codify white supremacy as a self-referential tautology at the heart of the sense of self.

The more unjustifiable the murder, the greater the frisson—and self-affirmation—when the murderer walks. The greater that gap, the greater the *jouissance*. Objecting to such a veritable sport—here we have George Zimmerman guffawing online over sixteen-year-old Trayvon Martin's body[469]—threatens a carefully cultivated cultural proprioception. Without it many white Americans wouldn't recognize themselves.

Kim Potter, Daunte Wright's killer convicted of first- and second-degree manslaughter, was sentenced to a light two years, to be cut to sixteen months, by a judge who local defense attorneys described as a harsh sentencer otherwise.[470] "This is a cop who made a tragic mistake," said an emotional Judge Regina Chu, who, up for reelection this year, received "hundreds and hundreds" of letters in support of Potter.

Each split second encounter is a cultural production the size of society.

WHEN IN UPTOWN MINNEAPOLIS a couple days ago, my kid and I visited the Wince Marie Peace Garden carved out as liberated space at the spot of Winston Smith and Deona Marie Knajdek Erickson's murders.[471] We placed flowers where Marie was killed by a white supremacist at the wheel.[472]

The lengths to which Mayor Jacob Frey and the MPD are pursuing a counterinsurgency against Black Lives Matter for such a small plot of land seems out of proportion.

But these efforts represent the danger of an example. Not a single square of land—here or up north along the Line 3 pipeline being built—is supposed to be involved in anything other than reproducing capital and the race and class character of the state. Even a lot left undeveloped for years.

If a busy city district—one about which Prince wrote a couple songs pre-gentrification—suffers the consequences, Frey and the rest of the state apparatus have only themselves to blame. The Smith murder, atop the nearby garage, has the stench of an assassination about it. And people are no longer letting such horrors slide, however booming the business in bodying Blacks has been.

Within hours of our visit, the city destroyed the garden (after giving only a three-minute dispersal warning). Making no bones about those lengths to which it was willing to go to void protest and public mourning.

According to the Garden on their now absent Instagram account, We Push for Peace claimed without evidence that the Smith family wanted the garden destroyed. Push for Peace is one of the POC community groups Frey's administration has paid off as collaborators, as it provides security for local businesses and advocates for more police.[473] Divide-and-conquer straight out of the COINTELPRO manual, rolled over today into IRON FIST.[474]

The balm of shopping isn't what Prince, who contributed thousands of dollars to BLM before he died,[475] had in mind for Minneapolis, where Uptown was a place *to set your mind free.* [476]

YES, FRACTURES THROUGH THE body politic.

While I appreciate being diagnosed as a neurasthenic by former political allies who have conflated the understandably painful damage of their own personal isolation during the pandemic and an anti-liberal socialist libertarianism—one, funny, also backed by Biden's CDC—the debate is already over.

Democrats and Republicans have greenlighted opening up, damn the consequences. My side's position has been refuted by U.S. political realities acted on with a swift abandon a year of wobbly interventions never approached. So why then the continued counterattack upon our side? Sore winners are a bore.

Opposed to our friends' mistaken epistemology and their preemptive strike of an accusation based on a recent *Times* article that any skepticism to official pronouncements is treated over on this side as irrefutable, the data from two studies presented in the midst of a fluid situation aren't the wooden stake in the COVID vampire that must die by happy hour.[477]

It's great the vaccines seem to be working. I advise everyone get stuck. But our friends here conflate individual immune reaction and antigenic cartography.[478] Pathogens evolve. And while perhaps not on influenza's annual schedule, many of the SARS-2 variants are already chipping away at vaccine effectiveness. Investor reports are showing pharmaceutical executives are banking on exactly that and, against the *Times* article's assurances, are planning lucrative boosters beyond the constraints of present pandemic pricing.

So the caveats are twofold. The strong immunity demonstrated here is directed at the strains that the patients tested happened to be attacked with (and may not persist for those who have not been infected with COVID directly). The potential scope of that protection across the burgeoning SARS-2 phylogeny was not tested. In other words, that the immunity might last for as long as decades doesn't matter once the virus evolves out from underneath that blanket.

The result accounts for Brian Orelli's caveat to his contention the vaccines are likely to be money losers:

> If they don't protect against the variants, then it doesn't really matter if you have B cells in your lymph nodes. If they're not going to protect against the variants then we're going to have to get a booster shot anyway.[479]

Second, seventy-seven subjects is a good number for a molecular study, as are the nineteen for the bone marrow aspirates, but such sample sizes still do not serve as grounds for the kind of population essentialism our friends appear to presume as the natural order of things and that somehow covers the inevitable dispersion in clinical and pathogenic responses.

The *Nature* study the *Times* reports on is clear-eyed about some of these issues the *Times* in contrast largely passed on:

> However, we do acknowledge several limitations. Although we detected anti-S IgG antibodies in serum at least 7 months after infection in all 19 of the convalescent donors from whom we obtained bone marrow aspirates, we failed to detect S-specific [long-lived bone marrow plasma cells] in four donors. Serum anti-S antibody titers in those four donors were low, suggesting that S-specific BMPCs may potentially be present at very low frequencies that are below our limit of detection.
>
> Another limitation is that we do not know the fraction of the S-binding BMPCs detected in our study that encodes neutralizing antibodies. SARS-CoV-2 S protein is the main target of neutralizing antibodies and correlation between serum anti-S IgG binding and neutralization titers has been documented. Further studies will be required to determine the epitopes targeted by BMPCs and MBCs as well as their clonal relatedness.[480]

That's all good and part of a typical line of research that requires development while we continue to engage in the kinds of multiple and synergistic interventions that have been documented to best control COVID. Except the United States effectively stopped pursuing nonpharmaceutical interventions entirely.

In other words, against another point raised by our friends, an anti-state state can be as Foucauldian as any medical panopticon.[481] As planned shrinkage, benign neglect, and the early days of AIDS demonstrated, a refusal to pursue governmental intervention into a public health crisis—let it burn!—acts as a negative placeholder against the kinds of effective responses that allowed other countries' populations to hit the bars COVID-free in a matter of months.[482]

The fiasco of the American COVID response is not something to toast. The irony is that I hope the live-free-or-die left is right, as in correct, if for all the wrong reasons. It would be a great relief to dodge

this COVID bullet. We would find no succor in proving live-free-
and-die wrong.

Indeed, their disturbance, cloistered away by a year-and-a-half of
misrule, is a long-recognized challenge. "The shutting up of houses,"
Defoe wrote,

> was at first counted a very cruel and Unchristian Method, and the
> poor People so confin'd made bitter Lamentations: Complaints
> of the Severity of it, were also daily brought to my Lord Mayor,
> of Houses causelessly, (and some maliciously) shut up.[483]

A London administration over 350 years ago made house inspec-
tions that nearly no U.S. jurisdiction undertook this pandemic to
check on the sick and comfort the well.

THIS IS HELL'S Chuck Mertz, on whose excellent show I've
appeared, followed up with a question about the *Nature* study. Citing
a commentary on the study,[484] a listener soothed:

> Chuck, please don't worry so much about unvaccinated people.
> After the last 2 years (which felt like 4), I think it's safe to assume
> that everyone you meet outside contracted the virus already.
> Which, in turn, means their immune system adapted to the point
> that they are literally protected by the infection as if they've had
> a vaccination.

I replied that the listener had conflated two topics.

First, there is the matter of strong immune reaction in the paper
the *Nature* commentary reviewed we discussed above. Long story
short, a strong reaction to one strain does not necessarily offer protection to the new variants now cycling in. The listener's contention
is such an essentialist position as it is. Not everyone produces such a
strong immune reaction.

There is also the matter of the fallacy of silent evidence.[485] Many of those people who died from COVID didn't produce that long-term immunity. Not just because they died, but autopsies showed lymph nodes with no germinal centers and at best capable of producing only low-affinity antibodies.[486]

Does that mean we've had a selection event and all those people have been removed? Not necessarily. There are still many millions out there who are likely unexposed to the virus. Who and where and when they might be, we have no idea. In other words, even if they wouldn't subsequently die, we presently don't know who would, and who wouldn't, produce such an immune reaction.

The listener conflates the duration of a natural immune reaction and its coverage (say, in comparison to vaccination). As Columbia University Professor of Virology Vincent Racaniello described in an interview in May, it's unclear whether a natural infection would offer what a vaccination does:

> So, on the one hand, yes, you make a lot of viral proteins [when naturally infected] and those are great epitopes for mainly T cells because I think most of the antibodies that are going to block infection are going to be [directed at the spike protein]. But any other viral protein could in theory be a T-cell target. So you'll get more epitopes.
>
> The counter view is that the virus may encode immune antagonists that could alter the immune response in some way that's not as good as, say, a vaccine. So it really depends. And we don't know enough yet. So I think if people are making a blanket statement that natural infection is always better, that's not always correct. It really depends on the virus.[487]

Yet Racaniello remains bullish on T-cell protection across variants, at least for the next couple years.

He reasons that the coronavirus evolves for rapid antigenic escape from neutralizing antibodies. That largely involves the spike protein evolving escape. On the other hand, the array of other epitopes T cells tag for destruction, from across all the other viral proteins, are unlikely to evolve at such a pace. That would give those naturally infected more protection from this second arm of the specific immune system until those proteins eventually evolve resistance.[488]

I am not convinced the putative protection is so clear-cut. Molecular geneticists Santiago Vilar and Daniel Isom show most SARS-2 proteins are indeed conservative in their mutational variation.[489] But several proteins other than the spike—the NSP12, NS9C, and the nucleocapside—are exhibiting respectable mutation rates.[490]

It's a population variation that increased over time as the virus infected more people across 2020 and, although proving global in its reach for the D614 replacement in the spike protein by December 2020, remained spatially heterogeneous across all the other replacements surveyed for the spike protein and the other proteins.[491]

So on the T-cell coverage, I think we're back at Racaniello's initial answer—it depends.

Modeling that Rodrick Wallace and I pursued in the early aughts applied Irun Cohen's notion that the immune system is a cognitive system.[492] Whether the immune system reacts, and how so, involves a series of decisions it makes: from no reaction to full-blown attack. It's a continuum dependent upon a variety of inputs that extend far beyond the model of immunity as a simple reflex and involving bodily systems other than the immune system itself.

So, it's not clear how the immune system will react to SARS-2's mutational combinatorials across proteins. There might be some parts of the cross-protein evolutionary space—defined by the stereochemical relationships across the proteins and an adjunct compensatory evolution—that will elicit strong immune responses.[493] Other parts of that space, on the other hand, might offer the virus immune escape.

We have no means by which to model those potential pathways beyond playing let's pretend *in silico* or by toying with some dangerous gain-of-function studies we've heard so much about lately, neither of which will capture the totality of what a coronavirus in the wild is capable.

Nor, as Vilar and Isam's maps suggest, is it clear whether such an

immune reaction will be the same from place-to-place or community-to-community. The immune system, in the argument Rod and
I arrive upon, is an open system exposed to the variety of social
determinants of health that structure disease outcome across all the
horrors of racism and classist deprivation.

What I'm doing here is asking people to let go of the essentialist pre
sumptions of viral evolution and clinical course. A *Gray's Immunology*
should not serve as the basis for public health policy. Think of immunity more in terms of Engels's *The Condition of the Working Class in
England* or Cedric Robinson on racial capitalism.[494] Another natural
science is possible.

FOR WE ALL WANT to exit the pandemic. Even I among those Public
Health Experts accused of championing a "never-ending lockdown"
while making millions of dollars off all those talks to the Connecticut
Green Party and the Landless Workers' Movement. I mean real Gates
Foundation money. With my real-world grant running out before the
year ends and no employment in sight for 2022.

Contrary to some leftists who claim objections to the CDC abandoning its mask recommendations are markers of said panopticon,
many of us oppositional epidemiologists aim to put ourselves out
of business. As trust is an epidemiological variable, recommending
practices that continue the business of the pall of the pandemic would
violate that objective. That's exactly why some of us are speaking out
against the CDC on the matter of the masks.

As I described in *Dead Epidemiologists,* the pandemic has been a
disaster for working people.

Certainly no socialist better object to workers attempting to survive the economy. And no one I know denounced as public health
pariahs the service and industrial workers who, abandoned by
employers and government alike, had to troop to work to pay their
bills. Indeed, quite the contrary. Although to limited success, a lot of
time and fight went into demanding them better protection and pay.
That is, the capitalist reality to which we must adhere at the moment

can also be condemned. We can, and should, object every step of the way. Otherwise we rubber stamp our own demise.

Handing over "the realm of political possibility" as both ontology and imaginary may fit with our present sense of impotence, but it offers no way out of the trap. Capital has successfully imposed its norms upon our epistemology as a form of labor discipline, but such opportunistic pragmatism isn't in the capitalist favor either. The system has turned into a phantasmagoria on borrowed environmental time.

In the other direction, many of the alternatives are either bat-shit crazy or abandoned wholesale or—as Salvatore Engel-Di Mauro, who we referenced earlier, describes in his new book—are at best caught out of practice.[495] So any first step toward parallel governance is no safe bet.

But we'll never get anywhere near that starting line presuming our very lives solely matters of our lords and masters or next month's rent due. The latter is real, of course, but kissing its ring is another thing entirely.

THE COVID VARIANTS—OR, as dismissed elsewhere, the *scariants*—aren't evolving on our news cycle schedule. The reports CDC itself summarized, however, show various strains emerging by interdemic selection out from underneath vaccines bit-by-bit. News reports are highlighting when and where the vaccines work across variants—a great thing!—but are omitting that not all vaccines control all strains. As the combinatorics increase, the logistics for matching vaccines to strains may extend beyond the institutional cognition of a system that couldn't even bother with contact tracing.

As we discussed, Pfizer is banking on exactly such antigenic cartography. So, lots of people, including rads exhausted by the liberal public health panopticon, are conflating the variants for archetypes rather than quasispecies evolving on the daily across millions of walking experiments.[496] The pharma executives know better and are betting accordingly.

I do believe we were on the right track getting people vaccinated, but any antimicrobial resistance researcher knows full well the out-come of half-ass efforts to complete population inoculation, while also ending all nonpharmaceutical interventions in the meantime.[497] There's nothing surprising about the likely outcome. I could be wrong, sure. Either way, we are choosing to run the not-so-natural experiment and will find out.

Boris Johnson, of all people, is (sorta) more on point on this problem. The Brits are reacting to the growing cases of the India strain B.1.617 by increasing the pace of vaccinations. B.1.617 appears threatening to outpace the British B.1.1.7 strain that itself had outcompeted the post-China strains across many countries, including the United States. B.1.1.7 expressed greater transmissibility and deadliness. The Brits are preparing that B.1.617 is even worse.

The *New York Times* reported mid-May:

Prime Minister Boris Johnson of Britain said on Friday that vaccination protocols would be changed to swiftly deliver second doses to people over 50 to combat the spread of a coronavirus variant first detected in India, a warning sign for countries that are easing restrictions even though their own vaccination campaigns are incomplete.

"We believe this variant is more transmissible than the previous ones," Mr. Johnson said at a news conference. What remained unclear, he said, was by how much. . . .

While he said that England would not delay plans to ease restrictions on Monday, before a full reopening in June [now mid-July], he warned that the variant could force a change of course. . . .

In Scotland, Nicola Sturgeon, the first minister, said on Friday that plans to ease restrictions in Glasgow would be delayed at least a week out of concern about an uptick in cases that officials said might be driven by the variant. . . .

Much is unknown about the new variant, but scientists fear it may have driven the rise of cases in India and could fuel outbreaks in neighboring countries.

Dr. Maria Van Kerkhove, the technical lead of the W.H.O.'s coronavirus response, said a study of a limited number of patients, which had not yet been peer-reviewed, suggested that antibodies from vaccines or infections with other variants might not be quite as effective against B.1.617. The agency said, however, that vaccines were likely to remain potent enough to provide protection from serious illness and death.[498]

By mid-June, the new variant turned out exactly as feared. Case rates went up exponentially.[499] Hospitalizations went up. It wasn't just some stochastic burp. Some of the new COVID variants, more infectious and deadlier both, are demonstrably beating a first vaccine dose that eight in ten Brits had received.

B.1.617.2, or the Delta variant, is now detected in all 50 U.S. states and the CDC has bumped it to a "variant of concern":

The CDC is concerned about the Delta variant mutating to a point where it evades the existing COVID-19 vaccines, according to [CDC director Rochelle] Walensky.[500]

"It's the fact," tweets @angryblkhoemo, "that [the CDC] knew about the Delta variant before they released those premature [mask] recommendations for vaccinated individuals for me."[501]

Now a Delta-plus variant (B.1.617.2.1) has emerged in India that, with a K417N amino acid replacement in the spike protein already associated with increased infectivity, appears to be resistant to monoculture antibody cocktails casirivimab and imdevimab.[502]

On the high heels of a series of scandals around their response—from paying politically connected companies for goods and services they couldn't deliver to a Health Secretary fucking the sister of a health executive and awarding contracts to his own sister's firm he owns shares in—the Brits are scheduled to open up for good July 19.[503]

"Opening up will make us healthier," Sajid Javid, the new Health Secretary, cheerily asserted.[504] Even with a comparatively strong vaccination campaign, British cases early July have spiked.[505] "We are

going to have to learn to accept the existence of Covid and find ways
to cope with it—just as we already do with flu."

SO THE BRITS HAVE circled back to the COVID-is-like-flu argu
ments with which Trump began the U.S. response to the pandemic.
Being social is now critical to health says the party that, despite Boris
Johnson's March 2020 walk-back, continues to act upon the nation's
modern founder, Margaret Thatcher, who contended that "there is no
society."[506]

Even a more appropriate response would be difficult in the present
moment. Think of public health as the *Evergreen* cargo ship. Its value
is in its large capacity, but it's slow and, if the support isn't available,
can get stuck in a proverbial Suez. That's on a good day. With governance that hasn't abandoned public health as a public commons.

So, reports (and CDC recommendations) signaling all is well aren't
intelligence enough. To reach a scale threshold, one has to choose a
future that may not pan out empirically. A precautionary principle
bears its costs in funding and attention and epistemological violation.

It perhaps may seem gauche to pile on the metaphors and compare
public health also to taking a dump, but this one we should embrace—
the metaphor, not the crap—given the Great Reform movement's
success in sewage and sanitation.[507] In any public health campaign,
including responding to a pandemic, we must wipe our ass twice to
learn that we must wipe a third time. And we must wipe our ass three
times to learn we only needed to wipe twice.

What I mean here is that we are responsible for investing effort into
a pandemic response the outcome of which we can't know until after-
ward. With a virus acting at scales (and speeds) we cannot track well
in real time—molecularly and across continents—such campaigns
are by definition temporally opaque. We must invest in interventions above and beyond what any transient data capture. We must
fight pandemics in multiple tenses as pathogens do not adhere to our
common understanding of cause and effect, repeatedly evolving solutions to problems they've yet to encounter.[508]

The United States has chosen otherwise, indeed taking a polar opposite heading. Now post-India, the country has returned to its initial standing post-China, all chips in on the side of a Type 1 error that we won't be prepared for a real risk. It's not quite the same spot. One doesn't step in the same river twice. But there's an element of the neurotic binger at which Ed Yong hinted, where Marx meets Lacan.[509]

THE PATHOLOGIES FOLD TOGETHER. The land use driving disease emergence and climate change alike weave together through the megamachine that killed George Floyd on that street corner.

Alleen Brown reports that Governor Walz's administration and local county sheriffs in northern Minnesota agreed to escrow funding from Enbridge—the Canadian company building the Line 3 pipeline through Native land and across the Mississippi River—that paid for repressing peaceful protests against the pipeline:

> As part of its permit to build Line 3, the Minnesota Public Utilities Commission, or PUC, created a special Enbridge-funded account that public safety officials could use to pay for policing Enbridge's political opponents. The police were concerned about who state officials would hire to decide which invoices to pay or reject.
>
> Last June, Kanabec County Sheriff Brian Smith wrote an email to other sheriffs along the pipeline route. "I think we need to let the PUC know that the person selected needs to be someone that we also agree upon," Smith wrote. "Not a member of the PUC, not a state, county or federal employee, but someone that has an understanding of rioting and MFF operations"—referring to mobile field force operations, or anti-riot policing.[510]

The counterinsurgency up north went full Israel on Minneapolis, arresting and strip-searching a reporter on assignment for the *Los Angeles Times* covering the Line 3 protests.[511]

Returning to the Twin Cities, and circling back to the point with which we began our travelogue, such invasive policing extends into science and medicine. Almost a year to the day after Floyd's murder, the *Star-Tribune* published a report on a petition Hennepin Hospital staff submitted objecting to the hospital's Tactical Emergency Medicine Peace Officer program.[512]

Under TEMPO, the hospital continues to train Minneapolis police to diagnose uncooperative detainees—almost exclusively of color—who require "medical force," including sedation and restraints, under the dubious syndrome of "excited delirium."

It's been three years since objections to the hospital's program, including preemptive use of ketamine, were registered as unethical at best and deadly at worst. Elijah McClain was killed by Aurora, Colorado, police upon injection of ketamine.[513] Several Minneapolis patients were documented as requiring medical intervention, including resuscitation, as a result of their ketamine injections.

The hospital's new CEO gestured at "dismantling institutional racism" but went on to defend the ketamine practice on the grounds Hennepin treats some of the county's most difficult patients.[514] She even passed the buck onto the 1,000-plus doctors, nurses, and staff who signed the petition. The employees should "roll up their sleeves and be part of the solution."

There is nothing more Minnesotan than that tennis return of a reply. Blame the people who point out the problem. And the diagnosis of Blackness as a medical condition to be controlled or cured, at a hospital where staff were later found wearing blackface, suggests that the nice apartheid that killed Floyd marches onward.[515]

This is the settler mentality—downstate and up north—that the regional political class is structurally incapable of abandoning even at this late date because, as we noted, it's only in the mirror of such practices that it can recognize itself.

Indeed, there's a direct line through Minnesota history. Upon the infamous mass hanging of thirty-eight Dakota in Mankato, Minnesota, on Abraham Lincoln's orders in 1862, William Mayo, the founder of the now internationally known Mayo Clinic, dug up at least one of the bodies for dissection.[516] He, and then the clinic, kept the bones of Marpiya Okinajin, one of the hanged, before the clinic returned them in 2000 to the Santee reservation in Nebraska, the Dakotas long driven from Minnesota.

There are synergies in a better direction. Across the street from the Third Precinct in Minneapolis, the Floyd riots also burned down the Indian restaurant Gandhi Mahal.[517] With its owner's approval, a local farmer rescued the restaurant's walk-in fridges to preserve veggies on his outstate farm. More broadly, BIPOC farmers are slowly starting to better stake their Minnesota claim.[518] Radical rural and urban getting together.

FRIENDS EXCAVATE OTHER THINGS lost in the fire. Leela Corman is a high school classmate of mine. She concocts poems in pen and ink. A very Jewish appreciation, my mother remarked once, when I kvelled over Ben Katchor's *Julian Knipl* the same way.[519] Or in a different tradition, Faith Ringgold's *Tar Beach*.[520]

Corman is finishing a graphic novel set in the 1940s. It includes women's wrestling of the Mildred Burke era, sushi committing harakiri, a waitress Holofernes, and the Holocaust as a series of psychedelic Busby Berkeley musical numbers by way of George Grosz and medieval depictions of hell.

Her most recent publication served as a shorter meditation on visiting her grandfather's village in Poland, which suffered a Nazi massacre.[521] Two panels spoke to me:

A few nights after I returned, a Jewish colleague told me, over dinner, "Jews need to stop talking about the Holocaust. It's so boring."

My feet remembered the sensation of my great-grandparents' bones beneath them. My eyes went to my boots, still dusted with dirt from their mass grave. My colleague's mouth continued to move.[522]

And, earlier, this:

Your grandfather and his brothers were called the flowers of town. They were modern, they were cleanshaven, they rode bicycles. And if anyone hurt a Jew, if a Jew was attacked and beaten up, they would come with REVENGE. Ve called them the flower of the town. THE FLOWER OF THE TOWN! And your grandfather was like a soldier, under order from only himself.[523]

I'm not a good soldier. But I suddenly feel the campaign I only previously suspected there. It's everyday and maybe for life. What about you? What are you feeling other than the confusion of our times?

Only later the second panel made me think of my shaved mustache. It also occurred to me that I haven't bought a single new item to wear in a year. I reject individualist interventions into climate change, but think on my infinite—our infinite—and indigestible comet of plastic waste. I think about the *Independent*'s report on police efforts *to train* the fascistic Oath Keepers.[524]

I think of commenters on Floyd family attorney Benjamin Crump's page who propose Kim Porter, the president of the Brooklyn Center police union, who shouted out "Taser! Taser!" only to cover her ass for the shot in Daunte Wright's back.[525] I confess to myself that I think that might be truer than I'm prepared to go. I think about how I should take my own advice when I counseled students this semester to learn to leap out of the trap of it all.

IN THE FACE OF THIS eschatology, we clutch at the Yūgen (幽玄) myth of the mustachioed samurai who fights against all odds and loses.

But as the dreamer plays all the parts in a dream, perhaps such a story shares no more with us than that we confuse what we tell ourselves about our struggles for liberation and the nature of our unattainable objects of desire.

Philosophers Walter Benjamin and Franco Berardi and the appropriately renamed sociologist Sylvain Lazarus suggest an otherwise.[526] In reality, alternate futures and liberatory possibilities are *always* imminent even in a history foisted upon us by the winner.

BARRY LOPEZ, THE TRAVEL writer who died last year, spent a career writing about emerging out of such imposition on lands near and far. Occupations are as much an idea as a garrison, he wrote. Where colonial materialism meets action and signification.

In his final full book, Lopez revisits the travels of his middle age to take stock—to use the unfortunate Americanism—of how he had changed as much as the landscapes he remembered.[527] Up in the high Arctic he thinks of the Navajo farther south:

> In my understanding, which is imperfect, Beautyway [or Blessingway] rites are conducted over a period of several days by a medicine person called a singer, in the home (usually a hogan) of a "patient," with his or her family present. The patient is referred to as "the one sung over" and is conceived of as someone who has "deteriorated" or is otherwise in a state of spiritual imperfection. The Navajo way to view this state of deterioration or incomplete integration with the world is to regard it as normal, a condition that develops over time in every person.[528]

Here in the United States, and now an Americanized Europe, that incoherence is celebrated. I wonder if I shaved because, like José Halloy I quoted earlier, I no longer wished to engage such a hellscape on its impossible terms even in opposition. There is no way to talk to people who feast upon themselves. So many defending murdering children. Or pols profiting off elderly deaths. Or the normal that caused the disaster. Corruption as a matter of concerted principle.

We need instead to find people—of any and all races and nations—prepared to make the journey out:

> Restoring a person to a state of "beauty" requires that the singer "make it incumbent upon the universe" to re-create in the *patient* those conditions in the natural world that signify—for Navajo people—coherence or harmony. . . . A beauty can be renewed in us through reintegrating ourselves with a world over which we have no control.[529]

No one need appropriate another's mysticism. Indeed, such acquis-
itive grasping represents part of the problem. But the core here may
model a portal out of a place that solemnly sanctions child sacrifice.
What a grotesquery of a can-can! Can it be replaced with the music
of the spheres, a bolero that crescendos to a vibration felt in a walk in
the woods or in the passing lift of the laughter of children at recess?

THE FRUITS ARE FOUND in more than transcendental projection
out into the fabric of all things. The benefits can be pragmatic to a
degree many a Midwesterner would appreciate.

Without placing anyone on a pedestal or fetishizing cultures themselves bent by historical time—people are still people—it'll take pivoting
around what even those who oppose the present death machine think
are our best features. "When I was young," Lopez continues,

> and just beginning to travel with Indigenous people, I imagined
> that they saw more and heard more than I did, that they were
> overall simply more aware than I was. They were. . . .
>
> The event I was cataloging in my mind as "encounter with
> a tundra grizzly," they were experiencing as an immersion in
> the current of a river. They were swimming in it, feeling its pull,
> noting the temperature of the water, the back eddies, and where
> the side streams entered. . . . They began gathering various pieces
> together that might later self-assemble into an event larger than
> "a bear feeding."
>
> My friends . . . had situated themselves within a *dynamic* event.
> Also, unlike me, they felt no immediate need to resolve it into
> meaning. . . . More often I was only *thinking* about the place I was
> in. . . . On occasion I would become so wedded to my thoughts,
> to some cascade of ideas, that I actually lost touch with the details
> that my body was *still gathering* from a place.[530]

Reinserting ourselves back into the ecological matrix and a
common humanity, yes, partly of our own making, will change us.

I've concluded that the mustache didn't matter. Grow one out. Shave it off. Head for a bar patio upon vaccination. Drink at home. Whatever. The key is something else. Are you and yours in a different constellation of mind, body, and meaning upon this historical precipice? Are you making ready for exodus? Out of which terminal are you departing Elon Musk's alienated Mars back for Earth?

Otherwise, from cop to COVID cough, it'll be a splatter of split seconds out of which humanity's last moments will spring. A spray too crowded together to interrupt and too spread apart to capture.

WHAT MIGHT THAT MEAN?

Whereas climate change and pandemics and other such hyperobjects—everywhere all at once—place the space of the globe inside each of our spinning little heads, the time clicks left for mitigating the damage also have compressed into something too finely numerous to parse.[531] Global capitalism has squished a wealth of geological processes into our historical time scale, with those who caused the wreck still calling the shots.

As @Merman_Melville waxed: "Kind of a bummer to have been born at the very end of the Fuck Around century just to live the rest of my life in the Find Out century."[532] Merman followed up with how disturbed he was by the number of scientists who retweeted the post.

One result, cause and effect can feel reversed. The loopholes automated into the social action of life—letting capital and the state get the best of us at work and out in the neighborhood—feel as if we're repeatedly shot down with our hands already up or back at work unmasked before we cycle out of the worst of the pandemic. A friend reported his wife was recently fired: supermarkets that punished employees who refused to wear masks are now punishing them for wearing them.

Defoe wrote of such an algorithmic lag—always a step behind—built into the system of a down:

I often reflected upon the unprovided Condition, that the whole Body of the People were in at the first coming of this Calamity

upon them, and how it was for Want of timely entering into
Measures, and Managements, as well publick as private, that all
the Confusions that followed were brought upon us; and that
such a prodigious Number of People sunk in that Disaster, which
if proper Steps had been taken, might, Providence concurring,
have been avoided, and which, if Posterity think fit, they may
take a Caution, and Warning from.[533]

WHAT TO DO? Upon what to draw our Caution and Warning?
We need more than slip out of the proverbial alleyway before the
cop arrives. The ShotSpotter of the megamachine is everywhere. The
gun (or email account or pesticide) we Camus-like protagonists find
in our hands is a structurally imposed compulsion. We seem to have
no choice as Things Fall Apart around us. In this we can agree regardless of our opinion of when, or if, to reopen.

So, okay then, what to do? First, we need to converge upon enough
shared objectives that we also understand are likely to change upon
our journey to meet them. One possibility is a world of many worlds,
as the Zapatistas demanded.[534] That offers a soul-saving subtraction
by addition. We can mitigate the ongoing extinction event by increasing both the agrobiodiversity and the variety of place-specific means
by which to place humanity back into the ecology and the virtuous
cycles on which we all depend.

Clean water. Nutritious food for everyone in a culturally appropriate way. Shared community at whatever stage of life we find ourselves.
In the bigger picture, a planet less swiftly tilting down upon our present environmental precipices. Healing all these metabolic rifts from
soil to community.

How to get there? The boundaries of the possible change as matters of necessity and goodwill. Liberation is an exercise in suddenly
shared revelation.

Angela Davis observed that the trans movement showed Black
Lives Matter and beyond that we can bend the very girders of our
categorical imperatives.[535] Not only does my son now no longer view

gender as a binary, it's not even a continuum. It's a scribble! More esoteric conjunctions see a trans Marxism firmly in anti-capitalism's camp *and* assimilated with the thrum of contradictions underway.[536] Paths in other domains also open up. Clearly a lively and environmentally friendly rural life makes for better city living (and vice versa).

Such transformations can be painful experiences. Millions may arrive only kicking and screaming. Millions more will likely fight us for their right to extinction. For the suicide by cop they paid for.

As journalist Sims Kern, spouse of a NASA flight controller, describes, even Musk and his ilk aren't escaping what they've wrought:

> Let me assure you that the rich escaping the earth for a space utopia is only a trope in fiction—at least in our lifetimes . . .
>
> Around half a dozen astronauts live up [in the International Space Station] at any given time, bouncing around a narrow tube with roommates they didn't choose and who can't properly bathe for months on end. The wi-fi is slow. The food is not Michelin starred, to say the least. Their sleeping situation is akin to a floating coffin. And pooping involves a complicated procedure in a port-o-potty where the door is a plastic curtain and everything *floats.* . . .
>
> Space-dwellers must exercise at least two hours a day to keep their bones from turning to goo. They spend a ton of time studying systems and conducting repairs on equipment that frequently breaks because *space wants to kill you.* . . .
>
> The pointlessness of it all is especially despicable when you understand that space tourism is funded with the hoarded wealth of billions of workers who are struggling to survive here on Earth. The space tourism industry will be built with the profits off supply chains that work people to death-by-exhaustion, literally enslave people, and are rapidly destroying the future habitability of our planet.[537]

Rats onto a sinking ship. Musk rats, to spoil the real rodents' good name.

ABOUT TWENTY YEAR AGO, an offbeat comic told a different joke
at the Poetry Project's annual New Year's Marathon reading in New
York City, another kind of space race. "I saw a slip of paper on the
street," she began; "It said 'The Human Condition.' I snatched it up for
a closer look. It read 'The Hunan Kitchen.'"

It'll be slips of paper, pub walls, oral lore passed down generations,
off-track journals, conversation in the street, minor presses, maybe
a few blog outposts, and—much more in our favor—the billions of
minds in various stages of liberation by which the neurototalitarian-
ism of the global machine that philosopher Franco Berardi claims can
be sabotaged:

> The present depression (both psychological and economic)
> obscures the consciousness that no determinist projection of the
> future is true. We feel trapped in the tangle of techno-linguistic
> automatisms: finance, global competition, military escalation.
> But the body of the general intellect (the social and erotic bodies
> of a million cognitarians) is richer than the connective brain.
> And the present reality is richer than the format imposed on it,
> as the multifold possibilities inscribed in the present have not
> been wholly cancelled, even if they may seem presently inert.[538]

One of political scientist Yekaterina Oziashvili's Sarah Lawrence
College undergrad students, not much older than Adam Toledo,
channeled philosopher Samo Tomšič on a final term paper with a
clarity of mind:

> Capitalist ideology hollows out human beings and defines them
> according to their exteriority: their pleasure, their suffering,
> their desires, their appearance and their utility. Identity takes all
> of these things, the specific pleasures, miseries, desires, uses and
> appearances and makes them into a soul. A capitalist spiritual-
> ity is a psychological egoism. The subject of "identity" screams,
> I am me! I am me! I am me! in order to prove to himself that he
> really does exist.

Reduced to objects, human beings can spend their entire lives seeking to be recognized as subjects. Frantically, he searches for evidence, and oh such evidence does he find. His own pain is handed to him like a trophy. Here, this is you, you are real, you are a person. Capitalism produces a human being who is constantly trying to prove what he already is. He tries to find himself as a thing he can hold, see, touch, feel and know. The abstract self is at war with the world because he wants to reproduce himself in everything that comes into view. The "identity" that defines the self today must be constantly asserted, relentlessly accounted for; an obsession that manifests in everything, always needing an outlet and never resting in its "expression."

There is no telling what a society that does not produce abstraction in human beings will look like. However, only an ideology that emerges out of suffering but does not become attached to it, will succeed in such a project.

No Blessingway that. A horror of a soul fracturing on repeat. If, however, the kids are figuring out the bounds of this suffering early on and, importantly, acting to circumvent it, then we might recover a path to the next seven generations Native Americans plan around.[539]

Not on their own, however. The sorrow of a children's crusade, with all its dissonant historical connotations, is that it can't and—as Greta Thunberg repeatedly points out—shouldn't have to win.[540] Kids—well beyond Zalia Avant-garde, Dara McAnulty, the Linda Lindas, Gev and Tata, Liv Harness, Nandi Bushell, Emer, and nine-year-old Emma singing Serge Lama's "Je Suis Malade" as if mourning a world already passed—should be given the room to be their brilliant selves. Indeed, against the specialized schools, all kids are Gifted and Talented if we allow them the play of their childhoods.

We all will still need to eat, of course. At least some of us will choose to raise the next generation in all that joy and hard work. Heartbreak will follow upon love's demise. *Je suis sale sans toi,* we will weep. Diseases will still arise, although with enough preparation to much less carnage. History and conflict will rumble on. And yet, if we can agree to act accordingly, (almost) all that seems so distressingly solid now can be made to melt into air. Or at the least offering us up a fighting chance for the better.

—PATREON, JULY 16, 2021

The Blind Weaponmaker

"Shouldn't I tell her about the puma?" asked the younger man.
"That's not my problem. Or yours," said the older man, still looking
away. "We're in this together."

— CHUCK KLOSTERMAN (2019)

IN A WORLD OF NEOLIBERALS and new-century Nazis, there
are few chances these days to get genuinely excited over an idea with
which one disagrees.

A couple months ago, Bioscience Resource Project's Jonathan
Latham and I compared notes over the origins of COVID-19. I left
room for *discussion* of the putative lab origins of the outbreak. As I
wrote in *Big Farms,* with *thousands* of BSL-3 and -4 labs built around
the world since 9/11 and H5N1—the first of the new celebrity pathogens—the rarity of an accidental release of a deadly pathogen under
study bends toward inevitability.[541]

But that doesn't mean any single outbreak is so determined. That's
a different issue. Such a conclusion depends on the preponderance of
evidence accumulating across a variety of explanations.

In May 2020, I provisionally concluded the genetics of SARS-CoV-2,
the COVID virus, supported the field origins hypothesis.[542] That is, I

backed the notion that SARS-2 emerged out of a series of recombination events across wild bats, wild food animals, industrial livestock,
and the labor that tend them across Central and South China.

Latham and Allison Wilson continued down the more difficult
path.[543] As they would come to note, the lab hypothesis has been quietly relegated as conspiracy theory by establishment science and the
mainstream press.

Certainly there are off-the-wall versions of the story. But the possibility is in and of itself too fraught otherwise. What would we all do if
one of the more cogent versions proved true? What aspersions would
it cast upon nation-states across the globe that endangered billions of
people in the name of protecting them? Must the lab theory be treated
as absurd by dint of necessity?

In mid-July, Latham and Wilson posted the next iteration in the
more sophisticated version of the hypothesis, revising their original
take.[544] In their first cut, the duo declared a bat coronavirus sampled
in 2013 escaped one of two governmental labs in Wuhan, China, the
apparent ground zero of the SARS-2 pandemic. A view perhaps parsimonious to a fault.

Latham and Wilson appear to agree. The team now proposes that
the spillover into humans actually took place in 2012, when six guano
miners were infected in a Yunnan cave, coming down with what
Latham and Wilson assert were COVID-like symptoms, as described,
they submit, in a Master's thesis written by a medical doctor in Chinese
that the Bioscience Resource Project team had someone translate.[545]

The pair proposes that it was when among the six miners—three of
whom would die—that the SARS-like (SL) virus evolved the adaptations to the human immune system we see now in SARS-2. It's those
miner samples, stored away since in Wuhan, that escaped some time
after the BSL-4 lab there went operational in 2018 and scientists began
dangerous "gain of function" studies that permitted the samples free-
range, including, accidentally, out the lab back door only miles from
the Wuhan wet market that served as the preliminary focus of investigations into SARS-2 origins.[546]

It certainly makes for a terrific story. Is it true? Maybe, maybe not.

The important point here is that taking the time to unpack the possibility marks the attention with which we should offer good faith efforts at widening our exploration of the origins of a seminal global crisis.

The Interrogation

My critique of this iteration of the lab theory of SARS-2 origins is by necessity terse and technical. If you're having a little trouble, I ask that you follow the links to patch together the details. Whatever my position, perhaps the take-home is that researchers, journalists, and officials should replicate following up, however likely we all might ultimately disagree with the hypothesis's plausibility. The stakes are too high to skip probing the possibility for expedience's sake.

1) To start, Latham and Wilson point out that while declaring the 2019 bat sample that never made it to Wuhan closer to SARS-2, epidemiologist Hong Zhou and colleagues' own SimPlot graph showed that the 2013 sample that was shipped to Wuhan, which was sampled from the *very* mineshaft where the miners got infected, proved genetically closest to SARS-2 across the *entire* genome.[547]

The question remains, however, whether this 2013 bat strain was more similar to SARS-2 than a *recombinant* of that 2019 bat strain. The recombominant appears more similar to SARS-2 across all genes except the spike gene that codes for attaching the virus to its human target. As South China Agricultural University's Kangpeng Xiao and colleagues show, the recombinant also sports a receptor binding domain or RBD of the spike gene from a pangolin strain also isolated in 2019 and closer to that of SARS-2.[548]

2) So it's unsurprising that Latham and Wilson would attack that pangolin sequence. They do so not on the basis of its genetics, but on procedural grounds. First, the 2019 pangolin sequence closest to the SARS-2 RBD has been repeatedly presented in the literature under the guise of additional pangolin sequences supporting the recombination event.[549] Second, pangolins don't appear to be a long-term reservoir for coronaviruses.[550]

Even should these objections hold water, they don't discount the original 2019 pangolin sample isolated in Guangdong. And even if pangolins aren't a steady reservoir, coronaviruses have been documented splattering across different host species—wild foods, traditional livestock, and humans—since 2002.[551] The wide range of infection is a marker of the geographic and taxonomic extent over which SARS-like strains have been circulating out there.

That is, as I proposed earlier, causality can be found in the field of relationships across the ecosystem, and not necessarily only in the object of any particular hosts.[552] It's a notion that field hypothesis proponents Roger Frutos and colleagues, although out-and-out rejecting pangolin as an intermediate host, still converge upon.[553] Indeed, we should add here, humans—the six miners included—weren't reservoirs for SARS before this pandemic either. Host species of a variety of taxonomies can still contribute to SARS origins even if they serve only as passing hosts.

3) SimPlot analyses—already models dependent upon how researchers parameterize them—aim to detect recombination events. They are not the basis of rooting a phylogenetic tree or the evolutionary relationships between all the samples involved here.

Such rooting depends on the ingroup included and the kind of rooting one does—molecular clock rooting, outgroup comparison, by coalescence, etc.[554] How do we weigh nucleotide transitions and transversions or codon position or back mutations or branch-specific variation in the molecular clock? Indeed, as evolutionary biologist Lenore Pipes and company show, some rooting methods place the 2019 bat sample as the closest outgroup (others the 2013 sample).[555]

Indeed, Peter Forster's group roots a subcluster in SARS-2 clade A represented by four Guangdong patients—far from Wuhan—as the ancestral clade.[556] Yes, the Guangdong patients were *tested* later than the beginning of the Wuhan outbreak, but their infections can still represent the ancestral genotype. Evolutionary geneticist Jesse Bloom later offered a practical explanation for the Guangdong connection:

Four GISAID sequences collected in Guangdong that fall in

a putative progenitor node are from two different clusters of patients who traveled to Wuhan in late December of 2019 and developed symptoms before or on the day that they returned to Guangdong, where their viruses were ultimately sequenced.[557]

Three research teams rejected Forster's approach on methodological grounds.[558] Other haplotype networks put Wuhan as the likely point of origin.[559] That possibility might still be a function of the greater number of samples taken there and the possibility any samples leading up to the Wuhan outbreak are presently unsampled. Latham and Wilson, placing origins in the Wuhan lab first, would summarily disagree such pre-Wuhan samples exist beyond the Yunnan cave in which the miners picked it up.

4) Meanwhile, the recently evolved traits or apomorphies—to use the old cladistics term—that SARS-2 shares with these bat outgroups make neither the 2013 nor the 2019 sample SARS-2's direct ancestor, a common enough error made by molecular biologists. Most phylogenies—even viral haplotype networks—are cladograms, in that they capture only relative evolutionary relationships. They are not necessarily family trees, as in Alfonse and Julia begot Rodrick, who with Deborah, begot Robert. Or, as in some criminal investigations, the hair found on the killer's coat was a genetic match for the victim's dog.

5) Indeed, Latham and Wilson present such a mode of investigating causality, within such a restricted scope of time, space, and connection—the epidemiological equivalent of the first 48 hours of a police investigation—as *in and of itself* evidence in favor of their lab hypothesis.

That is, the team leans upon a more forensics model, proposing a direct line between the relatives of the 2013 bat sequence and SARS-2 by way of adaption in the miners and ranking *a priori* the cryogenic spillover out of the Wuhan lab above the possibility that SARS-2 emerged out of recombination events across multiple host species. It wouldn't be the first time a pandemic arose out of a medical accident, with the relatively mild 1977 influenza strain likely emergent out of a vaccine trial or vaccine development gone wrong.[560]

To be sure, that way of thinking isn't unheard of in field hypotheses either. One team claimed to identify the putative tree from which roosting insectivore bats infected the index case for Ebola Makona in 2013 outside the village of Meliandou in Guinea, West Africa.[561]

But a scientific explanation encapsulating the many provinces and millions of animals and humans across decades—what counts for a virus as deep time—can offer *greater* explanatory power for SARS-2 emergence than what amounts to a police procedural, even as it will be harder, if at all possible, to reconstruct the exact specifics of SARS-2 emergence. The combinatorials available across place and species to test SARS-2 emergence far exceed the small closet of possibilities inside of which Latham and Wilson have locked themselves.

6) For one, coronaviruses are notorious for recombination events.[562] That the 2019 bat outgroup and the pangolin RBD got together that way is entirely plausible, a mechanism repeatedly documented in coronaviruses. Indeed, the 2013 bat isolate the lab proponents favor is no holotype, itself showing exactly such recombination, including in the spike gene.

Many other protopandemic viruses emerge by exactly such twists and turns. Highly pathogenic avian influenza H5N1, that first celebrity virus, evolved in a series of reassortment events trading genomic segments with a variety of other bird flu subtypes over many years across a wide swath of provinces in China.[563] That doesn't knock out the lab accident possibility for SARS-2, but a complex mode of origins doesn't knock out a field source either. Otherwise, it would behoove us to blame *every* outbreak on a simple lab accident to start.

7) That's a position to which Latham and Wilson unfortunately gravitate. In a passing paragraph, they raise the possibility that pandemic strain H1N1 (2009) arose as a vaccine accident too, citing commentary that makes similar claims that influenza can't possibly circulate far enough to engage in intercontinental reassortment.[564]

Gold-standard phylogeography work on H1N1 (2009) that followed showed that to be exactly the case, with the United States and Canada, the largest global exporters of hog and also the largest exporters of swine flu across all serotypes and genomic segments.[565]

Additional work showed H1N1's genomic segments reassorted out of multiple hog populations across the United States, Canada, and Eurasia before emerging in Mexico.[566]

8) That is, Latham and Wilson's vantage errs on the side of an incredulity about "natural" disease emergence (and a not undue distrust for industrial and governmental labs). It is as closely clutched a position as those held by lab accident skeptics who view the State—even upon the recent explosion in Lebanon's port—as somehow incapable of such catastrophic failure.[567] Among proponents of the lab hypothesis, nature is nigh on incapable of designing such a SARS.

Where geneticist Kristian Andersen's group screwed up contending a lab event possible only if SARS-2 looked exactly like SARS-1, in Latham and Wilson's version or that of Birger Sørensen's group, spillover still depends on a series of concerted experiments, however accidental in outcome, to arrive upon such an accelerated design.[568] After all, Latham and Wilson write, "Such exceptional affinities [for the human ACE2 receptor], ten to twenty times as great as that of the original SARS virus, do not arise at random."[569]

But there *is* another way. A "design without a designer" is exactly how evolutionary biologist Francisco Ayala summarized natural selection.[570] Richard Dawkins described the syllogism at the heart of natural selection—random mutation, adaptation, and differential reproduction—as a blind watchmaker by which the incredible in organic design can be, and is regularly, arrived upon.[571] It's a notion I have found some molecular biologists in the godlike position of running a series of experiments—however much they remain natural scientists and well informed of Darwin—can forsake.

9) From genetics to proteomics. Latham and Wilson note the 2013 bat sample's spike structure mimics SARS-2 (and so could very well have infected those miners). But its receptor binding domain or RBD misses five of the six contact sites shown necessary for efficient binding to the human ACE2 receptor through which SARS enters human cells.[572] In contrast, the pangolin sequence expressed all six contacts.

There are other features that permit easier human infection. The polybasic furin cleavage sites are open to host proteases snipping at the spike protein's S1/S2 juncture and enhancing cell-to-cell fusion.[573] Latham and Wilson spitball, but do not show, that the miner infections helped select for these cleavage sites in SARS-2.

And such sites repeatedly arise in nature. They may not be present in the 2019 bat sample as initially proposed, but have been inferred in SARS-2 ancestors, alongside SL strains expressing widespread spike conservation and recognizing both bat and human ACE2.[574] The furin cleavage sites have been identified in MERS, so these are not solely a function of putative genetic engineering or gain-of-function.[575]

In short, the polybasic sites in "natural" coronaviruses and the RBD in pangolin flag us that all the elements for making SARS-2 are circulating in animal populations out in the field, and—across thousands if not millions of bats, livestock, and undetected human infections combined—in all likelihood in great abundance. All the time and tools in the world to arrive at those "random" exceptional affinities that Latham and Wilson reject from the start.

10) Against Latham and Wilson's notion of rapid adaptation in those miners that took a 2013-like bat sample across fifty years of molecular clock in a matter of weeks, work by biodiversity researcher Shu-Miaw Chaw and colleagues shows very little positive selection in the SARS-2 genome, a result since replicated in different analyses.[576] Indeed, still other work indicates that whatever positive selection accrued in its lineage occurred *before* the divergence between the 2013 bat sample and SARS-2.[577]

On the basis of great divergence in nucleotide sequences at synonymous amino acid sites, Chaw's team also proposes that SARS-2 and the pangolin strain share the same amino acid residue in the RBD not by virtue of convergent evolution but of common ancestry.[578] Secondly, they show the "pangolin recombination event" in SARS-2, which didn't require an actual pangolin to host it, took place *forty years ago*.

Indeed, the Chaw team proposes that by purifying selection ever since, the progenitors of SARS-2 had been circulating in a similar form among humans *years* before Wuhan. So plenty of time—much more than a few weeks in a handful of miners—to evolve toward human adaptation. In other words, against the Sørensen team's incredulity, it's entirely reasonable that SARS-2 would be fully human-adapted upon the Wuhan outbreak. And against Latham and Wilson's hypothesis, a failure to evolve beyond a few amino acid replacements and a cloud of nonsynonymous mutations since the outbreak began needn't be a marker of a lab accident at all.

We see then that along the way Latham and Wilson play fast and loose with when and where the SARS-2 genome evolves. Fast in those six miners. Slow for the up to the fifty million infected since. As if a host switch is the only means by which SARS-like viruses adapt.

On the other hand, I'm not surprised that there appears little variation in SARS-2 post-Wuhan given how fast and furiously the pathogen spread across the globe in a matter of weeks, which can be as much placed on how integrated the global travel network is as the virus's infectiousness. At the same time, it's not like there's been *no* evolution. With infections numbering as high as 50 million at this point, multiple amino acid substitutions define each of the new SARS-2 clades.[579]

11) Meanwhile those damned pangolins keep getting in the way. Alongside the many intimations, but few open declarations, of a cover-up in China in their piece, Latham and Wilson imply the pangolin and 2019 bat sequences—which comprise the basis of alternate field hypotheses—are convenient to a fault. But presuming such sequences "fake news" would now require many multiple labs involved in those samples' collection and sequencing—in Beijing, Guangdong, Shandong, and Yunnan—involved in a national conspiracy. Not just Wuhan.

Latham and Wilson complain the lab theory is held to standards the field theory is not. But extraordinary claims require extraordinary evidence. Proponents of the lab accident—or at least the media in charge of helping us learn something about the world—are thereby on the hook for sifting for evidence for such a nationwide operation without resorting to knee-jerk Sinophobia. China covered up SARS-1 in that outbreak's early months. Lab theorists must now proclaim the same for SARS-2.[580]

And the putative SARS-2 in the six miners—originally reported as a pneumonia of no known cause with no pathogens identified in the cave at the time other than a new paramyxovirus in rats—must be backed by actual SARS-2-like sequences.[581] Especially as the clinical courses the Chinese Master's thesis describes could be any number of infections other than COVID-19, although the diagnoses of high fever, poor oxygenation index, acute respiratory distress syndrome, "ground-glass" exudation in the lungs, pulmonary thromboembolism, twenty-plus days ill, apparent dose effect, older patients dying sooner, a test order for SARS antibodies, confirmation miners were exposed to horseshoe bats, and a medical team's proposal to test bats and their feces are *all indeed* suggestive of a SARS infection.[582]

Is pointing out that the Zheng-Li Shi lab at the Wuhan Institute of Virology—experts in SARS, and not the paramyxovirus—subsequently took samples in that same cave in Mojiang, Yunnan, four times in 2012–13 enough circumstantial evidence that SARS-2 was sampled there? Will Latham and Wilson argue China's failure to produce such genetic sequences as part of the conspiracy? Or are we to be placed in the classic pseudoscientific position of declaiming that we can't prove it's not true either?

12) The Sørensen group effectively makes exactly such a charge of a cover-up, claiming China destroyed all relevant lab materials and blocks access to Chinese scientists.[583] But the group claims that by unpacking the scientific literature alone, it can reconstruct how SARS-2 receptors were (however unconsciously) built one EcoHealth Alliance-funded gain-of-function study upon another in series.[584]

The Sørensen white paper is worth reading, adding to Latham and Wilson's forensics, although the latter now err on a more "natural" lab accident from the miner samples than the "built from scratch" approach the Sørensen group favors.

But along with an omission of the extraordinary evidence it claims destroyed and appeals to the group's own authority, the Sørensen model suffers from an ironic fallacy. Although the Sørensen group are as vehement as Latham and Wilson in their rejection of Andersen's contention that SARS-2 isn't lab-based because it differs from SARS-1, the team redeploys Andersen's misstep for its own purposes. Now *because* SARS-2 differs from naturally emergent SARS-1, SARS-2 must therefore be lab-based.

Perhaps the series of gain-of-function studies *are* a smoking gun. I pointed out the dangers of a number of them myself.[585] They are certainly smoky enough to warrant a serious follow-up. But on that particular contention concerning SARS-2's essence, nature in all its variety, producing many biochemical roads to a pathogenic Rome over many decades, might snigger into its own sleeve.

13) In the meantime, the absence of (presently available) evidence does not constitute evidence of absence. That goes for both hypotheses. Latham and Wilson have knocked away the notion that the lab hypothesis is ridiculous in the way establishment researchers have claimed in order to shield the field hypothesis from serious critiques of its own.

On the other hand, in the face of Latham's now undue focus on the Andersen paper, efforts at investigating the field hypothesis are continuing apace. Indeed, the (provisional) failure to find reservoirs of pangolin SLs that Latham highlighted is part of the work field proponents are engaging to test the hypothesis. There is meanwhile a deepening vein of phylogenetic and coalescent analyses of SARS-2 and its taxonomic relatives.

There is the Chaw work we touched on, proposing SARS-2 circulating in humans for years preceding Wuhan. Indeed, it's a notion to which Latham and Wilson opened a door themselves, as their lab theory depends on SARS-2 circulating nearly fully formed in that Yunnan cave out in the wild by 2012.

Early SARS-2 may not have had the obvious affinity for human-to-human infection of the strain that emerged in mid-December and increasingly showed in the months to follow after infecting hundreds of thousands of humans, as represented, for instance, by the relatively recent amino acid replacement D614G in the spike protein.[586]

But Don't Blink

Other field teams appear to be converging on a similar position, but with a twist I did not see coming.

Computational epidemiologist Maciej Boni and colleagues at the Center for Infectious Disease Dynamics conducted recombination analyses and divergence time estimations on genetic sequences derived from human coronaviruses SARS-1, SARS-2, HCoV-OC43, and MERS.[587]

The team found that the sarbecoviruses—the clade with SARS-1 and -2, the SARS betacoronaviruses—undergo frequent recombination. Sixty-seven out of 68 samples the team tested showed genetic mosaicism at various temporal depths. As Latham and Wilson note, the 2013 bat sample and SARS-2 group together throughout the sequence, but that need not speak to the scale of spread the lab theory addresses. The Boni team did not include the 2019 bat sample in their analysis as it is.

As previously shown, the team did find the 2019 pangolin sample closer to SARS-2 in the variable-loop region of the spike gene. But here's the twist: the Boni group rejects a recombination event by way of that pangolin lineage. Instead, they support a *loss of function* in the 2013 bat sample—RaTG13—alone:

> On first examination this would suggest that that SARS-CoV-2 is a recombinant of an ancestor of Pangolin-2019 and RaTG13, as proposed by others. However, on closer inspection, the relative divergences in the phylogenetic tree show that SARS-CoV-2 is unlikely to have acquired the variable loop from an ancestor of Pangolin-2019 because these two sequences are approximately 10–15 percent divergent throughout the entire S protein (excluding the N-terminal domain). It is RaTG13 that is more divergent in the variable-loop region and thus likely to be the product of recombination, acquiring a divergent variable loop from a hitherto unsampled bat sarbecovirus.

This is notable because the variable-loop region contains the six key contact residues in the RBD that give SARS-CoV-2 its ACE2-binding specificity. These residues are also in the Pangolin Guangdong 2019 sequence. The most parsimonious explanation for these shared ACE2-specific residues is that they were present in the common ancestors of SARS-CoV-2, RaTG13, and Pangolin Guangdong 2019, and were lost through recombination in the lineage leading to RaTG13. This provides compelling support for the SARS-CoV-2 lineage being the consequence of a direct or nearly direct zoonotic jump from bats, because the key ACE2-binding residues were present in viruses circulating in bats.[588]

In other words, Boni's team comes out against a recombination event across livestock or wild animals other than bats, but also crosses out the 2013 bat outgroup as the kind of direct ancestor Latham and Wilson have proposed.

I would follow up with a few questions. On Latham and Wilson's behalf, I would ask, if the 2013 bat outgroup without the human-adapted RBD is the exception, does that mean the six miners could have been infected by a related bat SL virus *with* such a RBD? That might mean that SARS-2 entered the miners nearly fully formed and may have needed no accelerated adaptation.

On my behalf, I'll ask, Why upon describing the extent of recombination across multiple loci, including *within* the spike gene, would a recombination event involving the RBD be ruled out merely because the outlying segments differ 10–15 percent? The recombinant could have been negatively selected at the contact sites even as the side positions diverged over time. Or if not the 2019 pangolin strain, why not another source also with the six contact points? Or are such questions the field version of the forensics approach, demanding a specific genomic event account for SARS-2's emergence?

An alternate possibility is more chilling.

Boni's group declares the recombination event in the spike gene appears to have taken place with no known sarbecoviruses, suggesting the lineage leading to SARS-2 was singular in its expression of *this* ultimately human-specific phenotype. As SARS-1 and MERS represent, there are a variety of roads to such a phenotype.

And if the human-specific RBD has always been there in this lineage of bat SL viruses, and perhaps other lineages, then successful spillovers into humans must be ongoing at a rate *much* greater than assumed. And why not, given how similar the bat and human ACE2 receptors are?[589] Most human infections might not amount to much, if by luck alone, but we might be under far greater fire than three deadly SARS outbreaks indicate. Although three protopandemics in less than twenty years is perhaps *exactly* the right pace. Under that kind of barrage, we should expect more human SARS to come in rapid order. There's probably a new one circulating among humans right now. Whether it pops out as a human outbreak is an open question.

However these new studies twist and turn our thinking, many of the new field phylogenies in the literature are converging upon scenarios about COVID's origins that are plotted out across expansive swaths of time and space.

By three dating methods of differing conservativeness, the Boni team clocked divergence of the SARS-2 lineage from its bat sarbecovirus sister group in the years 1948 (95 percent highest posterior density, 1879–1999), 1969 (1930–2000), and 1982 (1948–2009). That is, the strain leading up to the beginning of the pandemic likely circulated for decades unnoticed, perhaps, as the team surmises, in bats. When the virus spilled over into humans, however, they leave unspecified.

The team offers a temporal version of the kind of pandemic gun under which we remain. As both SARS-1 and -2 appear 40 to 70 years divergent from their bat ancestors, *many* closely related but unsampled SLs in this clade in all likelihood are circulating out there across different species of bats—horseshoe or otherwise—and in different places across Central and South China.[590]

Indeed, the Boni group finds the sarbecovirus clade is genetically structured at the regional level across China, speaking to the expansive geographies in spread and recombination that I raised in May 2020 and upon which Chaw's team also converged.

The trope best suited for organizing our thinking here isn't necessarily a murder mystery. It may be better conceived as an alien invasion of our own making.

As Roger Frutos and colleagues put it:

Searching for a culprit in the wild is not realistic. According to the circulation model [as opposed to the spillover model] there is a broad circulation of viruses in different species, including humans, upon contact but with no epidemic to follow. This fits with the observation that humans have been a lot more exposed to various viruses than expected and without any related epidemic.[591]

A point well served as to the scope with which RNA viruses get to experiment with molecular evolution.

I do think the Frutos team takes the idea a step too far, cutting out causality at the level of socioecological damage in favor of framing emergence as entirely a matter of molecular stochastic terrorism:

Several RNA viruses, among which the Coronaviruses, including SARS-CoV and SARS-CoV-2, were shown to undergo a quasispecies evolutionary process. This process postulates that there is no specific preadaptation of the virus to the host but instead a post-exposure, host-driven selection of viruses displaying the best propensity to evade immune surveillance and replicate. Contact, low affinity receptor interaction and lack of molecular interference during replication are enough to establish productive infection after what the virus will follow in-host selection. This is compatible with the high diversity observed in the spike proteins of Coronaviruses which is under positive selection, i.e. host driven. In line with this model, the RBD from SARS-CoV-2 is not fully optimized for human ACE2. . . .

According to the circulation model, what really prepares the ground for the epidemic is simply an accidental event, i.e. a mutation, recombination or reassortment in the virus genome. The virus is already present in an animal population close to humans or even in humans, and this mutation makes it more invasive and/or pathogenic.[592]

There is no reason such processes can't be taking place or accelerating *in a context of* shifting agroeconomic exposures. SL circulation isn't panmictic—everywhere all at once—a conclusion the Frutos group strangely switches to suddenly, without connecting the dots the way we might wish:

> The real triggers for epidemic and pandemics are the societal organization and society-driven human/animal contacts and amplification loops provided by the modern human society, i.e. contacts, land conversion, markets, international trades, mobility, etc. A major positive effect of the circulation model is that the focus is put on these human activities and not on wildlife.[593]

Rogue Ones

In spite of my continued caution here, bordering upon skepticism, Latham and Wilson make a gallant effort at lining up a number of coincidences to match bats and miners with both SARS-2 and Wuhan. They aim to line up what the Sørensen group defines as the etiological criteria of "means, timing, agent and place."

Whether science will aim to test these possibilities, rather than leaving them unaddressed on the basis of a normative political economy based in power and prestige, remains an open question. Blocking such minority reports if by omission alone would catch establishment science in its own classic pseudoscientific maneuver.

One Facebook comment noted that Latham's Bioscience Resource Project is largely a one-man operation, as if the number of people involved offers a criterion for the character of his work. That's the kind of snooty ad hominem that cost Dean of Engineering Orson Krennic his life.[594]

We are only eight months out from COVID-19's emergence as a pandemic strain. We will likely hear more about the origins of the virus in the months, the years, nay, the decades to come. If I am perhaps less disturbed by explorations in (*this* version of) the lab hypothesis than some colleagues, it's because, as I noted above, I long joined others, including Pulitzer Prize–winner Laurie Garrett,

Princeton's Matt Keeling, Yale's Alison Galvani, and Harvard's Marc Lipsitch, in raising the alarm about just such a lab accident.[595]

Indeed, I see the field and lab hypotheses framed together. Big Ag's performative "biosecurity" and building all those labs post-H5N1 and -9/11 both represent efforts at avoiding addressing the economic model driving the emergence of virulent pathogens to begin with.[596] Cleaning up the mess only after it happens.

In other words, this may be less a matter of a clash of hypotheses, or a divergence in the values underlying the two theories' narrative paradigm, or even any detente that might be found in ontological pluralism.[597]

We may instead be witnessing what lucrative agnotology or groomed ignorance buys. Science is studiously investigating every-thing about COVID-19 but the money and power that helped bring on the pandemic and, it so happens, also allow researchers to continue to conduct their work. Now that's the kind of line that cost contract scientist Galen Erso *his* life.

—PATREON, AUGUST 25, 2020

The BoJo Strain

SEVERAL PEOPLE ASKED ME about the new SARS-CoV-2 variant in the UK. And, as it appears, another one in South Africa, following the Danish strain that spilled out of minks and back into humans.[598]

Here's how I responded to one such query with some bells and whistles added:

SARS-2 is an RNA virus. With high mutation rates and short generation times, these acute infections typically evolve like wild. It happens that the betacoronaviruses also have a "spellchecker" or "proofreader" that often corrects such mutations.[599]

That inherent characteristic hardly puts us in the clear, however, if the present pandemic doesn't offer us pause enough.

As we approach anything from 50 to 500 million people infected, a variety of strains are likely to emerge.[600] Most mutations that the spell-checking misses will have little effect or make matters *worse* for the virus. But we're trafficking in such numbers that rare improvements from the virus's vantage point bend toward inevitable.

The worry about the resulting fallout is twofold:

First, that the strains will engage in what's called "interdemic selec-tion."[601] The various strains emerging might compete at the level of host population until one beats all the rest and spreads out again from its point of origin, out from underneath whatever herd immunity we develop—natural or vaccine-derived.

Second, such selection so spatially arrayed selects for greater virulence, however small that likelihood.[602]

The BoJo strain—after Prime Minister Boris Johnson who let COVID-19 rage in Britain—is at this point only more infectious, as opposed to deadlier per case.[603] That offers little but cold comfort. The faster people are infected, the more will die in any given time period.

Transmissibility and inherent virulence are also interconnected.[604] The strains that better access new susceptibles could very well select for greater deadliness per infection too.[605] When there's no cap on susceptibles, it's those strains that burn through them fastest that win out. Along the way, replicating faster to the transmission threshold for the leap to the next host leaves more damage behind.

The crux is that widening variation across the globe provisions the virus with the fuel it needs to best explore its full evolutionary space.

So, the herd immunity, the kind of neoliberal neglect that pays out only $600 to people champions, not only kills more people than other more comprehensive interventions, but it also permits the virus free range to evolve solutions to whatever vaccines or drugs we innovate.[606]

Letting COVID cruise about may also serve as the basis of growing evidence for reinfection.[607] By antigenic drift, SARS-2 may be evolving out from under the umbrella of individual antibody coverage (and even innate immunity).[608] Those already infected may become susceptible again.

Should most COVID vaccines offer little sterilizing immunity and at least a few annual SARS-2 strains evolve out from host population immunity à la influenza, we may be in for an endemic infection.[609] Seasonal resurgences will require mapping out antigenic cartographies: tracking when a strain escapes any season's host population immunity.[610]

Eventually, enough people will be infected and, in combo with partially protective vaccines, the disease system should be driven toward attenuation and/or the kinds of chance extirpation to which smaller populations are subjected. The worst of the outbreak should pass. But how many people must be killed along the way?

The new orders of population-level evolution apparently now underway require global interventions the present world order is abandoning. Various centers of capital—bending toward new cold war divisions born in part out of an effort to lay blame elsewhere for the outbreak—appear much more interested in refusing to pay for public health if it comes at the cost of the billionaire class they serve.[611]

I explained some of these pathogen tricks in 2009, upon swine flu H1N1's emergence as a pandemic strain.[612]

It's remarkable how much that analysis retained its explanatory power. It's like causality extends beyond the biomolecular particularities of any single virus into the field of socioecological relationships capital imposes on land and labor alike.

Meanwhile, beyond what appears SARS-2's continuing experimentation, COVID-21, -22, and -23—representing different constellations of human-specific phenotypes—are almost certainly also in the works. They have long been emerging at a steady clip where put-upon bats meet capital-led deforestation.[613]

—PATREON, DECEMBER 21, 2020

To Live and Die in L.A.

Geoff Eley, reflecting on such struggles in his history of European socialism, accords the slum neighborhood equal weight with the factory in the formation of socialist consciousness: "No less vital were the complex ways neighborhoods spoke and fought back. If the workplace was one frontier of resistance, where collective agency could be imagined, the family—or more properly the neighborhood solidarities working-class women fashioned for survival—was the other . . . The challenge for the Left was to organize on both fronts of social dispossession."

— MIKE DAVIS (2018)

The following dispatch was produced by the PReP Neighborhoods working group for Pandemic Research for the People. I joined lead author Meleiza Figueroa of the Cooperative New School for Urban Studies and Social Justice, along with PReP interns Kaitlin Enouchs and Miguel Tinsay, Real Food Media co-director Tanya Kerssen, Pasadena Tenants Union's Allison Henry, Los Angeles Tenants Union's Fernando Ramirez, Alhambra Tenants Union's David Bond, and PReP organizer John Gulick.

COVID-19 CONTINUES TO surge in successive waves as new variants emerge while social restrictions are prematurely ended. As the ultra-infectious Delta variant increasingly affects younger and healthier populations, advanced age and medical comorbidities are no longer easy markers of new cases, disease severity, or deaths.

One marker remains in place beyond individual well-being. In practically all urban settings, the most socially vulnerable populations—workers with low or precarious incomes, communities of color, the uninsured and unhoused—are bearing the brunt of these infection surges, even in the face of universally free vaccination.

This PReP dispatch takes an in-depth look at how COVID-19 has affected Los Angeles County, one of the most populous and diverse urban centers in the United States.

Los Angeles became a national epicenter of the pandemic at the end of 2020 and into 2021. It is now experiencing yet another exponential surge in cases that started July 2021 as the highly infectious Delta variant gained dominance. These waves of COVID infections have collided head-on with multiple ongoing and deepening socioeconomic crises already present in L.A. County. Unaffordable housing and homelessness; worker insecurity; structural racism; and barriers to public assistance, health care, and other essential services are acting together to push the distribution of COVID cases across county demographics and geography.

As local, state, and national leaders push toward fully reopening the economy after a year and a half of pandemic lockdowns, with emergency protections such as shelter programs and eviction moratoriums ending shortly, efforts to address the continued spread of COVID-19 must consider the structural factors that compound the pandemic's effects on communities of color, working-class communities, and the unhoused.

The COVID-19 crisis has merged with and reinforced existing crises generated by a neoliberalized economy. Labor precarity, housing instability and homelessness, psychosocial stress, lack of access to essential health care services and social safety nets, and government (in)action represent the means by which the political class placed business priorities over people's health. Our analysis, rooted in the history of structural inequality, as well as personal and collective experiences on the ground, seeks to understand these factors in a more dynamic context. We examine the ways in which intensifying social and economic crises, at times exacerbated by pandemic response measures, feed off one another and compound the effects of the virus.

Addressing these structural inequalities is a political imperative for disrupting the repeated stress tests that the COVID-19 waves are administering to Los Angeles. There are no shortcuts or Hollywood endings. In the face of a recent ebb in COVID in California so celebrated in the press this past week, vaccines and mask mandates, however necessary, won't be enough.[614]

Los Angeles's Winter Wave

In December 2020, COVID-19's winter surge hit Los Angeles County like a tidal wave, as daily cases increased over 1,000 percent from the previous month.[615] By January 2021, a COVID-related death was occurring in Los Angeles County approximately every eight minutes, and on January 16, Los Angeles County became the first county in the nation to surpass one million cases.[616] The map of cases and deaths by neighborhood correlates strongly with the demographics of the city: case rates exploded in lower-income areas, as well as in historically redlined Black and Brown working-class neighborhoods.[617]

One of the worst-hit locales within the Los Angeles COVID-19 epicenter was the city of Pacoima, a working-class community in the San Fernando Valley whose case rate was over five times that of richer, whiter Santa Monica.[618] At the height of the COVID-19 winter wave, approximately one in five Pacoima residents had contracted the virus.

Pacoima is also 97 percent nonwhite, reflecting the fact that it is a historically redlined community of Black, Latinx, and immigrant industrial workers. Many are now essential service workers with little to no job security who cannot afford to skip work. "A lot of people in Pacoima are afraid to get tested for [this] reason," notes Elisa Avalos, president of the Pacoima Neighborhood Council, "God forbid if they come out positive, they will have to stay home for two weeks."[619]

Pacoima workers, Avalos continues, face a deadly dilemma: "Right now you're picking and choosing. . . . Is it food, water and power? Is it putting gas in your car? It's sad and frustrating to look at their kids and say they can't provide for you this month."

Few options to self-isolate exist in these communities, as many workers live in multigenerational households in densely populated neighborhoods dominated by apartment buildings. They often rely on their families and neighbors for daily survival.

Pacoima-based nonprofit Meet Each Need with Dignity (MEND) conducted a household survey in Pacoima and surrounding communities in July 2020 and found that 41 percent of those residents shared a household with another family, more than 30 percent lived in a back house, room, or mobile home, and approximately 8 percent lived in a garage.[620]

"Most live in some sort of substandard [housing]," says Janet Marinaccio, president of MEND, "There can be a family of six living in a garage. They'll double up and triple up. You might have four families, one in each bedroom and living room."

Melba Martinez, a Honduran immigrant and Pacoima resident who lost her job as a domestic worker at the start of the pandemic, describes the conditions, as well as the fear, that permeated her neighborhood as case rates neared historic highs:

> My neighbor upstairs lives with two other families, and she told me one of the people who lives there got everyone sick. . . . Downstairs from me are two families living in an apartment, and they've all gotten infected. . . . They've all told me, "Please don't tell anyone that I got COVID-19."[621]

Laura Hidalgo, an outreach team worker with MEND, notes that as cases and deaths soared in the community, "I see a lot more fear in people. . . . What we're seeing, still, is that a lot of families don't have any other choice but to continue business as usual."[622]

Undocumented workers, in particular, face barriers to health care and support services. They are not eligible for stimulus checks or pandemic-related federal unemployment assistance.

Low-income workers in Los Angeles and throughout California disproportionately face barriers to essential health and public services, exacerbating their vulnerability to infectious disease while eroding their ability to adequately address the situation.

A recent report from the Food Chain Workers Alliance notes that federal and state pandemic relief efforts "have also left too many workers behind."[623] Up to 15 percent of Los Angeles's labor force, many of them undocumented women, work in the informal economy as street and sidewalk vendors, who "found themselves literally pushed aside to make room for restaurants" that converted to outdoor dining.

While formal restaurants and businesses were given incentives and accommodations from the city government to continue operating, permits for street vendors were suspended, and "the majority of L.A.'s street and sidewalk vendors, most of whom are women of color who have been excluded for all income relief, remained banned for public safety until the fall."[624]

As one undocumented worker puts it:

> The pandemic has made big impacts because our children aren't going to school and they are missing a lot. We have to buy more food and we don't receive any programs because we are undocumented and we don't qualify. Even with the State help, not all of us qualify. . . . I'm undocumented, I don't qualify for any help, and I have a family that does need help, that worries me.[625]

Similar conditions exist in demographically comparable neighborhoods throughout the county and the state, highlighting the ways in which the structural inequalities of race and class have had a defining role in shaping the character and trajectory of the COVID-19 surge in Los Angeles County.

Media narratives that discuss the role of structural inequalities in the COVID-19 pandemic have tended to treat these factors as a matter of unfortunate circumstance at best. At worst, analyses of the disproportionate impacts on Black and Brown communities have laid blame on uneducated people and racialized caricatures of "ghetto" or immigrant culture.

Illustrating the disconnect between mainstream/public agency views of the pandemic and the experiences of those who live in the community, the same *Los Angeles Times* article that quoted MEND staff about the fear and helplessness among Pacoima residents also featured Barbara Ferrer, director of L.A. County Public Health. Ferrer attributes the high case rates to cultural practices and a false sense of security: "I think it may more reflect the gatherings and the parties, the mixing with people not in your household . . . once the rates go up, it can kind of feed on itself."[626]

Eight months later, the *L.A. Times* doubled down on the characterization of public health as merely the sum of individual behavior with the headline: "Unvaccinated people, riskier behavior: What is fueling L.A.'s coronavirus surge."[627]

Such a cognitive dissonance between how institutions understand the nature of the crisis and how it is experienced on the ground limits the effectiveness of public policy intervention at the community level. Structural inequalities that force many Black and Brown workers into a perilous balancing act between their families' economic survival and physical health are often downplayed entirely. When these inequalities are mentioned, they often serve as a scenic backdrop for a feel-bad story about the intrinsic nature of these urban communities.

Another story is often left untold. The pandemic and many of the approaches governments and employers are taking are contributing to increased social vulnerability, instability, chronic stress, and social and biological comorbidities that are disproportionately intensifying the impacts of COVID-19 in poor and working-class communities and communities of color.

These long-term impacts are making themselves felt beyond a pandemic that is slogging toward a third year. They make society as a whole more vulnerable in the face of the pandemics to follow, climate change, and other large-scale disaster events.

There Be No Shelter Here

As emergency quarantine and shelter-in-place orders rolled out across the United States in 2020, many poor and low-income workers and families found themselves stuck between the "rock" of the pandemic and the "hard place" of unaffordable housing or homelessness.

Even before the COVID-19 pandemic disrupted the economy, real estate speculation, gentrification, and skyrocketing rents in Los Angeles over the last several years had led to increased housing instability and unsustainable cost burdens. Seventy-three percent of L.A. renters spend more than 30 percent of income on rent and utilities, and nearly half of all renters are severely cost-burdened, spending more than 50 percent of their income on rent.[628]

According to the U.S. Census Household Pulse Survey, which tracks weekly demographic, social, and economic data during the pandemic, as of July 2020, 36 percent of Los Angeles metro area households reported having missed a rent payment, or had little to no confidence that their household could pay next month's rent or mortgage on time.[629] As of July 2021, 41 percent, or over 307,000 households, were not current on rent or faced likely eviction or foreclosure.

Before the onset of the pandemic, unaffordable housing had exacerbated overcrowding in low-income neighborhoods and set the conditions for community spread of COVID-19. To offset skyrocketing rents, and the increasingly insurmountable costs of living as a result, burdened renters have had to "double up"—taking in roommates or family members, or joining multiple families in a unit to share costs—increasing density within households as well as overcrowding in lower-income neighborhoods dominated by apartment buildings.

According to a University of Southern California study based on data from the 2018 American Community Survey, Los Angeles holds the distinction of having the most overcrowded rental housing in the nation, with 16 percent of households hosting occupancy of more than 1.5 people per room. Among Latinx households, this figure rises to over 23 percent, underscoring the racial disparities in housing density and increased risk of COVID-19 transmission.[630]

Housing instability also increases risk factors for COVID-19 complications and mortality, as the high cost of housing "is associated with difficulty affording health services . . . as well as higher rates of poor health, anxiety and stress disorder, depression" and other chronic conditions indicated as comorbidities influencing the severity of COVID-19 illness.[631] A recent cross-sectional analysis of U.S. counties during the pandemic found that in "households with poor housing conditions, there was a 50% higher risk of COVID-19 incidence . . . and a 42% higher risk of COVID-19 mortality."[632]

A tenant in L.A. suburb Monterey Park voices the acute stress experienced by rent-burdened individuals and families across the country in the face of skyrocketing rents: "Even though we had an understanding, they're raising the rent three times more than the agreement. I can't afford to pay that on my fixed income. I want to fight this, but if I refuse to pay the increase I'm afraid I'll get evicted. I feel hopeless."[633]

Claudia Ruiz, a twenty-three-year-old resident of the East L.A. neighborhood of Lincoln Heights, describes watching her mother's financial worries over their housing situation: "I would always see her really, really stressed out. She would tell me to go take out loans because she didn't have enough to pay the rent."[634]

A third tenant describes the anxiety produced by housing insecurity and poor living conditions before and during the pandemic:

> I was having some difficulty keeping my one-bedroom before COVID because the rents keep on going up, but once COVID hit I lost a work opportunity. . . . I owe my landlord $3500 which I plan to pay back with my stimulus check and having a payment plan. That I will probably be able to do, although it's added stress because my work situation is still uncertain. Also, while this has been going on, there have not been COVID precautions taken in the building; so we have bad ventilation and the resident manager doesn't wear a mask. . . . I appreciate the gov-

ernment-mandated reduction in rent, I do plan to pay it back but the services have not really come; also I've been threatened with eviction during COVID, so I've had a lot of anxiety and uncertainty and could really use government help.[635]

From Housing to the Body

The correlations across poverty, housing instability, and COVID-19 mortality are not simply environmental. They also are directly mapped onto individual bodies.

Symptomatic severity and mortality from COVID-19 have been linked to a cascade of systemic inflammatory responses, known as a "cytokine storm." Elevated levels of particular stress-related cytokines, such as IL-6, in combination with catalyzing agents such as C-reactive proteins (CRP), have been identified as reliable bioindicators or "red flags" of severe and life-threatening illness resulting from COVID-19 infection.[636]

These compounds form part of a complex stress-response mechanism that evolved in the human body to restore homeostasis after exposure to trauma or acute stress, including running from natural predators. In the modern world, socioeconomic factors such as financial instability and systemic racism trigger identical stress responses in the body. But now, as Rupa Marya and Raj Patel describe, "instead of the acute stress of a bear running after us, we are exposed to more chronic stressors, such as making house payments so we don't end up in the street, or going for a jog while Black in a racist society."[637]

Specifically, "in the face of acute psychological stress, pro-inflammatory markers, such as IL-1β and IL-6, rise, as does C-reactive protein. . . . When stress is systemic, IL-6 has a profoundly pro-inflammatory action, serving as a continuous alarm signal to the body" and can permanently alter the immune system, leading to "pathological manifestations, such as low-grade inflammation and decreased immune response to viral infections. This is one way chronic stress can make us more vulnerable to colds and other viruses such as COVID."[638]

Structural inequalities such as housing instability, poverty, and racism that are experienced over a lifetime can make this "toxic stress pathway" a permanent condition in the body, especially when trauma and stress are experienced during critical developmental stages in childhood.

A recent report from the California Surgeon General's office highlighted the biological effects of sustained Adverse Childhood Experiences (ACEs), including abuse, poverty, and housing instability on the toxic stress pathway, which alters the body on a molecular level and, especially for historically oppressed peoples, can be transferred intergenerationally through DNA.

According to the report, over 62 percent of California adults have experienced at least one ACE, and 16 percent have been exposed to ACEs on four or more occasions.[639] Toxic stress conditions are strongly linked to common chronic disease, including "nine of the 10 leading causes of death in the United States," and "increased risk of contracting or dying from COVID-19, either through dysregulation of the immune response and/or through increased burden of [ACE Related Health Conditions], which may predispose to a more severe COVID-19 disease course."[640]

Geographically, the spatial concentration of renter vulnerability in Los Angeles neighborhoods, which measures rent burden and housing instability, follows a now-familiar pattern, again correlating strongly with COVID-19 case rates.[641]

The unaffordability of housing in Los Angeles has also led to a dramatic explosion in homelessness, increasing 49 percent over the last five years, and 13 percent in 2019–20 alone.[642] In absolute numbers, Los Angeles County hosts the greatest concentration of people experiencing homelessness, with at least 66,000 unhoused people living on the streets. In the context of COVID-19, unhoused people experience the greatest risks to individual and public health, as they have no choice but to inhabit public spaces.[643] Many suffer from preexisting medical or mental health conditions that are greatly exacerbated by the lack of housing.

Only about 25 percent of the unhoused population in Los Angeles are sheltered or have access to shelter, which affects the incidence and mortality rate of COVID-19. Even then, deaths from COVID-19 across both sheltered and unsheltered populations are tragically high; with a 23 percent case fatality rate among sheltered people with the virus, and a staggering 37.5 percent among the unsheltered.[644] In other words, for the neglected among us, COVID cannot be dismissed as a "survivable disease" with only a 1 percent fatality rate.

Homelessness and housing instability, in particular, are so strongly linked to chronic disease, adverse impacts on childhood health, and COVID-19 mortality that Kaiser Permanente, one of the largest health care providers in Los Angeles, announced a $200 million social impact investment initiative to address homelessness and to preserve and create affordable housing in Los Angeles County.[645]

Housing Help to Housing Harm

Given the high risk of both transmission and mortality of COVID-19 among the unhoused, as well as the impact of job losses, furloughs, and closures of non-essential business on already overburdened renters, the state of California implemented several measures to protect tenants and stabilize the unhoused population.

Perhaps the most impactful of these measures was a state-level extension of the federal eviction moratorium issued by the Centers for Disease Control and Prevention, which alone may have prevented between 365,200 and 502,200 excess COVID-19 cases, and between 8,900 and 12,500 excess deaths.[646] More shelter options for the unhoused were established, including safe parking sites, sanctioned campgrounds, increased funding for temporary transitional housing, and Project Roomkey, which partnered with area motels losing business from travel restrictions to provide rooms for homeless seniors and those with special needs.[647]

The state's shelter-in-place order was also extended to the unhoused, and a moratorium was placed on police sweeps of homeless encampments, which would have dispersed the unhoused population into the wider community and increased COVID-19 transmission. But many of these much-touted state programs have been slow to materialize, much less at the scale needed to support the more than 60,000 people living without a roof in Los Angeles.

Rev. Andrew Bales, head of the Union Rescue Mission on Skid Row, lamented at the height of the L.A. surge in January 2021 that "the unexplainable protection that people who are homeless have had from COVID is disappearing. . . . All of Skid Row and many agencies/missions are hotspots. All are overwhelmed."[648]

One Skid Row resident says:

The city just forgot about us. Yeah, there's a lot of tough people down here, but there's a lot of good people too. It's as if they don't care about us at all, and while it's tough we have our community here on the streets.

Many Los Angeles residents continue to experience housing instability, homelessness, and toxic stress-related health risks as private landlords and local governments have pushed back on state-mandated COVID restrictions. In some cases, landlords and jurisdictions outright defy state orders, continuing with evictions and sweeps of homeless encampments.

One of the most notorious encampment sweeps during the moratorium occurred in March 2021 at Echo Park near downtown Los Angeles, which, according to local organizer David Busch-Lilly, "had become . . . a peaceful oasis during lockdown" for the unhoused under the shelter-in-place order but became the site of a highly charged standoff as hundreds of homeless campers, community organizers, and housing activists mobilized to block the eviction.[649]

In the spirit of a long history of aggressively policing the homeless, from Daryl Gates and William Bratton to the murder of Charley Keunang, L.A. police enclosed the park with chain-link fences and attempted to clear the area with rubber bullets and pepper spray, culminating in 182 arrests and four injuries to protesters, including "concussions and broken limbs."[650]

For one unhoused resident at the protest, this action confirmed his distrust of city government policies toward the unhoused: "We have to stop relying on a city that has criminalized us. . . . No matter the idea, it has led to more criminalization for us." [651]

Another encampment resident and protester said no one at the park had intended to go unhoused and remarked upon the city's absent planning that "if you want us out, you need to come with reliable, sustainable, long-lasting, permanent solutions, not dog scraps."[652]

Cruel Landlord Tactics

The Los Angeles Tenants' Union, which helps renters organize throughout the city to enforce tenants' rights and defend against illegal evictions, reports that private landlords are taking advantage of legal loopholes and renters' ignorance of the law to continue evicting renters during the pandemic. Landlords are sometimes resorting to lockouts, utility shutoffs, outright bullying tactics, and harassment to drive tenants out.

One tenant reports:

The landlord has turned off the water and electricity for almost a month during a heat wave to get us out. It was awful. The County finally sent the landlord the message he needed to turn the utilities back on. It is hard to move with the price of rent.[653]

Another tenant, in East L.A., was not only subjected to bullying, but also suffered the lack of information available to tenants about the eviction moratorium and their rights under pandemic protections:

The landlord said she's going to send her husband and cousin to come move me and my wife out of the unit today. I have nowhere to go, my wife is dealing with mental health issues, and the landlord doesn't care that I'm between jobs. This pandemic is making it impossible for me to find any stable work, and now I'm going to be kicked out. Is this legal, is there anything we can do to stay in our home?[654]

One popular loophole used by landlords to effect evictions during the moratorium was an allowance to move tenants out of buildings for "substantial remodel or repair." This prompted many landlords to leave problems unrepaired for months, rendering units practically unlivable and adding to the pressure on tenants to leave or be evicted.

One Alhambra neighborhood resident reports: "Our owner is a slumlord, they let our unit rot with mold, AC breaking down, and busted entranceway for 6 months. Our sewage backed up and they let it sit that way for over 2 weeks!"[655]

In the Mid-City district, renter Kim Moore notes how her landlord boarded up the windows with plywood and left debris all around the building's exterior, including bunches of exposed wiring: "He wants it to look abandoned out here . . . some of this wiring doesn't even go to anything . . . he wanted us out, like now."

Soon after, an eviction notice arrived, which Moore protested: "'But you can't do this. We're in the midst of a pandemic. Where are we going to go? I have my grandchildren. People have kids over here.... He was literally just going to throw us out in the street. It was hard."[656]

Landlords have also raised rents during the moratorium, adding to the total balance of back rent that is to be paid in full once the moratorium is lifted, and increasing the financial burden on renters to the point they struggle to find money for food, health care, and other basic needs.[657]

In the L.A. suburb of Monterey Park, one tenant notes:

Even though we had an understanding, they're raising the rent 3x more than the agreement. I can't afford to pay that on my fixed income. I want to fight this, but if I refuse to pay the increase I'm afraid I'll get evicted. I feel hopeless.[658]

An undocumented farmworker in California's San Joaquin Valley describes the complex of problems exacerbated by the pandemic:

We were out of work for two months and we were evicted and had to find another place to live. We visit churches to also receive food from some organizations. It's worrisome to have children studying at home because they can get behind and the cost of childcare has increased too.[659]

Ultimately, the lack of robust policies or initiatives to address the underlying problems of unaffordable housing and an overheated rental market means that relief measures can only delay, not prevent, a looming catastrophe. As landlords continue to use every trick in the book to conduct illegal evictions and maximize rent burdens, and the federal government pushes toward a return to "normal" and a reopening of the economy despite the persistent spread of COVID-19, the eventual lifting of California's eviction moratorium will leave over half a million households in particularly precarious positions.

The economic "pause" engendered by the pandemic could have been, and still can be, an opportunity to systematically address the housing crisis, increase oversight of landlord practices, and implement solutions for safe and affordable housing for all. Even experimenting with ending rent as a concept is possible. Unfortunately, the pause appears to have deepened and complicated the housing crisis with consequences as yet unforeseen.

Pandemic Disrupting Work Regimens

Housing isn't the only sector affected by the outbreak. The emergency stay-at-home orders implemented at the onset of the pandemic disrupted the nature of work as we know it.

Schools and white-collar workplaces, assisted by technologies such as Zoom, were able to adapt to a work-from-home environment. A new category of "essential workers" meanwhile emerged as pandemic "heroes," including frontline health care workers, grocery store and restaurant employees, public works staff, and emergency responders. Millions of other workers were meanwhile thrown overnight into uncertain and unstable situations. As a result of this unprecedented mass job displacement event, millions of workers found themselves out of a job, furloughed without pay, or pressured to continue working in unsafe conditions.

According to a study in the *American Journal of Public Health*, only about 25 percent of the American workforce—approximately 35.6 million workers—are employed in occupations that can be pursued from home: technology, administrative, financial, engineering, and the like.[660]

The vast majority of workers—75 percent of the labor force, or approximately 108.4 million workers—toil in occupations that are challenging or impossible to do from home. Only a fraction of those workers—mostly health care staff, emergency responders, retail clerks, and some service workers—are considered "essential workers" eligible for hazard pay or other benefits.

The balance of the workforce that must circulate in the community to do their jobs—as transportation workers, delivery drivers, construction laborers, warehouse and factory workers, and workers all along the food chain—are more essential than ever to move goods and services in the pandemic economy, but they also carry the highest risk of death due to COVID-19.[661] Yet these workers remain virtually invisible, out of view of most consumers, corporate publicists, and policymakers who spin sentimental narratives about the heroism of essential workers for public consumption.

Extended unemployment benefits brought temporary relief to workers in certain sectors. But problems with applications and disbursement delays also brought added stress and uncertainty to many, like this Pasadena resident:

> I have been waiting for my unemployment benefits since February. . . . In July, I applied for the state rent relief program and have not yet heard anything. I borrowed money for August and September rent. But I am worried that technically I don't qualify for it. And looking for a job has been discouraging—so many cover letters and resumés and very little response. And the number of $14 and $15/hour jobs out there is depressing.[662]

Still others have had no choice but to figure it out themselves, combining multiple jobs and "side hustles" in the gig economy to make ends meet.

As traditional workplaces became high-risk factors for pandemic disease, the nature of work itself has become increasingly precarious and contingent. More workers than ever are operating as independent contractors, with no benefits, no security of tenure, and degradation or elimination of their rights and protections as workers.

Job insecurity has become the norm, with no indication that conditions will improve after pandemic restrictions have eased. Those who must continue working in essential sectors of the economy "risk increased exposure to disease and potential increases in job stress attributable to changes in job practices and duties to meet an increase in demand for services."[663]

Lax government oversight over the food and service sectors, as well as the lack of regulatory frameworks for the emerging gig economy, has accelerated crisis trends for labor that, like housing, predated the pandemic itself. The failure of the state is felt disproportionately by low-wage service and food chain workers, people of color, and undocumented workers who live in the neighborhoods most affected by COVID-19.

"They should give those of us who work in agriculture wage support," Martin, an agricultural worker in Southern California, shares:

> We're exposing ourselves every day to this virus and we don't have the good fortune to be able to work from home. You can't harvest from a computer. Nothing would make me happier than to know that my health isn't in danger.[664]

As non-essential businesses closed down or laid off their employees, many people who found themselves financially unstable also turned to highly precarious "gig" work during the pandemic, such as driving deliveries for DoorDash, Uber Eats, and Amazon, or performing various kinds of freelance work online. The gig economy grew 33 percent in 2020, now including anywhere between 16 and 36 percent of all U.S. workers.[665]

Employers Use Pandemic

Employers are taking advantage. Conventional companies are increasingly turning to freelancers and independent contracting as the new norm for employment in general.[666] As so-called "independent contractors," gig workers have none of the rights and benefits they might otherwise receive as employees. Wages and schedules change constantly, making it difficult to predict and plan around a consistent income.

A 2019 UCLA study found that after compensating for unreimbursed expenses, rideshare drivers end up being paid as little as $5.64 an hour, well below the federal minimum wage.[667] The "gamification" of app-based gig work, controlled by computer algorithms, compels workers to squeeze out maximum productivity for minimum pay.

Los Angeles gig worker Peter Young describes the impacts of his working conditions:

> I can't plan for the future. I can't be confident in what income I will have in six months, and that is really stressful. . . . They control the flow of my day through an app. They can pay different amounts at different times a day. They can get me to work when they want me to work. And rather than having more control of my job, I feel like I have no control over my job.[668]

Originally touted as a part-time "side hustle" that promoted freedom and flexibility for workers, up to 72 percent of gig workers, disproportionately Black and Latinx, rely on these jobs to support themselves and their families.[669] Working long hours in isolation under harsh and unpredictable conditions just to make ends meet, with no ability to negotiate the terms of their work with human co-workers or supervisors, many app-based gig workers suffer the psychological toll of their precarious working conditions.

"I'm just tired of the situation," says Rosa, a rideshare driver in Los Angeles:

> I'm so scared to come home and bring a disease or get infected. I have to wait four hours for a passenger. I'm always behind, I don't have enough earnings. What if I get sick? Who's going to take care of me? What about other drivers with a family, with people they're taking care of?[670]

Among rideshare and delivery drivers, in particular, the stress of responding to algorithmic management on the job to earn what little wages they can get, combined with the physical degradation from sitting in a car for long periods of time, takes a toll on their bodies. But as independent contractors, they have no access to health insurance or related benefits:

> More hours means less time to take care of yourself, which means a higher likelihood the driver could get sick. Being an independent contractor means drivers don't get sick days, though, so taking any time off means less money coming in.[671]

Fed Up with the Food Industry

Workers all along the food chain, from the farm to the fast-food window, often operate under systems of contracting and subcontracting that likewise create "a layer of separation, or 'fissure,' between workers and the companies responsible for their working conditions."[672]

Labor and workplace safety violations were already widespread and unaccountable in the food industry even before the pandemic. Wage theft and unpaid overtime, as well as injury from workplace hazards, were routine. With the onset of the COVID-19 pandemic, these routine violations have turned into a deadly catastrophe for food workers. One farmworker describes these harrowing conditions at his workplace:

The foreman just yells at us that the work must continue and that he doesn't care if one has COVID-19 or not. They don't even wear face masks. The employer kept quiet and didn't tell anyone until some died. They never pay attention.[673]

The deregulation of the food industry under the Trump administration gutted the oversight powers of the Occupational Safety and Health Administration (OSHA). In what experts have called a "regulatory boycott," the agency actually stopped tracking COVID-19 cases as the virus ripped through meatpacking plants, grocery suppliers, and fast food restaurants across the country.[674]

In California, the death rate for food system workers due to COVID-19 is a staggering 40 percent higher than the state average, and up to 59 percent among Latinx food and agriculture workers.[675] One Farmer John's plant in Los Angeles has endured over a year of continuous COVID-19 outbreaks that have killed at least five, and infected more than 780 workers, nearly half of its total workforce.[676]

Eliseo, a farmworker in the San Joaquin Valley, reports:

[The bosses] did not give us face masks, in other words, we asked them for face masks, and they just laughed. And we asked for soap to wash our hands, because there were many places where we could not wash our hands, and [the bosses] just laughed. And several of my co-workers and I called Cal/OSHA, and we got together to ask for help before we could get infected. And [Cal/OSHA] told us that they were going to send letters and that they were going to talk to our boss but they never did anything.[677]

For undocumented farmworkers, the fear is multiplied, especially at a time when racist and xenophobic social attitudes, as well as oppressive government policies, have made structural barriers to health care even worse. One Kern County worker speaks to this complex of fears: "I would be afraid to go to the hospital with my daughters because I could be blamed for neglect if I didn't take them soon enough. Then, they would separate us and deport us."

For a Coachella Valley farmworker, economic fears compounded the challenge posed by the virus itself: "I don't have insurance and it's very expensive to get treatment or be hospitalized. I don't have a large amount of income and in case of death by coronavirus the costs would be larger. This is a scary situation."[678]

Most of the workers who continue to keep the economy running during the pandemic, especially food chain workers, do not receive the token thanks and accolades given to "essential" workers, even as they put their bodies on the line in jobs that often put them at the most risk of infectious disease.

"We're supposedly indispensable and essential," Eliseo puts it, "but it feels like we're not essential, as if we are useless trash that you can throw away and then they'll just hire more people. That's how I feel."[679]

While grocery stores and fast-food chains make record profits during the pandemic, food chain work is highly precarious, sites have minimal regulatory oversight, and workers are overwhelmingly Black and Latinx.[680] Nine out of ten fast food workers in Los Angeles are people of color, who live with their families in densely populated low-income neighborhoods.[681] The risks they are exposed to in the workplace continue to be carried home with them, including COVID-19.

Just like housing instability, the sustained psychological stress of precarious employment is strongly associated with COVID-19 comorbidities stemming from toxic stress, chronic disease, inflammation, and dysregulated immune responses. Studies show that poor working conditions—particularly the low wages, long hours, lack of agency and uncertainty common to precarious gig work—contribute to toxic stress-related mental health issues such as anxiety, depression, insomnia, and fatigue, as well as physical manifestations like stomach issues, high blood pressure, sleep disorders, and chronic pain.[682]

The connections from political economy to cellular immunity are well documented. In a review of studies examining biomarkers of work stress specifically related to factors of "job demand-control," "effort-reward imbalance," and "organizational injustice," elevated levels of

IL-6 and C-reactive proteins—molecular inputs for severe COVID-19—strongly correlated with these workplace-based stressors.[683]

One study that examined the allostatic load index associated with abnormal stress response found that the physiological impact of precarious employment and poor working conditions was actually worse than having no job at all.[684]

As the economy reopens amid new waves of COVID infections, and the "Uber-ization" of work exports the precarity experienced by gig and food chain workers to the wider labor market, defending worker rights and protections becomes a public health issue for the vast majority of Black, Brown, immigrant, and low-income workers who cannot afford to stay at home. And ultimately, for all workers.

Another Round with Delta

By this summer, COVID-19 cases were again on the rise in Los Angeles and urban centers across the nation, driven by the Delta variant that emerged in India and already ravaged cities across the Global South. In the last week of July 2021, cases went up 80 percent in Los Angeles County, topping 3,000 new daily cases for the first time since February. Hospitalization rates have doubled, as ICU beds are once again filling across the county. The American Academy of Pediatrics reports that over one-fifth of new cases have appeared among children, up from a mere 3 percent of cases just one year ago, shattering expectations of COVID resilience among younger, healthier people.[685]

Disasters are colliding. With California's increasingly catastrophic wildfire season well underway, Harvard researchers reported 20,000 extra COVID-19 infections and 750 COVID deaths associated with smoke pollution, suggesting that the climate crisis is yet another compounding factor threatening communities on the front lines of environmental injustice.[686]

In strictly public health terms, L.A. County does appear to have taken some prudent steps toward discouraging unchecked community spread of the virus this time around. While other cities in California and states across the country are dropping mask requirements to prepare for a full reopening, Los Angeles County was the first jurisdiction in the country to independently reinstitute an indoor mask mandate, regardless of vaccination status, as a precaution against Delta's fast rate of spread.

Still, many experts and health care workers worry about the role of "disease fatigue" among younger people eager to resume their normal lives after a year and a half of lockdown. Despite the Delta variant's increased virulence among children, L.A. schools are still on track to reopen, albeit with a new mandate that teachers must either be vaccinated or undergo weekly testing to continue working.

Nearly 69 percent of L.A. County's residents have been fully vaccinated.[687] While a conspicuous number of breakthrough cases in vaccinated people have been documented, most cases, and nearly all hospitalizations, are occurring among the unvaccinated population, regardless of race or income status. Even so, dynamics of structural racism persist within that subset.

Vaccine hesitancy is portrayed in popular critique as a largely white conservative phenomenon, even given the history of racial medical abuse and distrust of health care institutions among Black communities that have contributed to lower vaccination rates and a disproportionate number of new infections. L.A.'s Black population began with the highest per capita case rates in the county during the first few weeks of the Delta surge.[688] And though a third of unvaccinated Latinx workers have expressed their desire to get vaccinated, access barriers still contribute to higher case rates in low-wage and undocumented Latinx communities.[689]

Despite these characteristic outcomes, vaccination rates in L.A. County appear to be the only variable that does not follow previous statistical patterns strongly correlating COVID-19 impacts with income and racial disparities. Unlike nearly all other factors related to the pandemic, the scatter plot we published in our original dispatch shows no significant relationship between race, income, or access barriers and the proportion of vaccinated individuals.[690]

Given the severity of the first wave and its disproportionate impact on low-income communities of color, this result can be attributed to the success of political will. L.A. County waged an aggressive campaign to encourage vaccinations, concentrating outreach campaigns and efforts on disproportionately impacted communities. The county offered free vaccination services to the general public at Dodger Stadium, a centralized location that was easily accessible for all residents. The success shows that local governments are in fact capable of addressing unequal public health outcomes and improving equity in access to an essential tool for combating the pandemic.

This is only one part of a larger story, however, when it comes to effectively containing the dangers posed—and exposed—by the pandemic. Though mass vaccinations may immediately protect people against the virus, the structural inequalities that lie at the root of COVID-19's social and physiological comorbidities must also be addressed. As we've described, housing instability, precarious work, systemic racism, and toxic stress are all factors that amplified the pandemic's cataclysmic effects among communities of color, the working class, and the unhoused. They remain critically important indicators of social vulnerability to future disasters.

Evicting the Eviction Moratorium

The ever-deepening housing crisis remains a critical linchpin in the complex of economic and public health hazards unleashed by the pandemic, and it continues to disproportionately affect Black and Latinx workers with no relief in sight. The Biden administration first allowed the federal eviction moratorium imposed by the CDC to expire on June 30, just days before the Delta variant propelled a surge of new cases in Los Angeles and across the country. The administration reversed course but the Supreme Court, legislating from the bench in a way the Democratic Party refuses to from Congress, placed a stay on continuing the moratorium.[691]

A new UCLA study linked the lapse in state eviction moratoriums to a doubling of COVID case rates and a five-fold increase in mortality.[692] With over four million renters at risk of eviction nationally, just 17 states, including California, elected to extend the moratorium until September. Landlords are pushing back against extended eviction moratoriums, including launching a $100 million lawsuit against the city of Los Angeles for extending local ordinances aimed at keeping renters in their homes.[693]

Even with the extended moratorium in place, renters in Los Angeles County alone now owe more than $3 billion in back rent, and 41 percent of all Los Angeles renters—over 307,000 residents and their families—face eviction once the moratorium is lifted.[694] CalMatters reports that even with the moratorium, at least 1,600 households have been evicted in several California counties since emergency shelter-in-place orders were announced in March 2020 (excluding Los Angeles County, whose sheriff's department declined to report numbers for the study). As of August 7, the L.A. sheriff's department resumed serving its backlog of over 1,000 eviction lockouts despite the extension of the state eviction moratorium and surging case rates in L.A. County.[695]

Rental assistance programs, including an ambitious and much-touted California initiative to pay 100 percent of back rent for troubled renters, have been impractically slow in implementation, adding to renters' anxiety and toxic stress levels.

Jenise Dixon, an L.A. resident who fell behind in rent after she lost work in the film industry and applied for rental assistance in April, told *The Guardian* in early August that she has yet to see her aid checks arrive, despite already receiving an eviction notice from her landlord:

> I'm just doing what I can to survive. . . . We didn't ask for this pandemic, we didn't ask to lose our jobs. We didn't ask for all this turmoil. Taking months to distribute these funds is just unacceptable.[696]

Isa Tabora, an East L.A. resident who owes an estimated $12,000 in back rent and had to reapply for rental assistance in June, lamented:

> What am I going to do? I cannot allow my kids to be on the street . . . We try to keep up, but we can't, because we're so behind. If I

have to sleep in the car, I will. But I can't let that happen to my kids.[697]

Christopher Flynn, a disabled and immunocompromised former film industry worker, echoed these anxieties in a recent local news interview:

> I have to check the door several times a day to see if there's an eviction notice because even though technically [the landlord] can't do it, I don't put anything past them at this point. . . . LA has a bad enough problem with homelessness. If you're going to throw another million people out on the street in California, where are we supposed to go? What are we gonna do? This is not a game. This is very real and I have no margin of error with this thing.[698]

Renewed state and local protection mandates prompted by the Delta surge have also become targets of partisan political battles, including the Republican-led recall effort against California Governor Gavin Newsom, further eroding the effectiveness of efforts to contain the pandemic in its new, more virulent form, and battering hopes of reaching herd immunity through vaccination, despite a recent contraction in the outbreak.

Updated workplace protections have pitted government agencies, unions, and industry associations against one another, making implementation and communications to workers haphazard and confusing.

Conservative groups have launched lawsuits against the L.A. Unified School District for its vaccine-or-testing mandates for teachers and mask requirements for students.[699] Police unions throughout California have pushed back on vaccine mandates for law enforcement and public sector staff.[700]

Meanwhile, the National Nurses United union demonstrated in front of UCLA Medical Center for better protections for health care workers on the front lines of the pandemic. As one University of California nurse explained, "We have had to continuously fight university management for the safe staffing, workplace protections, PPE, and access to testing that we deserve."[701]

The dilemmas posed by this latest wave of infections underscored the increasingly evident point that effectively tackling the pandemic also means addressing underlying inequalities in housing, employment, and access to essential services that exacerbate social vulnerability to disruptive shocks.

"Doesn't the government understand," one Canadian nurse put it earlier this month, "that when they cut education, mental health, housing, & social supports, it all ends up in the ER?"[702]

The ever-changing nature of the ongoing COVID-19 crisis, as well as the magnitude and seemingly intractable nature of its compounded effects, also presents an opportunity for community leaders, social movements, and progressive policymakers to rethink approaches to public health and safety, based not only on science, but also on the lived experiences and demands coming out of the communities that are most affected.

Exiting Out of the Trap

Housing insecurity and barriers to essential services
Community organizations such as the L.A. Tenants' Union, Housing Now, and L.A. Community Action Network have proposed solutions to the crisis of affordable housing and homelessness that can build community resiliency against the next pandemic or disaster.

Effective enforcement of tenant rights and protections, as well as rent and vacancy control measures can bring some accountability to curb the aggressive actions of landlords and defend against illegal evictions. Better mechanisms to ensure the development and sustainability of affordable housing, up to and including public provision of housing, can be implemented to replace the Low Income Housing Tax Credit, which has proven ineffective at curbing developers' intentions to maximize profit on new construction of multi-family units.

Local governments can adopt a Housing First approach to tackling homelessness as a cheaper, more humane alternative to law enforcement sweeps of homeless encampments.[703]

In Oakland and Philadelphia, unhoused and housing-insecure mothers have teamed up to mount direct-action campaigns by taking over and occupying empty houses to provide for themselves and highlight the needs of families for permanent, stable, and affordable housing.[704]

Providing affordable, safe, and stable housing is "both a moral imperative and a public health necessity" both in the context of the COVID-19 pandemic and to build long-term community resilience as a mitigation measure against future shocks.[705] Addressing the affordable housing shortfall for low-income and very low-income populations with innovative community-based solutions such as tiny home villages and repurposing of surplus vacant building stock and public green spaces are quick, relatively inexpensive forms of transitional housing that can relieve overcrowding in low-income neighborhoods and allow people in need to shelter in place safely and access essential services.

Conventional market-based approaches to institutional and social impact housing initiatives, such as developer tax credits, rent vouchers, and large capital projects, can be limited in effectiveness and scope if communities are not thoroughly and meaningfully engaged as primary stakeholders.

Community organizations and families on the ground who navigate these conditions on a day-to-day basis have built critical relationships of trust and, in many instances, have developed innovative, place-based ideas for housing solutions that work for them. Public agencies should allow these ideas to expand the scope of their bureaucratic imagination and be willing to mobilize public financial and in-kind resources in creative ways to be responsive to community needs.[706]

Worker precarity and unsafe conditions along the food chain

The frontline workers that maintain our food supply, from farm to table, must be recognized as "essential workers" in pandemic-related policies, and afforded the same respect and protection given to health care and other frontline workers.

While President Biden has issued an executive order to reverse Trump's actions at OSHA and restore the agency's regulatory oversight powers, the "emergency temporary standards" created to ensure workplace safety and prevent the spread of COVID-19 in health care settings "continues to exclude frontline workers in the food system and other sectors who have advocated for similar protections since the start of the pandemic."[707]

Food and agriculture workers, as well as those in many other essential sectors excluded from these policies, are disproportionately Black, Brown, poor, and most vulnerable to COVID-19 in the workplace and in their communities.

Risky conditions remain in large part unchanged for low-income immigrant workers. A recent study from UC Berkeley's Labor and Occupational Health Program and the Asian Law Caucus has revealed that one in five low-wage service workers received no information from their employer about workplace protections. Nearly half were afraid to speak up about the issue due to fears of retaliation, many of which were driven by immigrant status. Almost one in five workers were being paid less than the state minimum wage. In workplaces where concerns about COVID protections were raised, nearly half of workers reported that the employer did nothing at all to address the issue, or only partly addressed it.[708]

Unions and worker advocacy organizations continue to take actions to address these disparities and demand worker protections and equitable pay. Fast food workers in Los Angeles, Oakland, Sacramento, and thirteen other cities across the nation held a one-day strike in January 2021 for a federal $15 minimum wage and worker protections, pushing legislators to adopt an industry-wide standard for better working conditions.[709] Potentially hundreds more fast food and retail workers have participated informally in a de facto strike wave by simply quitting hostile workplaces en masse, many such actions going viral on social media and prompting complaints of labor shortages throughout the service sector.[710]

The United Food and Commercial Workers (UFCW) successfully organized to persuade the Los Angeles City Council to mandate an additional $5 per hour in hazard pay for grocery store workers.[711] The Food Chain Workers' Alliance calls for the inclusion of food supply workers in the new OSHA emergency standards, and supports a host of food worker organizations in their demands for better wages, working conditions, and protections from COVID-19 and other workplace hazards.[712]

Strengthening workers' rights and protections, as well as supporting workers' right to organize, are some of the most powerful bulwarks against the wholesale transition of the labor market to a gig economy as the nation reopens and transitions out of COVID-19 lockdown.

In California, gig workers and union advocates are mounting strike actions and suing to repeal Prop 22 and close the loopholes that allow gig companies like Uber, Lyft, and DoorDash to continue misclassifying workers as independent contractors.[713] Other gig workers who have been unable to find adequate work are organizing to qualify for the pandemic-related unemployment assistance they need and deserve.

It is not too late to call on the federal government to do much more to support all workers whose livelihoods have been disrupted during the pandemic. The danger to essential workers presented by the new Delta wave can also serve as a catalyst to reverse course in the transformation of work, away from the domination of the gig economy and casualization of labor. Worker precarity is also a public health matter. It can be best addressed by preserving the hard-won gains of over 150 years of labor activism, and making informed policy interventions that are responsive to the needs of workers today.

What COVID Teaches Us about Resilience

The COVID-19 pandemic has turned into an object lesson in the feedback dynamics of a compounding crisis.

The catastrophic impacts of COVID transmission and disease on workers and marginalized communities in Los Angeles, and across the nation, not only reflect historical inequalities that persist in our society, but also deepen structural race and class inequalities. Given the health impacts of inflammatory disorders from chronic toxic stress, these inequalities literally become a matter of life and death for the people and families that live in low-income communities and communities of color.

From government inaction and mishandling of the pandemic at the federal level to the individual actions of employers and landlords, COVID-19 has accelerated decades-long processes of economic neoliberalization to the point where extreme inequality, housing instability, economic precarity, and lack of accountability have become the norm. As Rupa Marya and Raj Patel put it in their 2021 book *Inflamed*:

> Your body is part of a society inflamed. COVID has exposed the combustible injustices of systemic racism and global capitalism. . . . Inflammation is a biological, social, economic, and ecological pathway, all of which intersect, and whose contours were made by the modern world.[714]

This will not be the last pandemic, nor will it be the last disaster we will encounter as a society. Climate change, ecological degradation, economic volatility, and reactionary political movements pose many current and future threats to social stability at local, national, and global levels.

With each disruption, long-lasting impacts accumulate in familiar patterns of structural inequality, falling disproportionately on the most marginalized and vulnerable among us. Overcrowding in low-income neighborhoods and homelessness will worsen from rising rents and evictions, as well as influxes of climate refugees from wildfires, hurricanes, and floods.

Chronic toxic stress will continue to accumulate in Black, Brown, and working-class bodies from the unrelenting pressure and anxiety of maintaining precarious housing and livelihoods while living under heat domes, cold snaps, and the shadow of deadly pathogens. Inadequate aid and protection policies that favor business interests over public health concerns exacerbate all of these conditions.

Indeed, such profit-first policies may already have allowed COVID-19 to establish itself as a permanent fixture in our society for years to come.

Yet this bleak new "Age of Crises" also gives us an opportunity to mobilize political will to propose, demand, and implement transformative solutions—not just to beat COVID-19 in the near term, but to finally address the long-standing vulnerabilities the virus has exposed in our society.

As global phenomena, COVID and climate change have made us painfully aware of our shared fate on this planet, as well as our shared responsibility to step up to the challenges of the moment. We need to rethink justice as extending out from courts and into our streets and landscapes. We must create more supportive, resilient communities and social systems that can weather the coming storms. Communities that are left behind, and the grassroots organizations that support them, are beginning to articulate alternate frameworks of community care and resiliency that could mitigate, and ultimately reverse, the dynamics of social vulnerability that underlie COVID-19's damage.

L.A. County's mass vaccination program, which delivered nearly ten million doses to local residents over the last several months, can be looked to as an example of what local and state governments are capable of in terms of tackling access barriers and delivering services equitably to diverse communities. Ultimately, universal health care overall is not only achievable, but could become a much more powerful grassroots policy demand, as the pandemic continues to illustrate the need for a robust, coordinated, and accessible public health system.

Even so, we should be wary of narratives that treat vaccination and biomedical interventions as a simple panacea for the complex of problems that have driven the pandemic's continued persistence and growth. Given the access barriers, distrust of institutions, and other social forces that have slowed vaccination rates and driven significant levels of vaccine hesitancy, it may already be impossible to achieve herd immunity through vaccination alone.

To truly defeat COVID-19, we need to shift to a treatment paradigm that encompasses the concept of *community immunity*, which, following Marya and Patel, is based on an understanding that "immunity is not a problem that can be solved merely at the level of individual choice."[715] Community immunity is derived from "social immunity," a zoological term that refers to "what happens when an immune response is beneficial not only to the individual mounting it but also to others in the community."[716]

We must break the cycles of trauma and toxic stress that harm marginalized communities. We must reestablish those vital functions in our individual and social bodies that move us all toward greater stability, security, and equity.

Institutional interventions can stop the pain and provide immediate relief by prioritizing stability for vulnerable people and families, defense of worker protections, and ensuring the human right to basic needs. Long-term recovery, however, is not possible without justice. A post-COVID "new normal" must shift the burden of responsibility off struggling individuals, facilitate the reconstruction of the vital social bonds that sustain us, and cultivate networks of mutual aid and "community care" long advocated by social movements and trauma-informed public health organizations.[717]

"The healing process," according to Marya and Patel, "must involve restructuring the world to make it a safe place for survivors to flourish—in other words, deep wounds require deep medicine."

To make ourselves and our society whole again, we must dig deep and repair our relationships with each other, our environments, and society as a whole. The exploitative relations that underpin our current neoliberal society have not only contributed to the emergence of multiple and compounded crises, but they have also critically weakened the very bonds upon which the whole society relies, rendering us all vulnerable to compounded injury.

In the context of a global pandemic like COVID-19, even complex, technologically advanced, and wealthy societies in the Global North are only as strong as their weakest links. In many ways, communities of the Global South have long understood this lesson. We need to listen and learn from such leadership. From South America to South Central and back again.

Resilient communities in nature are characterized by biodiversity, symbiotic relationships of mutual benefit, and efficient distribution of resource flows that make the whole greater than the sum of its parts. In the face of current and future challenges, building resilient communities means, Marya and Patel conclude, "recognizing the current state of emergency and simultaneously imagining a radically different future."[718] It is a future that is fundamentally rooted in valuing our interdependence. It is steeped in recognizing the fundamental public health principle that an injury to one is an injury to all.

—PANDEMIC RESEARCH FOR THE PEOPLE
SEPTEMBER 21, 2021

Homegrown

The Pandemic Research for the People dispatch about COVID-19 and Los Angeles included this sidebar. The U.S. lag in sequencing SARS-CoV-2 genomes helps feed nativist folklore from the Boogaloo Bois to the CDC that terrible diseases—and new variants thereof—emerge only from abroad.[719]

THIS DISPATCH LARGELY FOCUSES on the housing and work conditions that concentrate COVID in Black, Brown, and low-income neighborhoods. The success of the virus, however, also depends on a parallel history in economic geography.

Following up historian Mike Davis, political scientist Charmaine Chua reviews a switcheroo by which L.A. came to service the global supply chain instead of the other way around.[720] The regional economy became organized around finding global commodities their American consumers of last resort in all that tonnage arriving in the city port at San Pedro Bay. As the Empire Logistics Collective describes the resulting supply chain infrastructure across rail, ports, and distribution centers:

This global "factory without walls" allows capitalists to scour the planet for the cheapest and most compliant labor, externalizing costs of its maintenance onto the working class. These networks generate flows of commodities and information with ever-increasing speed, as the system strives for just-in-time production and inventory-less distribution for a unified global market. . . .

An astonishing 40-plus percent of all the goods that enter the United States move through the Inland Empire, making it one of the largest distribution hubs in the country.[721]

Such a capitalist geography also imposes itself upon L.A.'s "domestic" spatial organization. From the Port of Los Angeles to the corporate farms of the Central Valley, millions of vehicles and their passengers ping-pong to work and back on an expanding daily commute, likely introducing any new viral outbreak to the whole of Los Angeles.

The regional elbow room likely selects for both new viral recombinants that suddenly find each other in ways they couldn't before. It also selects for greater viral deadliness.[722] Above a critical level of spatial connectivity, the deadlier strains that usually burn out their local supply of susceptibles, cutting themselves off their transmission supply line, suddenly can now always find new patients to infect however quickly they kill them. The deadlier strains can now beat out the less deadly strains across the whole region.

Alongside many new COVID variants arriving from abroad, from the original Wuhan variant to Mu from Colombia and Lambda from Peru, Los Angeles has grown its own variants. In July 2020, the B.1.427 and B.1.429 lineages, what the World Health Organization renamed Epsilon, first emerged in Los Angeles, detected at the Cedars-Sinai Medical Center on Beverly Boulevard.[723]

Epsilon—between rock stars Delta and Omicron—was characterized by amino acid replacements S13I in the signal peptide, W152C in the N-terminal domain, and L452R in the spike protein.[724] The replacements may have helped make the variant more infectious, with patients hosting virus twice the level as other infected people.[725]

Molecular work showed blood plasma from people previously infected or vaccinated now had their antibodies reduced 2 to 3.5-fold when infected with Epsilon.[726] Other work showed that the new variant was also deadlier to patients.

Epsilon wasn't detected again until September 2020, but by January 2021 it was found in half the COVID cases in Los Angeles and spreading up into Northern California. By February, Epsilon was outcompeting other variants in cities as far as Houston.[727] By May, Epsilon was detected in thirty-four other countries. It would be subsequently outcompeted in California by the more contagious Alpha and Delta variants from Great Britain and India respectively, with the last cases of Epsilon detected there in June.

But clearly Los Angeles's social ecology doesn't make it just a sink for COVID variants arriving from abroad. It's also a source:

"The devil is already here," said Dr. Charles Chiu, who led the UCSF team of geneticists, epidemiologists, statisticians and other scientists in a wide-ranging analysis of the new variant.[728]

—PANDEMIC RESEARCH FOR THE PEOPLE
SEPTEMBER 21, 2021

Mo BoJo

I've often thought we were wrong to confuse American directness with an aversion to the non-linear.

—JONATHAN HICKMAN (2014)

I WAS HOPING TODAY would be my first vacation since the COVID outbreak began. But the virus never sleeps, and, with the outbreak's social and biomolecular disruptions, increasingly neither do people.[729]

A friend of mine passed on some local medical doctor's anti-lockdown harangue. Perhaps not as egregious as the celebrated Van Morrison, tellin' us what we're supposed to feel about lockdowns and crooked Imperial College scientists and their crooked facts.[730]

Or Morrison's follow-up with Eric Clapton to stand and deliver against fear and the bandit Dick Turpins still wearing their masks.[731]

In something of a similar vein, the doctor dubiously claims that along with being more transmissible, the new British SARS-CoV-2 variant everyone's all a-Twitter about, is also less pathogenic.[732]

So, we should let it spread, he says, "burning through the dry wood in the forest," to build the herd immunity ineffectual vaccines can't. That the lockdowns themselves have caused excess non-COVID-19 deaths.

That's the way to go, the good doctor says, sworn to do no harm. Millions more potentially killed—"dry wood"—for an elusive herd immunity that nowhere near approaches the specificity an effective vaccine offers, even one unable to offer sterilizing immunity.[733]

The determinate attenuation the doctor champions is a notion forty years out of date.[734] Models of the evolution of virulence since show when pathogens gain access to more susceptibles, as repeated bouts of global spread permit, *increases* in virulence could very well be selected for.[735]

Swells in non-outbreak mortality during a pandemic are meanwhile a function of for-profit health care systems that confuse gouging people for every pretty penny with public health.[736] Or of British Conservatives aiming to model their National Health Service after "shithole countries" that monetize health insurance.

Countries that stayed open during the pandemic had more deaths *and* worse economic outcomes.[737] Economy or health is a false dichotomy of these regimes' own imposition. Countries that slammed down on their outbreaks with suppression campaigns now boast greater economic output.[738] With their populations free to walk around or attend the rugby match at the stadium unmasked.[739]

The oath I'd use is something other than Hippocratic: "Stay the fuck away from my kid, doc."

Herd as Laboratory

Biomolecular researchers report the new British variant (B.1.1.7, VUI-202012/01, or Alpha) appears to have evolved an unprecedented fourteen nonsynonymous mutations, including an amino acid replacement—N501Y in the receptor binding domain of the spike gene—associated with better binding to target cells. [740]

The strain also hosts three deletions and an additional stop codon in the ORF8 locus, a gene previously shown in SARS-2, but not SARS-1, involved in downregulating MHC class 1 immunity.[741] The stop codon allows additional mutations downstream in the ORF8 sequence.

What's the source of the rapid shifts in this south England lineage? Other host species perhaps. The WHO reports the strain may have converged upon molecular phenotypes found in SARS-2 that spilled back into humans off mink farms.[742] Intrapatient evolution, particularly in immunodeficient patients suffering high viral loads or long-term COVID patients, can also drive rapid molecular evolution.[743]

But to make a point about the impact of governance on these dynamics, earlier I named the variant the BoJo strain, after Boris Johnson, whose government's cronyist negligence allowed the virus to engage in the kind of interdemic selection that permits pathogens the workspace for such evolutionary experimentation.[744]

So, alongside herd immunity, we need now introduce the notion of *herd multiplicity*. The more people infected, the greater the chance the virus has to evolve solutions to our various interventions. Minimizing spread, then, should help reduce the evolutionary combinatorials over which the virus can play lab scientist.

Epidemiologist Andrew Lover, for one, tweeted a hypothesis that the virus—still causing symptoms—could evolve to skirt biomedical detection:

Most malaria rapid tests ("RDTs") target a protein called HRP-2 (histidine rich-protein 2).

Way back in 2010, some "oddball" parasites were found that were missing this protein, and therefore "invisible" to the rapid tests. . . .

Head-scratching and sequencing found they didn't express the target protein (which was considered "essential"). . . .

Subsequent work suggest[ed] strong evolutionary pressure.

Undetected parasites . . . aren't treated, & thus far more likely to be transmitted onward.

If detection [of COVID-19] decreases, then people with these infections are less likely to be "captured" and into isolation, and contacts not followed up.[745]

There may be other ways of getting out from underneath detection.

Our team's latest paper, first-authored by University of St. Thomas evolutionary biologist Kenichi Okamoto, offers a second, if related, possibility.[746] Stealth is selected for at the level of infection life history—in the stage-specific attributes of the infection's development, growth, maturation, reproduction, survival, and life span.

Indeed, it's my interpretation that our model may offer exactly an explanation for the emergence of the BoJo strain: shoddy, neoliberal quarantines allow the virus time to evolve in a way China-Vietnam-New Zealand suppression campaigns do not.

Although our model doesn't explicitly address full-out lockdowns that reduce the supply of susceptibles, focusing on early-days interventions that we model as instantaneously pursued, we conclude:

> Generally, increasing isolation effort selects for a novel [asymptomatic] strain to spread in the host population, until the isolation efficacy is sufficiently high that disease control occurs before an asymptomatic mutant can evolve.[747]

The parameter space defined by isolation, quarantine, viral spread, and the evolution of infection life history can be convoluted:

> When quarantining also affects viral evolution and spread, we find increasing quarantine efforts can have divergent effects. At times, increased removal of symptomatic hosts selects for an asymptomatic strain, but this can be mitigated by more effective quarantining. . . . By contrast, [we can also see] the opposite effect: higher quarantining efforts interact with levels of isolation that select for asymptomatic viruses to drive high prevalence.

The convolutions can include twists and turns in how public health interventions interact:

> Even within the latter scenarios, the joint effects of isolation and quarantining are not always consistent. For instance . . . the

interaction between high quarantine levels and isolation dimin-
ishes as isolation efficacy increases.[748]

Under a scenario modeling more *dynamic interventions* that
change with the number of symptomatic cases:

> Although very subtle, in some cases modest to intermediate levels
> of isolation coupled with low quarantining modestly reduced
> the prevalence of the novel strain, while in others increasing iso-
> lation efforts are what reduced the strain's prevalence.[749]

Social Structure of COVID Evolution

The models practically recapitulate the Anglo-American approach
to toggling in and out of quarantines that produced the BoJo strain,
whether among pub attendees in Britain or, in the agribusiness version, in Danish mink:

> When intervention intensity tracks the prevalence of symptomatic
> infections, the more symptomatic strain is quite readily removed
> as isolation efforts increase, and as quarantine efforts are relaxed
> following a reduction in the prevalence of symptomatic infections,
> the novel [asymptomatic] virus can then escape suppression.[750]

The models even account for the issue of detection Lover raised.
The Okamoto team writes:

> When the ability to detect asymptomatic infections is limited,
> higher quarantining efforts promote the evolution and spread of
> an asymptomatic strain. . . . A key result [of modeling dynamic
> interventions] is that in comparison to the case where interven-
> tion efforts are constant through time, the qualitative differences
> in dynamical behaviors are driven much more by the detection
> ability of the novel strain rather than by different likelihoods of
> the novel virus causing asymptomatic infections.[751]

That failure to detect might be a matter of the pathogen's own evolution, as Lover offers, but—our contribution here—might be situated
entirely out in the field. Perhaps in the failure to launch a public health
campaign that tests everyone, including poor people who can't afford
the test, or, as public health ecologists Deborah Wallace and Rodrick
Wallace describe, people who are marginalized out of community
interventions before COVID and its tests ever arrived:

> Our data here show that in present New York City, the old ene-
> mies of public health and long life exert their force with renewed
> vigor: poverty, unemployment, lack of education, substandard
> housing, and segregation. This intertwined context of [socioeco-
> nomic] factors and public health forms the stage onto which the
> COVID-19 pandemic entered.
>
> The public policies at federal, state, and municipal levels
> that set this stage gathered steam from Nixon through Barack
> Obama and Donald Trump at the federal level; from Nelson
> Rockefeller through Andrew Cuomo at the state level; and from
> Lindsay through Bill de Blasio at the municipal level—with the
> cooperation of the legislatures.[752]

These calculated failures in governance long structured COVID
outcomes in a socially (and spatially) uneven way across the five bor-
oughs of New York City:

> Manhattan and Brooklyn were . . . the two boroughs with the
> tightest connections between socioeconomic (SE) factors and
> between SE factors and public health markers, including prema-
> ture mortality rate, COVID indicators, and diabetes mortality
> rate. . . . Tight connections indicate brittle, fragile rigidity, a
> system that cannot adapt with flexibility to an impact. . . .
>
> Although a clear pattern of premature mortality concentra-
> tion in the south central Bronx emerges . . . , the entire borough
> suffers from elevated rates of premature mortality. . . . the entire
> borough suffers from elevated rates of COVID mortality, even

though the geographic pattern may underestimate the full affliction because of undertesting of corpses. This very undertesting,
which explains the strange associations of COVID case rates
with SE factors (opposite direction from the associations in
Manhattan) and the lack of association of death rates and SE
factors, reflects the lack of responsibility of the authorities to the
Bronx.[753]

Indeed, Reuters tracked an analogous historiography underlying
the BoJo strain's emergence, of loose lockdowns, poverty, prisons, and
Jaws mayor Larry Vaughn tourism. Angela Harrison, a local council-
lor responsible for health,

said it became clear in late October that a new wave of infections
had hit the [Isle of Sheppey] particularly hard. "Everyone was
asking the same question: Why—what have we done?" she said.
Some islanders blamed outsiders for bringing in the virus, she
said, or blamed each other for not wearing face masks. Sheppey
was vulnerable because many people work in food distribution
centres, care homes or the holiday parks—jobs they can't do
while sheltering at home. . . .
    The bridge links Sheppey to the rest of Kent, known as the
"Garden of England" for its past abundance of orchards and
hops gardens, and for its beaches, castles and postcard-perfect
English villages. But Kent is less idyllic than its image suggests.
"There's a big class divide, a big geographical divide," said Jackie
Cassell, a public health expert at Brighton and Sussex Medical
School who grew up on Sheppey. "Most of the money is in the
middle of the county and most of the poverty is at the edges."
    One of those edges is Sheppey's main town of Sheerness. It
ranks among the most deprived areas in Britain; about half of
its children live in poverty. Many people trace Sheppey's decline
to the closure of the Sheerness Naval Dockyard in 1960, which
threw thousands out of work. Hundreds more lost their jobs
when the steelworks shut in 2011.[754]

Much as in rural communities in the United States that are dependent upon prison economies in the face of declines in regional agriculture, COVID swept through the local prison:

> Mike Rolfe, who worked with Tottman at HMP Elmley, is the founder of the Criminal Justice Workers' Union, which says it represents about 450 staff across Sheppey's three prisons. "It was really just a free-for-all once we had that disease in prison," he said. "Even those who were really careful were catching it quite easily." Rolfe estimates that 75% of HMP Elmley's 500 staff tested positive for Covid during the recent surge. At one point, he said, about 100 staff were off work.[755]

The Okamoto models track the impacts of these social disparities on the combinations of public health interventions likely driving SARS-2's evolution:

> When the ability to detect asymptomatic cases is low, as the evolved virus becomes increasingly asymptomatic (particularly towards the [immunologically] resilient [or more socially affluent] host), the effect of increasing quarantine efforts changes from successful suppression to facilitating the evolution of the asymptomatic strain at intermediate isolation efforts.
>
> This shift occurs because strains that cause more asymptomatic infections are harder to suppress even when quarantine efforts are high, whereas viruses less likely to cause asymptomatic infections are more readily controlled by increasing quarantine efforts. Once more, we see how these effects are magnified when the probability of being asymptomatic is high for resilient hosts, because the resilient host is also likelier to be subject to increased isolation and quarantine efforts.[756]

Without full-spectrum disease suppression, such newly evolved asymptomatic strains can blow back out into populations both more susceptible to the worst clinical courses and disconnected from healthcare, testing, and, by dint of being forced to commute, self-quarantine. But as the Wallaces observe, the wealthy aren't protected either:

> Prospero's castle, the affluent regions of Manhattan, together with Putnam and Hunterdon counties, is, at the date of this writing, locked down and telecommuting during only the very first stages of the COVID-19 pandemic.
>
> Experience of the last century, from the second wave of the "Spanish flu"—better described as Kansas hog influenza—through the many subsequent influenza outbreaks, suggests that, over time, the walls of that castle will indeed by breached, that the dynamic mixmaster indexed by the commuting field links every geographic entity of the New York Metropolitan Region with every other at much less than six degrees of separation. "Telecommuting" by the declining number of affluent US workers can only slow, but not halt, that dynamic process.[757]

Other Tunes

The Okamoto models show big-picture that when more socialistic interventions are pursued—evenly distributed and diligent in their isolation and quarantine interventions—they can squelch such surprises:

> In general, we find that more uniformity in transmission risk and isolation and quarantining efforts between vulnerable and resilient hosts usually reduces the prevalence of the more asymptomatic virus.[758]

There are complications and caveats as one expects in such a complicated parameter space, especially under dynamic interventions, but it's a take-home the Wallaces converge on in terms specific to U.S. political economy:

> The Great Reform did not gain traction until after the Triangle

Shirtwaist Fire. It did not gain ascendance until the New Deal programs to buffer effects of the Great Depression. Bringing another Reform to reality will likewise be a lengthy, laborious, dangerous, often-tedious, and demoralizingly frustrating piece of work.

Without this new Great Reform, the old enemies of public health and well-being will leave the people of NYC and of America sitting ducks for pandemics and premature mortality between pandemics: poverty, unemployment, low educational attainment, substandard and insufficient housing, and the war on countervailing forces such as labor unions, public health and environmental scientists, human rights groups, and voters.[759]

Even now, the greater culture is bristling at the caustic failures of the political class, with the new administration following up Trumpist incompetence with bipartisan austerity.[760]

From treacle to dark humor and hard-ass, a different COVID soundtrack is loading.[761] Iggy Pop stands and delivers, singing of the sassy little virus, which, only nineteen, can still kill you.[762]

In summing up the year, the rapper Curren$y sketches the public space in a very different way than Morrison and Clapton.[763] His Dick Turpin has the sense to mask up when surviving the superspreader events called the United States and England.

—PATREON, DECEMBER 24, 2020

Guilty Bystanders

MOLECULAR BIOLOGIST AND "bat woman" Zheng-Li Shi gave a presentation to a joint session of the National Academy of Medicine and the Veterinary Academy of France this morning.[764]

I hear there was some handwaving around placing SARS-2's origins in India and blaming the rest of the world for exporting COVID into China by frozen food.[765] All fodder for the political officers back home. And not her first time at it.[766]

But her team's latest paper appears to be solid stuff.[767] If it's an unfair comparison, my apologies, but very Rudolph Giuliani that, making up all sorts of stool about a stolen election for the press and offering no such evidence in the court where perjury is rewarded with a jail sentence.

In some sense, the paper offers the molecular equivalent of what phylogenetic analyses earlier this year indicated: SARS has been dancing across the bat-human interface for decades and will likely continue to do so.

Specifically, the team shows a variety of allelotypes in the spike protein in multiple SARSr-CoV strains hosted by Chinese horseshoe bats, a major reservoir of betacoronaviruses or sarbecovirus.[768]

The variants, collected across four provinces and Hong Kong, differed in their binding affinities with angiotensin-converting enzyme 2 (ACE2), the SARS-2 target, in human HeLa cells.[769] Their Figure 1 shows some variants did very well attaching to ACE2, others not so.[770]

With some amino acid residues under positive selection, the group proposes there's an evolutionary arms race between SARS and the bats' AEC2, modulating the resulting virulence not only in bats, but, with repeated spillovers, in humans as well.[771]

The phylogenies I reviewed as of late August—and which you read here first—showed that SARS-like (SL) coronaviruses have had decades of opportunity to spill over into human populations many multiple times:

> By three dating methods of differing conservativeness, the Boni team clocked divergence of the SARS-2 lineage from its bat sarbecovirus sister group at 1948 (95% Highest Posterior Density, 1879–1999), 1969 (1930-2000), and 1982 (1948–2009). That is, the strain leading up to the beginning of the pandemic likely circulated for decades unnoticed, perhaps, as the team surmises, in bats. When the virus spilled over into humans, however, they leave unspecified.
>
> The team offers a temporal version of the kind of pandemic gun under which we remain. As both SARS-1 and -2 appear 40–70 years divergent from their bat ancestors, many closely related but unsampled SLs in this clade in all likelihood are circulating out there across different species of bats—horseshoe or otherwise—and in different places across Central and South China.[772]

The Chaw analysis I also described places SARS-2 circulating in humans *for years,* long before Wuhan.[773]

The resulting splatter isn't just SARS-1, MERS, and SARS-2—three major deadly phenotypes in 17 years—but several other less virulent outbreaks documented in humans: 229E, HKU1, NL63, and OC43. The Zheng-Li Shi paper unpacks some of the molecular mechanisms by which we are placed under the gun.

In effect, the SLs are using our shared evolutionary histories with bats to their epidemiological advantage. Not that this is consciously so, of course, but our disease webs are more Epimethean in nature—harking back to deep histories—than they are Promethean or merely dependent upon our present immunities and biomedical innovations.

As Deborah Wallace and I wrote in "To the Back Cave" in *Dead Epidemiologists*:

> SARS may be mining our symplesiomorphies, the ancestral character states we share with the horseshoe bat, to attack us in turn. Deep evolution is a resource upon which animals across very different taxa may draw.[774]

In short, with governments and capital driving the deforestation that is increasing spillover events, humans appear here not-so-innocent bystanders killed in an ongoing fight between bats and their SARS viruses.

The Zheng-Li Shi team wraps its results in this bow: the work offers the possibility of predicting when a strain might go human-specific. But is that the lesson to draw here? It's very much in the vein of the EcoHealth Alliance and other establishment research outfits promising to fix disease crises without having to change anything.[775]

Instead, how about we back out of the bar and stop getting in between bat and virus? Rewild parts of central and southern China, and—for Ebola, Zika, avian influenza, and the like—sub-Saharan Africa, Latin America, and the Global North.[776] Turn agriculture back to the food forests local Indigenous and smallholders tended to for centuries and can continue today.

We can still feed the world without getting killed in what appears an escalating fusillade.

—PATREON, DECEMBER 3, 2020

Vic Berger's American Public Health

Florida Republican calls for review of all vaccine mandates, including polio, mumps and rubella.
— GUSTAF KILANDER (2021)

There is a reason, after all, that some people wish to colonize the moon, and others dance before it as an ancient friend.
— JAMES BALDWIN (1972)

DALE HARRISON IS A biotech consultant. I believe his recent commentary, more than the linked article he unpacks, is a cogent projection for U.S. COVID through the fall season.[777] It's also an excellent summary of the nature of the present vaccine coverage.

Yes, anti-COVID vaccines are *much* better than nothing, at both the personal and population levels. It's why we must break Bill Gates's stranglehold on COVAX and end the vaccine producers' intellectual property rights.[778] We need to stick billions of people in rapid order to have a shot at driving SARS-2 below its replacement rate.

The vaccines are *not* categorical in their coverage, however. They're statistical. That is, they vastly increase your likelihood of avoiding serious illness should you be infected. And, less so, they increase the likelihood you'll avoid infection (and infecting others). But, as Harrison describes, that latter protection is both conditional and—with the Delta variant needing fewer virions to break through—slowly falling out of the sky.

Our present trajectory was a well-described outcome. The Biden administration pretended otherwise, reversing the mask mandate in May knowing full well that Delta was on its way. It's as mendacious a decision as anything the mass murderers of the previous administration undertook.

Didn't the new administration declare it would follow the science? It said it would, but it has not done so. Against the Swiss cheese model of public health nearly every public health expert outside Atlanta supports—using a variety of interventions to cover for the holes in each intervention—the Biden White House abandoned every intervention save the vaccine.[779]

Now scientism, a kind of liberal magical thinking, is being wielded to protect this nicer set of perpetrators. I've taken to calling CDC officials and their R1 university supporters "Imperial droids" or "R1-D2s". They are offering post-hoc technical support for every one of the administration's ill-thought pandemic policies however much these positions ping across contradictory stances.

Castigating people who haven't gotten vaccinated misses the point. As science writer Ed Yong described, the Biden administration went all-in on making vaccination a matter of individual choice.[780] Doing to the red states what Trump did to the blue, when the virus started on the coasts, is not public health. It's indictable.

THE SPECIFICS OF SARS-2 and its origins, treatment, and prevention are puzzles very much worth the enormous attention the world is paying them. If I find myself swiveling to broader themes these days, it's because all that accumulating knowledge appears off-angle on every entry. Too many pins of actionable understanding remain standing rack after rack.

Writing on another crisis, the *New Yorker*'s Jelani Cobb remarked on the failure to heed systemic alerts or even act on them once the damage arrives: "The common theme in these warnings is our collective unwillingness to address them beforehand."[781] It's like the core defect is in the way we insist on rebuffing the problem as below our neoliberal divinity.

"Philosopher István Mészáros," I wrote in *Big Farms Make Big Flu*,

> differentiates between episodic or periodic crises resolved within the established framework and foundational crises that affect the framework itself. In the latter structural crises, unfolding in an epochal fashion through the very limits of a given order, the systemic contradictions start to run up against one another.[782]

Philosopher Donatella Di Cesare placed the matter in COVID's terms:

> This is where the defeat of politics becomes fully apparent. Listless and concentrated on a tomorrowless present, politics bounces from one emergency to the next, attempting to keep up with events and ride the wave. Irresponsibility—a lack of answers for the future generations—seems to be this politics' most particular trait.[783]

Insisting, then, upon the bright idea (almost) no one recommended that billionaires and corporations should be given total leeway in "solving" the problems they caused in the first place isn't the panacea by this point instinctively presumed.[784] That would add to what historian Adam Tooze calls the "organized irresponsibility."[785]

Where once chiefs and dictators developed cults of personalities that democracies (and Karl Marx, who coined the term) denounced, capitalism sticks such fallacies beyond even gestures to the collective. And the billionaires, richer than ever in the pandemic, insist their childish egos are humanity's saviors.[786] One wag described Jeff Bezos in his spacesuit and cowboy hat as the nine-year-old who couldn't decide upon the theme of his birthday party.[787]

Academic ethics, political theorist Fredric Jameson writes, designed for individual struggles over good and evil, are at best only fitfully applicable to large-scale groups.[788] In other approaches, say, the *Lebensweisheit* ("life wisdom") or the paradoxes of the *moralistes*,

> the relationships between the personal and the collective is reversed; and while so much political thought involves the illicit transfer of individualistic categories to the collective, this other kind of discourse sees the personal-ethical as the political, and focuses the new categories of a late feudal or raison-d'état politics on the complexities of human relations, particularly in the court situations of absolute monarchy. [789]

Not that that works either, but it's Marxist critic Walter Benjamin's insistence, Jameson continues, that other ethoses are possible: "Benjamin's sense of the timeliness of older theological categories is therefore symptomatic and prophetic all at once."[790]

Rocker Phoebe Bridgers more recently sung of finding such new places to be from—haunted houses with picket fences, to float around and ghost our friends.[791]

Yes, an end is near, another Bridgers line. "The disaster that has now been announced," Di Cesare continues,

> only feeds the sense of impotence. Is it already too late? All this alarm may be the expression—who knows?—of a premature catastrophism. Maybe science has a last-minute surprise in store? Perhaps. But the very functioning of techno-scientific society does not leave much space for illusions, with its standards of well-being and its canons of prosperity.

An alternate public health, placing people's health front-and-center, needn't be either-or. We can explore the connections between pathogens' molecular call signs and these stumbling political economies. We can work to disconnect them.

WHY TACK INTO THESE deeper waters? The daily roil around COVID is marked by waters so choppy as to force any epidemiology boat crew—dinghy community scientist to an aircraft carrier of a school of public health—into bailing out the diarrhetic inundation. One is so sealioned by the demands of debunking that not only can't you get any work of worth done, but the attention hole sets the falsehoods we aim to refute as our organizational principle. It serves as a work event horizon from which we can never return.

And it's coming in from all directions of the twitterverse's political compass.

Doctors can make good-faith efforts at prescribing off-label in the face of declining options. Even iffy at best ivermectin, the anti-parasitical, if, for instance, the drug acts as a general anti-inflammatory or anti-coagulant.[792] The FDA disagrees, as the modality of molecular action isn't established and the dangers of abuse are legion. A large, double-blind, randomized, and placebo-controlled study eventually showed ivermectin useless for COVID infections.[793] You may have heard, there's also a vaccine alternative with documented prophylactic effects.[794]

Debate over its action doesn't explain the sweep of ivermectin through the Trumpist right and some of the natural health left. NBC's Ben Collins identified the fad's origins in the same octopus that championed hydroxychloroquine:

> Antivaxx groups on Facebook and Reddit wanted ivermectin. Doctors wouldn't prescribe it. Members did whack-a-mole with telehealth providers, trying to get doctors to sign off on scripts. But one reliably obliged: SpeakWithAnMD, who partners with . . . America's Frontline Doctors.[795]

You might recall AFD starring in that press conference for the ages that Breitbart staged, in which fringe doctors, including one who claimed sex with demons makes you sick, denounced wearing masks and championed hydroxychloroquine.[796] Naturally Trump retweeted the video to his 84 million followers.

Indeed, so pressed were medical skeptics for access to miracle drug ivermectin that many adherents went way off-label:

> Of the 14 recent ivermectin-related calls received by the Mississippi Poison Control Center, at least 70% were related to the ingestion of livestock or animal formulations of ivermectin purchased at livestock supply centers.[797]

As the livestock version is often administered as a paste, at a thousand times the strength for human use, getting the dosage right wouldn't be easy even for a professional.[798] Its taste was enough to inspire some online converts to ask if the drug could be self-applied as a suppository.[799] And the electronic dance music left thought recreational use of ketamine was courageous, or, as the kids say, based.

This is something different from the scams of a growing list of snake oil cures for COVID, a long American tradition.[800] We have here a faith-based scientism centered in agribusiness—a rural powerhouse—deployed to cover an extreme distrust in evidence-based public health. And what does it say when people treat themselves like their commodity livestock? Or that it was administered to Arkansas inmates without consent?[801] Some of the ivermectin pastes even carry the kind of microchips conspiracy theorists claim are in the vaccine.[802] Foiled by antifa again!

A faith strong enough to take some patients, denying their infections to the very end, through the shadow of the valley of death:

> CNN reporter just quoted a doctor as referring to many COVID patients as "the talking dead": they have lost so much lung function that they will die as soon as their life support is removed, but they are awake and able to discuss with their doctors.[803]

In getting one of the first citations from Trump's FDA for fraud, pastor Jim Bakker—a favorite target of video satirist Vic Berger—beat Anthony Fauci by a month in taking COVID seriously.[804] Bakker now wanders the land a fractal shade, a historical persona adapted in the millions, ghosting his friends in ways Phoebe Bridgers hadn't intended.

In April 2022, the Tennessee legislature passed a law making ivermectin available for treatment of COVID-19 without a prescription.[805]

THE CARTOON RIGHT AREN'T the only faith healers.

While Jamelle Bouie argued Republican pols are pushing policies that will continue the pandemic to Joe Biden's political misfortune,[806] and a doctor running for governor on Minnesota's Republican line called for "civil disobedience" against vaccines and masks,[807] the *New York Times* covered the present administration's failures in a guise of the usual difficulties of scientific investigation:

> Scientific understanding of the virus changes by the hour, it seems. The virus spreads only by close contact or on contaminated surfaces, then turns out to be airborne. The virus mutates slowly, but then emerges in a series of dangerous new forms. Americans don't need to wear masks. Wait, they do. . . .
>
> Americans are living with science as it unfolds in real time. The process has always been fluid, unpredictable. But rarely has it moved at this speed, leaving citizens to confront research findings as soon as they land at the front door, a stream of deliveries that no one ordered and no one wants.
>
> Living with a capricious enemy has been unsettling even for researchers, public health officials and journalists who are used to the mutable nature of science. They, too, have frequently agonized over the best way to keep themselves and their loved ones safe.[808]

The failure to get a handle on the outbreak isn't a matter of the provisional nature of science, but the concerted refusal to engage in the kind of public health campaigns many countries successfully undertook around the world before the vaccine.

But against all the evidence to the contrary, the *Times,* patting its readers on the head, insists otherwise:

The public disagreements and debates played out in public, instead of at obscure conferences, give the false impression that science is arbitrary or that scientists are making things up as they go along.

"What a non-scientist or the layperson doesn't realize is that there is a huge bolus of information and consensus that the two people who are arguing will agree upon," Dr. [Richard Sever, a co-founder of two preprint websites, bioRxiv and medRxiv,] said.[809]

Is it really so surprising, then, that Americans feel bewildered and bamboozled, even enraged, by rapidly changing rules that have profound implications for their lives?

Other countries also faced the tumult of science in real time. They chose to invest in the kind of public health response such uncertainty requires. The United States continues to choose differently.

What little contact tracing was pursued here in Minnesota has been largely abandoned, even now at a new COVID peak, with the Department of Health's statewide tracer team reduced from nearly 2,000 in December 2020 to 522 this September.[810] Last year, I used a Fitzhugh Mullan Institute for Health Workforce Equity calculator to estimate that at the time the Twin Cities alone needed 6,000 contact tracers to adequately track transmission chains.[811]

UNDETERRED BY THE PROOF of 700,000-plus dead Americans— the far majority put in the ground before a single vaccine was administered—neckbeard skeptics continue to rattle on about the supposed fallacies pharmaceutical companies are perpetrating. The companies are monetizing a harmless virus, skeptics claim.

Certainly the companies are guilty of profiting off a fictitious commodity. Health, like clean water, is part of the commons. It's not like a bag of potato chips. But that doesn't mean the COVID vaccines don't work or that the virus isn't real. In the footsteps of a long history on the left, one can both object to health profiteering and demand that the latest medical innovations be made available to all.[812]

Skeptics have lasered in on the differences between reductions in relative risk and absolute risk the vaccines represent. The skeptics repeatedly cite a commentary published earlier in the year in *The Lancet* underscoring the difference:

> Vaccine efficacy is generally reported as a relative risk reduction (RRR). It uses the relative risk (RR)—i.e., the ratio of attack rates with and without a vaccine—which is expressed as 1–RR. Ranking by reported efficacy gives relative risk reductions of 95% for the Pfizer–BioNTech, 94% for the Moderna–NIH, 91% for the Gamaleya, 67% for the J&J, and 67% for the AstraZeneca–Oxford vaccines.
>
> However, RRR should be seen against the background risk of being infected and becoming ill with COVID-19, which varies between populations and over time. Although the RRR considers only participants who could benefit from the vaccine, the absolute risk reduction (ARR), which is the difference between attack rates with and without a vaccine, considers the whole population. ARRs tend to be ignored because they give a much less impressive effect size than RRRs: 1·3% for the AstraZeneca–Oxford, 1·2% for the Moderna–NIH, 1·2% for the J&J, 0·93% for the Gamaleya, and 0·84% for the Pfizer–BioNTech vaccines.[813]

Absolute risk reduction and the number needed to be vaccinated to prevent one more COVID case (NNV) are dependent upon what's going on out there in the general population:

> ARR (and NNV) are sensitive to background risk—the higher the risk, the higher the effectiveness—as exemplified by the analyses of the J&J's vaccine on centrally confirmed cases compared with all cases: both the numerator and denominator change, RRR does not change (66–67%), but the one-third increase in attack rates in the unvaccinated group (from 1·8% to 2·4%) translates in a one-fourth decrease in NNV (from 84 to 64).

The skeptics have gone on to claim that the deaths prevented by the vaccines are by orders of magnitude outweighed by the (unsourced) deaths *caused* by the vaccine.

The authors of the *Lancet* commentary have publicly rejected the way the internet twisted their commentary:

> When asked [by Reuters] about the claim, [Piero] Olliaro, professor of poverty-related infectious diseases at the Centre for Tropical Medicine and Global Health of Oxford University, told Reuters via email it was "extremely disappointing to see how information can be twisted." He also said, "Bottom line: these vaccines are good public health interventions," and added that in the commentary, "We do not say vaccines do not work."[814]

The skeptics' argument depends on the low percentage of those infected who die from the disease. So, the absolute relative risk is by definition going to be low. The Reuters fact-check continues, quoting Meedan Health Desk:

> Let's say a study enrolled 20,000 patients into the control group and 20,000 in the vaccine group. In that study, 200 people in the control group got sick and 0 people in the vaccine group got sick. Even though the vaccine efficacy would be a whopping 100%, the ARR would show that vaccines reduce the absolute risk by just 1 percent (200/20,000=1 percent). For the ARR to increase to 20% in our example study with a vaccine with 100 percent efficacy, 4,000 of the 20,000 people in the control group would have to get sick (4,000/20,000=20%).[815]

In absolute terms, however, a small proportion of those killed by the virus out of a large number of unvaccinated is still a large number. Especially compared to the minuscule numbers of vaccinated killed by COVID.

As reported in the CDC's *Morbidity and Mortality Weekly Report,* we find the disparity reproduced in cases and hospitalizations in New York City as elsewhere:

> During May 3–July 25, a total of 9,664 new cases (1.31 per 100,000 person-days) occurred among fully vaccinated adults, compared with 42,507 (9.80 per 100,000 person-days) among unvaccinated adults. . . . A total of 1,285 new COVID-19 hospitalizations (0.17 per 100,000 person-days) occurred among fully vaccinated adults, compared with 7,288 (1.68 per 100,000 person-days) among unvaccinated adults.[816]

That all may change as the virus evolves. It has the room to evolve vaccine resistance in part because we haven't gotten enough people vaccinated around the world to drop the infection below its rate of replacement. A wince of an irony to which we will return.

ABROAD, CHINA'S OWN CONSPIRACY theorists launched what was clearly a redundant disinformation campaign. The United States appears dunning itself. Pushing back against all the evidence that COVID began in China, the Chinese government now claims the outbreak started at Fort Detrick in Maryland:

> Wang Wenbin, a Chinese Foreign Ministry spokesman, has used routine news briefings this week to air baseless speculation that the virus had emerged in the United States before the first cases were reported in China. He cited an outbreak of lung disease in July 2019 in Wisconsin that American health authorities have already connected to vaping, not Covid.
> On Wednesday, he said the W.H.O. should investigate labs in Fort Detrick and elsewhere in the United States that research coronaviruses.[817]

Trump's rap supporters included, famously, Kanye, but also Lil

Wayne, 50 Cent, 6ix9ine, Ice Cube, Lil Pump, Waka Flocka Flame, and Fivio Foreign, among others. China now deploys its own crews:

> Officials and state media have promoted a rap song by a patriotic Chinese hip-hop group that touted the same claim, with the lyrics: "How many plots came out of your labs? How many dead bodies hanging a tag?"[818]

In reality, both the United States and China are detracting from accumulating evidence that the New York–based EcoHealth Alliance and the Wuhan Institute of Virology together conducted gain-of-function studies on coronaviruses, even if those experiments may not have served as the origins of the outbreak.[819] Externalizing blame serves as an attempt to absolve a fifteen-year-long collaboration between the countries.

So, from ivermectin suppositories through Chinese rappers, we took the long way around to the possibility that disengaging from the ludicrous nature of the storytelling now firing out of both imperial ports may make more room in the way of understanding how we arrived at our COVID moment.

PHILOSOPHER SLAVOJ ŽIŽEK DESCRIBED our reaction to climate change in terms of the cycle of grief: denial, anger, bargaining, depression, and, not necessarily a good thing here, acceptance.[820]

U.S. COVID—and the imposition of its own epidemiological image upon the world—is proving more Oedipal. Our one-party state—which, as Julius Nyerere described, indulges in the typical American extravagance of two parties—is sacrificing its ostensible constituents upon one ICU bed at a time.

Characteristically, the Democrats are snatching defeat from the jaws of victory. Despite warnings that vaccine success was more circumstantial than intrinsic, the Biden White House ceased all other public health interventions the Trump administration never really began.

So intent on saving the day it is losing, liberals are foisting blame for the next COVID wave upon the unvaccinated they abandoned. Are the worst of Trumpist denialists out of their minds? Yes, as a cultural archetype, they are. But as commentator Yasmin Nair puts it, scientific illiteracy is widespread and represents a kind of failure of vaccine access.[821] Successful governance demands finding ways to administer to even those who presently reject intervention.

Public health is a shared commons. There is no alternative. No rugged individualism or monetized clinic visit is enough. Scaling up consistently competent governmental intervention neighborhood by neighborhood cures distrust. It's the kind of campaign the feds haven't practiced at such a scale for decades, save perhaps against smoking.

The institutional cognition to do so is long absent. And the impulse to start is aimed in the wrong direction. Quietly handing over another $25 billion to the Pentagon the other day—enough to pay for global vaccination instead and atop the DoD's record-breaking budget this past December—assures no such domestic campaign is even operationally possible were the impetus present.[822]

As conservative Bret Stephens's *New York Times* column in September typifies, the present failure, as much structural as a matter of daily administration, is reopening the electoral door for a party that not much more than half-a-year ago put half-a-million Americans in the ground and attacked the Capitol.[823]

The damage also blows back upon a putative strength—science itself.

Those Nerdy Girls are typical of liberal scientism.[824] They're a group of epidemiologists who are posting memes refuting denialist claims. It's good work that is also unable to assimilate the basics of a political economy reversing some of their page's basic assumptions.

I responded to their early September post on the CDC's pivot back to recommending masks for the vaccinated to that effect, including:

I appreciate the efforts this page is making to debunk denialist disinformation around COVID.

But its response to the CDC's sudden reversal from its ill-considered mask recommendations in May also situates the page as itself a purveyor of disinformation. . . .

Our present trajectories around masking and the vaccines were entirely expected outcomes. A full spectrum of public health practitioners, from nurse unions to deans of schools of public health, denounced the CDC's May recommendations in no uncertain terms (and offered evidence-based chapter and verse why).

In contrast, this page did not object. It largely offered a "scientific" rationale for the CDC's position, even as it joined the CDC in knowing full well that the Delta variant was on its way. Most epidemiological projections are at best provisional. Delta's arrival was not. . . .

The philosophically idealist scientism this page practices— a liberal magical thinking of science as justification enough whatever its recommendations—is apparently being wielded to protect this nicer set of perpetrators. After all, the page appears to assume loony Trumpists are our only alternative. . . .

I've taken to calling CDC-NIAID officials and many of their more public-facing university grantees "Imperial droids" or "R1-D2s." The latter are offering post-hoc technical support for every one of the administration's ill-thought pandemic policies however much these positions ping across contradictory stances.

Yes, circumstances change. Yes, new data emerge. Adapting our understanding is both necessary and laudable. This drunken dance in political epistemology is nothing of the sort. . . .

Little different from the Trump administration in this way, our Foucauldian claque is aiming to protect itself from blame by dumping it elsewhere. Shitting on people who haven't gotten vaccinated misses the point. As science writer Ed Yong described, the Biden administration, washing its hands of responsibility, went all-in on making vaccination a matter of individual choice. . . .

The U.S. is on the far side of its cycle of accumulation. Its bourgeoisie is cashing out, turning capital back into money and liquidating imperial infrastructure, including public health. The political class and its scientific cadre—conveniently unaware of their identities as historical subjects—are along for the ride, justifying every step in the abandonment of the commons.

Do the epidemiologists behind this page have the courage to refute their funders with the rigor they refute anti-vaxx wingnuts?[825]

A recent inspection showed my comments had been removed from the post.

OTHER SCIENTISTS HAVE TAKEN a different tack. Many of you may remember spatial disease ecologist Marius Gilbert, my colleague, who in the early days of the COVID outbreak became a TV star in Belgium, spending hours addressing questions from anchors and audiences alike.

After months of working closely with the government on, he admits, its uneven response, he bailed to return back to his lab. He also wrote a book about his experiences, from which all of us can draw understanding.[826]

Here's a link to a new interview.[827] Here are some excerpts Google-translated from the article and Gilbert's Twitter book announcement:

> **On researchers:** "In the end, our job was to do everything so that a pandemic did not start. Coming from China, Thailand, Vietnam, the United States, Italy, we met at conferences, workshops, field visits. It was the daily life that animated us and which still animates us."
> **Scientism:** "The error of political communication may have been to seek to use scientific argumentation to justify the choice of measures which combine science and politics."
> **Culture:** "By depriving us of social contact, the pandemic temporarily deprived us of a little of our humanity. And in a period dominated by fear, what better way to reconnect us, to escape,

to dream, than live shows? What a missed opportunity for the government not to have understood it!"

His anxieties: "Sometimes I have to cut myself, protect myself. I have outbursts of anxiety linked to the strong and intense exposure to this information and these images." Or again: "Yes, the epidemiologist in me is satisfied with the decisions that were inevitable. But the father, the brother, the friend, the companion, the son, the one who takes the measure of what is busy happening in his life, he who trembles with others in the face of an invisible threat, he is as helpless as those who listen to him."

His role: "I realize that the best thing I can do to contribute to the fight against this epidemic will be to help as many people as possible to understand what is happening. My role will be there. Give meaning to the measures, explain what you are trying to do, say what you know and be frank about what you do not know, confront everyone with the same dilemmas as those who have to make decisions, show how they are the result of difficult trade-offs between different options, none of which is without impact, that there is not a 'good solution' unambiguous and obvious to all."

What's next: "Finally, I am trying to develop some avenues for meeting the challenges of tomorrow: participatory democracy, diversification and debate on expertise, taking into account the systemic nature of crises and increasing openness of science to citizens."

The excerpts evoke Wolfram Eilenberger's insight on one of Walter Benjamin's early leaps:

Benjamin derived conclusions in his dissertation that would revolutionize not only his image of himself as a critic but also the way art criticism has understood itself since. First and foremost among these is the conclusion that the function of art criticism lies "not in judgment, but on the one hand [in] completion, consummation, systematicization."[828]

Gilbert appears on his own journey of mutual discovery with the virus to the benefit of us all.

"Are we a part of the experience we analyze?" is more than a matter of pop existentialism. From Plato's cave to Wittgenstein's closed window, to Turing's test developed cruising the bars of homophobic England, to Philip K. Dick's is-he-or-isn't-he Rick Deckard, and to MC Hammer himself, it's a long, if also in establishment science, deeply neglected pursuit.[829] While we in the United States are stuck with the likes of the utterly unselfconscious imperial droid FAUCi.

The rewards of Gilbert's personal suffering are borne back to the community he serves. Novelist Benjamín Labatut placed one wellspring of Erwin Schrödinger's wave function of quantum mechanics in a dream of a Hindu deity:

> In his nightmare, the goddess Kali would sit on his chest like an enormous beetle, crushing him so that he could not move. With her necklace of human heads, and brandishing swords, axes and knives in her many arms, she would bathe him in drops of blood that fell from the tip of her tongue and jets of milk from her swollen breasts, rubbing his groin until he was no longer capable of bearing the arousal, at which point she would decapitate him and swallow his genitals.
>
> Miss Herwig listened to him impassively and told him his dream was not a nightmare, but a blessing: of all the forms taken on by the female aspect of the divine, Kali was the most compassionate, because she granted *moksha*—liberation—to her children, and her love for them extended beyond all human comprehension.
>
> Her black skin, she said, was the symbol of the void that transcends all form, the cosmic uterus in which all phenomena gestated, while her necklace of skulls comprised the egos she had freed from the principal object of their identification, which was nothing less than the body itself. The castration Schrödinger suffered at the Dark Mother's hands was the greatest gift he could receive, a mutilation necessary so that his new consciousness could be born.[830]

A tightly wound Werner Heisenberg, meanwhile, stumbles into a fetid saloon and is forced by a hilarious composite of Benjamin, Charles Baudelaire, and Marcel Proust—the subconscious of the age—to imbibe a quaff of absinthe that happens to help Heisenberg hallucinate his uncertainty principle on his way home.

And you, scientist, who are you? Do you find inspiration in traditions other than the departmental retreat, corporate R&D, its labor discipline, and other neoliberal Vedas?

THE LATTER SCRIPTURES PRODUCE hallucinations no less frightening than Kali, perhaps more so as they are imprinted upon a landscape they also deny exists.

In *Dead Epidemiologists*, we described the construction of thirteen-storey hog hotels, with a thousand head per floor.[831] Now such hotels are being built into campuses. One such farm comprises twenty-one buildings that Muyuan Foods opened in September 2020.[832]

"In the race to take share," Reuters reports,

companies like Muyuan are designing higher-density automated farms, betting they can keep disease out while increasing efficiency to satisfy the country's huge appetite for pork.

Muyuan's new mega farm near Nanyang, which will eventually house 84,000 sows and their offspring, is by far the largest in the world, roughly 10 times the size of a typical breeding facility in the United States. It aims to produce around 2.1 million pigs a year. . . .

"We will employ fewer people and use more technology," [Qin Jun, Muyuan's vice general manager] said, pointing to "intelligent" feeding systems, manure cleaning robots, and infrared cameras to detect when pigs have a fever.

High-rise facilities are increasingly popular in China amid a scarcity of suitable land. Though corporate producers have an edge in winning land deals with local governments thanks to their clout and promises to create jobs by building slaughterhouses too, Muyuan recently attracted controversy for planning 55 pig farms on 1,000 hectares of Henan's cropland.[833]

It's hilarious the way Muyuan's American competitors pushed back:

"Large farrow-to-finish projects with high animal density are a long-term concern because once a pathogen enters, it's very difficult to control or eliminate," said Gordon Spronk, chairman of Pipestone Holdings, a Minnesota-based pig producer and veterinary services company.[834]

Pipestone's own critics in Minnesota and the Dakotas have said the same about the operations from which the company draws its own hog.[835]

More recently, Pipestone set up Wholestone, a new consortium of conventional hog farmers from Minnesota and South Dakota. From Hormel, one of the world's largest meat companies, also based in Minnesota, Wholestone bought an industrially sized processing plant in Fremont, Nebraska.[836]

Wholestone declares it aims to capture a greater proportion of hog commodity value for source producers. That sounds righteous, but, as Land O'Lakes and Crystal Sugar already show, economies of scale pursued by corporatized cooperatives across supply lines of hundreds of miles can still reproduce the damage privately held firms impose.[837] Even now, under the guise of "sustainable intensification" and "eco-efficiencies."[838]

Back in Nanyang, the nuclear plant mid-horizon beyond the hog campus is a *Simpsons* touch. Sidestepping facile equivalences, China and the United States appear metamodernisms in the mirror, both, as Bridgers sings again, with country-first rap songs and slaughterhouses and outlet malls and a fear of God.[839]

ALL TO CONSIDERABLE EPIDEMIOLOGICAL damage. The rate of new disease emergence picked up through the turn-of-the-century across outbreaks, kinds of disease, host type, pathogen taxonomy, and transmission mode, all with the neoliberal turn in agriculture worldwide.[840]

The socioecology of disease emergence folds together with the pathogens' evolutionary mechanics.

Interdemic selection—natural selection across populations adding hundreds of thousands of new infections a day—embodies parallel computing extraordinaire.[841] Pathogen solutions to our prophylaxes are swiftly arrived upon.

Now add a RNA virus, even one with a replication spellchecker, and we increase the speed of the pathogen computer at which it solves our vaccine equations. Indeed, so fast, I argued in *Big Farms,* that solutions to vaccines not even deployed yet are daily evolved upon.[842] As if reversing cause and effect!

Next, add vaccines that appear on their way to letting SARS-2 transmit at times as well across the population as between the unvaccinated.

Finally, add Bill Gates's hold on COVAX—the WHO's effort to distribute vaccines globally and cheaply—placing intellectual property rights before speedy distribution. By that intervention, we've already dropped out of the race between herd immunity and vaccine escape, leaving SARS-2 the field.

Instead, as I described in my previous Patreon piece, we've settled on a different (and more lucrative) drag race between variants and booster shots for the few: "What the variants win from a host system intent upon profitably denying itself herd immunity, the industry wins from the variants' proliferation."[843]

I quoted Matt Stoller: "The current price for a Covid vaccine, [Pfizer CEO Frank] D'Amelio noted, is $19.50 per dose. He told analysts of his hope Pfizer could get to a more normal price, '$150, $175 per dose,' instead of what he called 'pandemic pricing.'"[844]

The resulting calculation appears nigh on mechanistic, with a clanking much like the rotors of Turing's machine breaking the Nazi Enigma cipher.[845] CNN reports:

An analysis by British academics, published by the UK Government's official scientific advisory group, says that they believe it is "almost certain" that a SARS-Cov-2 variant will emerge that "leads to current vaccine failure." SARS-CoV-2 is the virus that causes Covid-19. . . .

The scientists write that because eradication of the virus is "unlikely," they have "high confidence" that variants will continue to emerge. They say it is "almost certain" that there will be "a gradual or punctuated accumulation of antigenic variation that eventually leads to current vaccine failure." . . .

In minutes from its July 7 meeting, SAGE scientists wrote that "the combination of high prevalence and high levels of vaccination creates the conditions in which an immune escape variant is most likely to emerge." It said at the time that "the likelihood of this happening is unknown, but such a variant would present a significant risk both in the UK and internationally."[846]

EVENTUAL VACCINE FAILURE APPEARS algorithmic beyond the virus representing a difficult biomolecular problem. Why?

A month ago, I participated in the *Review of African Political Economy*'s webinar on vaccine imperialism.[847] Three take-home points:

1) I provocatively proposed that the World Health Organization's objectives had little to do with stopping the COVID-19 pandemic. For if that weren't the case, WHO, now complaining that 80 percent of 5.5 billion vaccine shots were administered in the Global North, would never have switched out the open medicine model of sharing any and all SARS-2 knowledge and antivirals with which it began the pandemic for Bill Gates's Covid-19 ACT-Accelerator.[848]

The Accelerator, premised on protecting pharmaceutical intellectual property rights first, now serves as the underlying model for the COVAX program aimed at supplying 20 percent of the populations of low-income countries with discounted vaccine. That effort largely has failed, and NATO countries and the companies have fallen back on bilateral deals, with the companies setting their own prices, prioritizing wealthier countries, and inhibiting licensing.

In other words, what should have been a race between the pathogen and a humanity aimed at vaccinating the world before vaccine escape set in was replaced by a race between the pathogen and booster shots for a fusillade of variants only a few countries can afford. Despite involving the pathogen, vaccines, and people the world over, the two races are categorically different. The first would have made a real run at driving SARS-2 to extirpation. The second places profits (and the pathogen) before people.

I concluded that the variants and pharmaceutical industry together prosper from a model that *chose* to turn vaccines into a scarcity economy.

2) Marlise Richter of the Health Justice Initiative in South Africa detailed the resulting vaccine gap in Africa.[849] Her slides tracked many of the key specifics:

- Even with many of the countries of the Global North struggling to meet their vaccine goals, Africa clearly represents a vaccine donut hole.
- The few vaccines that have found their place in Africa represent minuscule proportions of the total population. Morocco, doing better than most African countries, has vaccinated only a third of its population. Africa overall has administered two-thirds of its available supply, fully vaccinating less than 2 percent of its total population.
- With its present supply, South Africa will be able to vaccinate 67 percent of its population only by 2023.
- One Health Justice Initiative chart showed the commitments companies made to South Africa and what they delivered. The U.S. government and Pfizer delivered on its 5 million doses, as did Johnson & Johnson, through the Sisonke Program, inoculating frontline health workers.[850] But direct deliveries of 30 million-plus doses remain largely unfilled.

- As of June, against widespread support from governments around the world, the EU, Australia, Israel, Malaysia, and Costa Rica opposed waiving WTO TRIPS protections for COVID drugs and vaccines. The United States uncharacteristically appeared in favor of the waiver.
- Richter's next diagram showed huge gaps between the vaccines countries of the Global North purchased above and beyond their population sizes and the huge deficits between population and vaccines in Africa.

Fully acknowledging the terrible moment, Richter did draw comfort from a political lay of the land that was not unprecedented. In the short term, a path to victory could follow the program of global grassroots efforts against the WTO's Trade-Related Aspects of Intellectual Property Rights, which, until enough pressure was brought to bear, permitted pharmaceutical companies to fend off the production of anti-HIV generics.

Certainly leftists of the Global North must make supporting such an effort against TRIPS a major part of any COVID opposition. Pharmaceutical multinationals and home governments need to be inundated with demands and disobedience that punish them for their murderous program.

As an audience member noted, the long term would have to be marked by a broader redirection in global political economy. We simply cannot afford to leave the world epidemiological stage to—my words—expropriative sociopaths.

3) Tetteh Hormeku-Ajei of the Third World Network-Africa, based in Ghana, sketched out the contribution Africa could make to the path out.[851] He described growing momentum toward working with, and following in the footsteps of, Cuba in founding domestic vaccine production. Hormeku-Ajei made the explicit distinction between domestic and "local" production, with the latter little else but satellites beholden to knowledge and supply lines controlled by multinational headquarters abroad.

Hormeku-Ajei's model harks back to Samir Amin's notion of delinking, whereby the Global South begins to unplug itself out of the colonial economy.[852] This present Gates moment, arguably fouler than partying with Jeffrey Epstein, underscores the point that countries outside NATO must strike out on their own to produce their own antivirals in shorter order, if for the very lives of their own people.[853]

Beyond the present COVID crisis, other pandemics are assuredly to follow, and pivoting from dependence and domination to decolonization and developmental convergence will protect us all. Keeping much of the world unvaccinated endangers even those presently vaccinated.

That's why punching down on individual Trumpists refusing the vaccine misses much of the plot line.

YES, THINKING GLOBALLY, September 14 marked the 154th year of the publication of Karl Marx's *Capital I*. It isn't the fossilized dreck an exhausted race of academics claim. It is an extraordinary book (including Marx's own copy on which he added notes incorporated in the 1872 edition).[854]

Along with helping us get a handle on the rudimentary natures of capitalism—as opposed to its boosterist depictions elsewhere—the book, its second half, one short page-turner of a chapter after another, also offers a history of capitalism that would make any Howard Zinn green with envy.

For instance, in two paragraphs in chapter 29, Marx places the genesis of capitalism on English agricultural middlemen who by the middle of the fourteenth century served as administrative mediators between peasants and feudal landlords. Bailiffs and sharecroppers who employed wage-laborers began to parlay their outputs from ground rent to surplus value they controlled. And while the rents owed to landlords depreciated across their 99-year leases, demand inflated food prices.

The resulting surpluses transformed the new farmers' political power, which in turn drove the expropriation of the commons and subsequent rounds of accumulation: "Thus [the farmer] grew rich at the expense of both his labourers and landlords."

Or take this passage from chapter 27, a short eighteen-page history of serial primitive accumulation in Britain, prefiguring indigent pluriactivity in the Global South and NGO-led expropriation in the name of saving the environment:

> By 1825 the 15,000 Gaels had already been replaced by 131,000 sheep. The remnant of the original inhabitants, who had been flung onto the sea-shore, tried to live by catching fish. They became amphibious, and lived, as an English writer says, half on land and half on water, and withal only half on both. But the splendid Gaels had now to suffer still more bitterly for their romantic mountain idolization of the "great men" of the clan. The smell of their fish rose to the noses of the great men. They scented some profit in it, and let the sea-shore to the big London fishmongers. For the second time the Gaels were driven out.

Timothy Morton, the dark ecologist of a philosopher, complained about the MATTs—those who declare Marx Already Thought That.[855]

Agreed, capitalism continues to permutate into new orders, including, maybe, as McKenzie Wark provocatively argues, unto something worse than its own death.[856] So, yes, new characterizations are always both necessary and appreciated, even as writer Reuben Dendinger concludes Wark can't stick to her own anti-communist thesis, which, Dendinger continues, is also debunked by the work of the likes of sociologist Intan Suwandi.[857]

But anyone in agriculture and environment reading through these pages—whatever their political inclinations—will be taken by Marx's capacity to clearly explain the ways by which the precepts of our modern and officially elevated smash-and-grabs arose out of a contingent history.

Against the claims of the powerful, such primitive accumulation and its financialized abstraction since are not the natural order of things or our very species-being.

There's always been another humanity steeped in kindness and acuity. And even now, out there already walking among us, a better world offers us its arm. Do we have the wherewithal to take it for the grand adventure it proposes?

OTHER PATHWAYS ARE LESS grand. An unvaccinated friend posted a misguided if erudite defense of the rights of the unvaccinated.[858]

One should raise an eyebrow at comparisons, whatever their superficial verve, of vaccination campaigns and ancient human sacrifice or the Rwandan genocide. Alex Jones in Giorgio Agamben dress-up, a comparison unbeknownst to me which Benjamin Bratton also converged upon, albeit served with an overreach of a smear against radical Romanticism that the record does not support.[859]

The posted piece went on to place any incipient vaccine escape on the head of the vaccinated, as if other deadly variants, nasty Delta included, didn't already evolve when we were all unvaccinated. Or as if the death cult wasn't in part actualizing itself: *Ninety-nine* percent of those Americans killed by COVID in June were unvaccinated.[860] Are the vaccinated to blame for those proportions?

Yes, the vaccines increasingly appear to offer little in the way of sterilizing immunity—the vaccinated can infect others. But a full-spectrum campaign—vaccination plus masking; testing, tracing, and isolation; rent and utilities moratoriums; and community health visits other countries pursue as a matter of course—would drive down the pathogen population. Many of the anti-vaxers, however, *also* object to all those other interventions.

It's an old story. When there's an outbreak, it's argued we don't need vaccines. When we don't have an outbreak, we don't need vaccines either. Anti-vaxers make this stuff up as they go along. "Doing their own research" is a Gish gallop through disinformation cascades ranging from Children's Health Defense to Fox News amplified by social media algorithms. It couldn't be clearer what McLuhan meant about the medium and the message.

In the 2010s, those seeking exemptions on measles vaccination—

from natural health types to orthodox religiosos—claimed that they didn't need the vaccine because infectious diseases such as measles were virtually eliminated.

But the epidemiological state of things isn't categorical. For measles and COVID alike, it was, and remains, circumstantial. As the outbreaks that followed in France and the West Coast indicated, measles was locally extirpated *because* of the vaccines.[861] Once enough people refused vaccination, pop-up outbreaks were inevitable.

Freedom, a loaded concept stateside, may reach beyond other people's hurt feelings, but does not supersede the damage of the deadlier rapid contagions. Philosopher Donatella Di Cesare places such a *noli me tangere* ("do not touch me") formula as at best a "negative conception of liberty" that "confuses guarantees with liberty" and "does not reach the places where the losers of globalization live."[862]

She later pivots to finding the "muns" in "immunity" and "municipality," falling, however, on the side of immunity—severing off undesirables or diseased—as an opposition to the community (which is by definition "constitutively open"). It's a dichotomy too far, I think, as public health should be pursued to such a degree, and humane care, as to permit the town square to reopen.

But even so, nearly nothing of the present denialism is a matter of principle, save, perhaps, expediency. Many of the present refuseniks took all their compulsory vaccines to go to school (and by dint of those are alive long enough to refuse this vaccine). Many put on their seat belts instinctively without a second thought to body autonomy or the Constitution. Another friend proposed that putting on headlights is a better metaphor given the danger to others involved in refusing to do so.

Those who have been cheering this pillory so far may be missing the point, however. Yes, COVID denialism and vaccine refusal aren't blows against the system anti-vaxers think they are. They're *symptoms* of a system that over the past forty years abandoned public health as concept and practice, spinning off health as a matter of monetizable choice. Structures of thought, all the way to their carnivalistic margins, bubble out of the financial base and its power struggles (and back again).

So, in the other direction, scorning the unvaccinated, as the Biden administration spearheaded as a response, is only a recapitulation of an individualized public health that is a contradiction in terms.

Social pressure, from family and friends, and concerted public health campaigns door-to-door to convince holdouts are reasonable responses. They're not the mob rule that the vaccine refuseniks claim. At the same time, verbally bludgeoning the unvaccinated is as much a reflex of that slumping system as that awful anti-vax rally at New York's City Hall in August. It's a reactionary response that escalated last week on multiple fronts:

- Reversing its ill-thought mask recommendations in May letting the vaccinated—and effectively everyone else—forgo masks, the CDC now has failed to push for universal masking despite its own reports describing such practices to be "essential."[863]
- In early August, congressional Democrats slashed back a $30 billion infusion of pandemic preparedness funds slated in the $3.5 trillion infrastructure bill.[864] The money was to restock medical and mask stockpiles and proactively develop vaccines. A limited notion of public health, but a step forward nonetheless.
- The bill's failure continued what a 2018 Trust for America's Health report documented was the long decline of such funding.[865] CDC's budget then was $7.15 billion, which, adjusting for inflation, was flat for the previous decade despite increasing threats: weather disasters, flooding, wildfires, extreme drought, hurricanes, infectious disease outbreaks, and deaths of despair. The latter emerge out of racial disparities, opioids, and the regional disparities that both cost Hillary Clinton the 2016 election and continue to drive governmental distrust.
- The Democratic-led government of Illinois privatized its vaccination verification system in such a way as to punish the poor: "The state is using Experian, a credit reporting company, to handle identity verification, and residents who have frozen their credit reports though Experian will have to unfreeze them, then wait 24 hours, to access the vaccination records."[866]

- *The Atlantic's* science writer Ed Yong argued against a Zero COVID campaign aimed at driving COVID to extirpation, which the United States never bothered starting.[867] It seems our Kantian duty is to avoid trying what we don't wish to do. Yong argued against such an effort—already nineteen months late—as the kind of *real épidémiologie* many a liberal in power embraces, waving the white flag on any progressive notion that threatens business as usual. Turns out anti-vaxers aren't the only ones who object to a full-spectrum intervention.

- Those Nerdy Girls, fighting anti-vax disinformation on Instagram, continue to pretend the CDC doesn't make mistakes, broadcasting every one of the agency's wayward policy pivots as if it were the plan all along.[868] The establishment epidemiologists behind the account earnestly argue the scientific rationale for every contradictory CDC position without a whit of self-consciousness.

- Mike Osterholm, the disease expert of choice here in Minnesota, pursues the same. Days after public health faculty here published an op-ed objecting to the University of Minnesota's refusal to mandate vaccination, Osterholm, advising both the UM and Biden administrations, co-authored a counterpoint arguing against the mandate.[869] A month later, Osterholm was suddenly quoted in the establishment *Star-Tribune* in favor of the mandate the university is now pursuing, without any allusion to his role in initially blocking the effort.[870] The dithering, now a national sport, left thousands of students who needed a month between shots in the lurch with the semester soon starting.

  Changing our minds on policy isn't anything to be ashamed about. It's choosing the clearly wrong one as a matter of political expediency that's deplorable. The dearth of principle is the order of the day—pro- and anti-vax. Indeed, the earlier Osterholm used one of my lines to the effect that epidemiology is a matter of trust (and so, he argued, vaccines shouldn't be mandated).[871] But conflating earning trust and pandering is a telling proposition.

- Perhaps the most shocking realization for some is that letting the unvaccinated die appeared an implicit part of the Biden COVID plan.[872] That's no less a genocidal impulse than Trump's negligent massacre, killing half-a-million Americans. Two hundred thousand Americans have since been killed, with one September week accumulating a *million* new cases, a rate now back in decline.[873]

The presumption that death is message enough misses the depths to which American despair has plumbed. Some of those now dying—or at the very least their family members—might undergo a change of heart, but nurses report many patients are in denial right to the end, a marker of the sociopathic individualism the Biden administration helped cultivate.[874] If the dead do speak beyond the fallacy of silent evidence, they say a lot of things other than that maybe I was wrong.

Others are finding a spite-your-face glory in a lost cause that sociologists identified even before the outbreak: Better to deny health care for all in favor of a spreading *Bittereinderism*.[875] The Afghans falling off those last C-17 jets out of Kabul aren't the only beatific suicides at empire's end.

The other side of anti-vaxers who refuse vaccines to which people the world over wish they had access are the liberals berating vaccine skepticism who won't roll back intellectual property rights to share the vaccines they champion. Bill Gates's Covid-19 ACT-Accelerator turned the WHO's initial model of open medicine to a proprietary system *designed* to deny access to those worldwide who can't pay.[876] To SARS-2's cladogenetic glee.

That is, COVID denialism extends to refusing to grasp that the lazy, sloppy, and chronically cruel nature of the U.S. response to the pandemic is a structural problem extending out of capitalist realism and the two political parties that service it.

A FARMER DOWN SOUTH I know, able to speak to hog and turkey, shared that she doesn't understand Minnesotans. If I finally learned anything in my time here, it was the locals' jouissance, their existential delight and power, in refusing direct communication.

I speak of white Minnesotans, who, with Somalis I've spotted sharing uproarious sake along with their off-duty Japanese waiters on Franklin Avenue, are no longer one and the same. It took me a decade, the swarthy and gesticulating New Yorker, to learn I wouldn't ever pass either.

The doomed Oklahoman John Berryman, who taught poetry at the University of Minnesota, didn't have a chance: "He died in 1972, by jumping from the Washington Avenue Bridge in Minneapolis," Anthony Lane writes. "To the appalled gratification of posterity, his fall was witnessed by somebody named Art Hitman."[877] Prince, claimed by the city lords only upon his success, overdosed alone in his capacious mansion a few miles away.

In contrast, at the pandemic's start, the tightly closed-off inner circles in the music scene here shocked themselves with the extent to which they circled-within-circles their wagons around what proved their favorite hometown sexual abusers.[878] Weirdo Berryman, undeniably a racist, tried something different, writing of giving birth in Anne Bradstreet's seventeenth-century voice: "drencht & powerful" in the "unforbidding Majesty"![879]

Or better yet, there's the utterly un-Minnesotan illiberality—the anti-missionary position—of the recently passed Diane di Prima:

> a few of us tried it, we tried to stop it with printing / we tried to protect you with mimeograph machines / green posters LUMUMBA LIVES flooded Harlem in those days / well, the best thing to do with a mimeograph is to drop it / from a five story window, on a head of a cop.[880]

Perhaps on one of the several officers here in Minneapolis recorded "hunting" protesters a few days after four of their own killed George Floyd.[881]

we buy the arms and the armed men,

Di Prima continues,

we have placed them / on all the thrones of South America / we are burning the jungles, the beasts will rise up against us / even now those small jungle people with black eyes / look calmly at us out of their photographs / and it is their calm that will finish us, it is the calm / of the earth itself.[882]

That's 1966, a half-century before the Institute on the Environment here at the University of Minnesota, without a speck of shame, took money from a Cargill company that cuts into an Amazonia the Institute maps to protect, leaving in its bulldozers' fumes a trail of assassinated Indigenous leaders.[883]

Jim Crow North, routinely patting itself on its humble back, is one vile mascot.

HERE'S BIOTECH CONSULTANT Dale Harrison's summary of a recent Dutch paper encapsulating what offers better protection to COVID: natural infection or vaccine or both?[884]

Long story short, by way of the Dutch paper and Harrison's commentary:

1. You have to get really ill—like hospitalization ill—for a natural infection to produce the immunological oomph for adequate protection in the next exposure. A vaccine inoculation produces that oomph (without the hospitalization). An infection *and* vaccine is best.
2. The new variants are escaping both vaccine and the protection produced in fighting off earlier variants. So, the immune memory of my no-hospital March 2020 infection would likely be useless on its own at this point.
3. It isn't the antibody titers produced that many studies record that matters, but *which* antibodies produced against *which* variants in the body. It's about what neutralizes the virus.
4. Most of the antibodies produced in a natural infection—producing a greater scope of attack than just a vaccine—are likely useless

because they don't target what's exposed in an active virion.

5. With the infectivities involved, we're all likely to be hit by COVID multiple times.

6. And the size of SARS-2's genome will likely lead to a rise of auto-immune diseases whereby our immune system attacks protein presentations our bodies share with the virus if only by chance.

You should read through the comments under Harrison's post for more commentary, including the structural epistemology involved:

• what counts as rigorous molecular science
• the different confounders built into population surveys vs. molecular studies
• the way SARS-2 is evolving ahead of even our sped-up research output

DOCTORS COMPLAINING THAT INJURIES from the milk crate craze are adding to the burdens of ERs hammered by COVID are punching down to displace an existential impotence.[885]

Docs (and nurses and other health professionals) are certainly bearing the brunt of an abandonment of the now passé policy of flattening the curve. As well as the very notion of public health. But they'd do better than blaming the Black joy found in a backyard game of walking up and over a wobbly pyramid of milk crates.

Why not organize resistance to a Biden-led death drive opening up everything at the start of a wave of a more infectious COVID variant we knew was emerging out of India months ago?

Why not blame Governor Tim Walz here in Minnesota for letting the officially sanctioned joy of the State Fair go on unvaccinated and without masks?[886] As one mailed-in seed art entry at the Fair put it: "The Great MN Superspreader: COVID on a Stick. See You at the ICU." Subsequent surveillance showed a small but demonstrable Fair-associated bump in COVID cases.[887] Minnesota COVID hospitalizations are presently matching last winter's terrible peak.[888]

When the Walzes of the world take a Tory line that we'll have to live with COVID here on out—with evictions starting up again to place people back into unsafe COVID exposure—they've long stepped beyond the lesson of limits the crates teach us.[889]

OTHER STUNTS DESERVE CENSURE. It's unfortunate I received the series of screenshots secondhand, as left business observer Doug Henwood unfriended me a couple years ago when I pushed back against his juvenile ecomodernism.

The posts in the shots are a form of climate denialism. By their arguments, worry over our present environmental circumstances—documented increases in extinction rates and such—is just symptomatic of a fundamentalist catastrophism.[890] Efforts to heal the metabolic rifts between human civilization and the ecological substrate upon which we necessarily depend are presented as no more than Malthusian ecoprimitivism.[891]

Here, hiding behind a scarecrow Marx of their own making, Henwood and his gang, attacking ag writer Wendell Berry, mock farmers and peasants as "rural idiocy."[892]

Three immediate reactions:

The first is visceral. There's the irony in Berry's lifetime effort making sure these gourmands are supplied the *petits goûts* they celebrate—I kid you not—in repeated posts and food selfies. Where do they think ingredients come from? How are these commodities produced? Who labors to grow them? Out of what soil and waters do these emerge? The unselfconsciousness is tellingly indulgent.

Second, I may be no Marxologist, but the Moor wrote sympathetically of peasants from the get-go, from "Thefts of Wood" through *German Ideology, Grundrisse,* the second half of *Capital I,* all the way to the "Critique of the Gotha Program" and *Capital III.*[893] From the Neolithic to the modern era. Even the urbanite Engels argued that the Deutscher Landarbeiter-Verband should have organized East Elbian agricultural workers across Prussian commercial estates.

Indeed, sociologist John Bellamy Foster showed Marx effectively originated what would become critical agrarian studies, writing on the now common notion of shifts in food regime, the metabolic rifts in capital-led agriculture, the resulting nutrition budgets by occupation, the effects of commodification (and class structure) on oft-poisonous food alteration, and intensified husbandry's impact in both driving out rural populations and reducing locally available food for the urban underclass.[894]

Kristin Ross traces how Marx—what Foster and Kohei Saito document was an ecological Marx—drew from his readings of, and conversations with, Elisabeth Dmitrieff, Nikolay Chernyshevsky, and Vera Zasulich on agriculture to arrive upon the notion there were multiple paths to socialism.[895] Historian Eric Hobsbawm was scathing on the matter: "No misinterpretation of Marx is more grotesque than the one that suggests that he expected a revolution exclusively from the advanced industrial countries of the West."[896]

Third, denigrating rural communities, huh. And, as agrarian sociologist Max Ajl describes, this ilk has an inside track on the various politicos, publishers, and their staff spearheading the push for a Green New Deal.[897] I would advise anyone associated with those efforts to keep an arm's length from these not-so-useful idiots, who have positioned themselves to the right of General Mills. If only for the GND's sake.

SUCH SINS OF COMMISSION are complemented by sins of omission. Pulitzer Prize–winning Ed Yong posted another think piece in *The Atlantic,* this one on the near certainty other pandemics are on their way.[898] Yong declares the United States unprepared. In many ways, it's as good an article as establishment America can produce.

But as City University of New York anthropologist Marc Edelman noted on Twitter:

Why, in this otherwise excellent article, is there no mention of industrial poultry and hog farms, where zoonotic diseases fester and potentially jump to humans? Without restructuring industrial ag, new pandemics are inevitable.[899]

Absolutely. I think, however, the problem is much more fundamental than the eerie of a missing topic. The superstructure of neoliberalism's swoon—here, the COVID failure across administrations—is confused for its base (however much both are interrelated). There's little grasp of the way the collapse of what smidge of public health was pursued post–Second World War is woven into the cycle of accumulation, with the 1946-founded CDC in effect a Bretton Woods institution aimed at cleaning up the U.S. world system of its own damage.[900] The failure of the American political class to deal with the present pestilence even on its own shores is at this point, as geographer Eric Sheppard describes, nigh on deterministic.[901]

Yong's complaints about the state of the American pandemic response are more sophisticated than the *New York Times*'s twist, which bent Biden's Trumpian disregard for science into good intentions gone awry: "Biden Vowed to Follow the Science. But Sometimes He Gets Ahead of Experts."[902] Or the *Star-Tribune* editorial board's notion of a bad day out in the field: "Biden's unforced COVID miscues."[903] But Yong, channeling Jeff Daniels's *Newsroom* monologue beat for beat, still can't reach beyond getting the liberal empire back on track.[904]

It's as if American political economy, across its albeit limited spectrum, is the Phineas Gage of the world, stumbling around inside a compulsive persona it can't recognize with a piece of its brain missing.

The lost institutional cognition appears much the case for what passes here as the left: from ecomodernists to the libertarians play-acting Marxists who subtweeted angrily at my appearance on Rania Khalek's show.[905] I had the temerity to suggest that people the world over should be given free access to the latest medical innovation—specifically, COVID vaccines—in the face of Bill Gates's efforts to deny them in favor of pharmaceutical companies' intellectual property rights.

Clearly that makes me a tool of the companies. I mean, who cares that the overwhelming proportion of COVID deaths were found summer 2021 in the unvaccinated? Freedom! And so on, the herd of tweets sprinting off into the discursive horizon.

If I haven't posted much on COVID lately on social media, it isn't just that I'm under deadline for several projects. The derangement syndrome on display is so astonishing that I dash past these Weimarian grotesques to get a few more things done before it all collapses. It's like religiously posting a series of *Times* and *Guardian* articles from a university bunker won't be counterattack enough.

Yes, there are these hideously loyal oppositions the world over. But millions elsewhere also grasp that the history of capitalist development and other structural processes are driving our COVID moment—from South America to South Los Angeles.[906] That army isn't just a source of hope. It's an indictment of the American archetype that, however brilliant, however left, insists on failing to assimilate what the rest of the world already knows.

Earlier I posted a link to a preprint by a team led by disease ecologist Luis Chaves and geographer Luke Bergmann that applied theories of underdevelopment from the likes of Milton Santos and Samir Amin to analyzing COVID outcomes in the Global South.[907]

Among other results, the team maps out two cluster analyses across Mesoamerica and the Caribbean. The color of the upweave across its map of the region differentiates country clusters by epidemiological variables such as exponential COVID growth rate, rate of COVID deceleration, COVID cases n days after detection of first case, and number of mitigation policies in place before and after the first case was detected, among other factors.

The color of the downweave on the map marks country clusters differentiated by variables of uneven development, including the human development index, the WHO Universal Health Coverage index, foreign direct investment, and a concentration of exports index.

The team found that trade openness increased COVID cases and deaths. The number of international cities connected at main airports increased COVID growth rates, cases, and deaths. Increases in concentration of imports, a marker of uneven development, correlated with increases in early epidemic growth and deaths.

The paper suggests that stopping the next pandemic or climate change might have something to do with our very mode of social reproduction rather than just failures in political persona or jostling on the Hill or resetting America to pre-Reagan, as Yong suggested. That might be worth talking through even if, or rather because, our best and brightest are sociopolitically committed to their epistemological seizures. Like a tamping iron blasted through their skull. And as if the way the hat doesn't fit now is the problem.

In early October, human geographer Fábio Pitta of the University of São Paulo and I joined the Fórum Popular da Natureza for just such a conversation.[908] Other such discussions elsewhere are ongoing. There's a whole world beyond Beltway banter.

REBUKES ARE ARRIVING HERE at home along other spectra. The emerald ash borer—an insect whose larvae eat through ash trees of the *Fraxinus* genus to the trees' death—arrived in Minnesota in 2009.[909] With fewer cold days to staunch larvae, there is a climate component to the borer's arrival.[910]

Insecticidal treatment can slow infestation, but structured removal, removing whole stands of the tree, appears the sole barrier to subsequent spread.[911]

The city of St Paul removed several blocks of ash trees along a street not far from my house. A University of Minnesota report explored the means by which to best converse with the public about such damage in terms far ahead of anything I've seen discussed and enacted around COVID.[912]

Yes, there are the economic impacts upon property values and the loss of canopy cooling. But the report goes further:

> Surprisingly, while scientists, resource managers, and some interested groups with a particular interest in conservation and the environment are very attuned to the potential ecological impact of EAB's continuing spread, many other interested groups and most of the members of the public focus groups barely mentioned the impacts on ash trees as a population, their associated species and habitats, or the water table.

Less referenced [is] the cultural importance of ash to American Indian communities; we did not get data about this one way or another, but the Minnesota EAB management plan (2006) suggests that collection of ash from native forests is not considered a vital part of acquiring the requisite materials by people practicing the craft.

For me, I found myself a walking wound at such a loss, suffering through a neighborhood version of the cycle of environmental grief Žižek identified.

The neighbors are trying their best to build gardens great and small around the stumps, eventually to be replaced with a wider diversity of new trees. There is the kinesthesia of dressing up a phantom limb about them. Neighbor and tree alike.

There are too the decades of tree loss poorer neighborhoods have suffered north of University Avenue. Killed by the redlining borer infesting City Hall downtown.[913]

And, again, by Jim Crow North from all points of the compass nearby. Under the Fox News report of local efforts to plant trees in Black neighborhoods, viewers commented:

> **Thundering Applause:** NEXT they will demand you rake the leaves and prune them.
> **LikeTalkingTo aWall:** If I was a tree . . . I WOULD LEAVE THE AREA nome sayin homies?
> **Mike Nelson:** I've also heard trees have been targeting minority housing when uprooting and falling over in severe weather. So not sure this tree planting equity initiative will really achieve overall arboreal justice.
> **Brown Green:** Why didn't people living there plant trees themselves? That's what the rest of us do.[914]

COVID APPEARS TO HAVE transformed into a serendipitous bio-economic weapon in a global hybrid war on the very notion of the commons. "Why didn't people living there plant trees themselves?"

In the first year of the pandemic, countries as different as Uruguay, Vietnam, and, famously, New Zealand engaged in the full-spectrum interventions that controlled their outbreaks.[915] Testing, tracing, and isolation—the Tetris program—along with timed shelter-in-place orders, state wage support, and eviction moratoriums permitted countries to ride out the worst of the pandemic even before the vaccine arrived.

All three countries, among many others, have since lapsed in the face of the evolution of the more infectious Delta variant and other new variants that were allowed to circulate and evolve in countries that refused to engage public health interventions in the name of protecting the capitalist economy.

Populations in many of the countries that had acted in good faith, including now New Zealand, have grown exhausted from the lockdowns.[916] Perhaps by its initial success, but also because of its place in Global North economics, New Zealand finds itself at the back-of-the-line in the affluent vaccine market as well. Economic elites elsewhere—in Uruguay and Costa Rica, for instance—have bent their home countries back to reopening. COVID spikes proved the unsurprising result.

Only a few countries remain on track. China and Panama, according to my colleague disease ecologist Luis Chaves, are two examples.[917] They continue to engage in the strange notion that controlling local outbreaks with full-spectrum interventions *protects* your economy.

But the failure of so many (particularly neoliberal) governments around the world to even bother with such efforts permitted COVID to evolve around concerted public health plans and national resolve elsewhere. In effect, sociopathic policy laid medieval siege upon everyone else, catapulting diseased bodies over the walls of recalcitrant towns.

The insistence that the capitalist economy is realer than people's health served to break what was long only a wavering sense of global solidarity to the virus's advantage.[918] One result is to extend the pandemic for the foreseeable future. Another is to weaponize SARS-2 as a means of burrowing under the notion that anything other than a market of commodities is an ontological possibility.

From a *New York Times* article:

> For a year and a half, New Zealand has pursued a strategy of "Covid zero," closing its borders and quickly enforcing lockdowns to keep the coronavirus in check, a policy it maintained even as other Asia-Pacific countries transitioned to coexisting with the viral threat.
>
> On Monday, New Zealand gave in. . . .
>
> Overall, New Zealand's approach to the virus has been a spectacular success, giving it one of the lowest rates of cases and deaths in the world, and allowing its people to live without restrictions during most of the pandemic.
>
> But the mood among many in Auckland has soured as the most recent lockdown has stretched on, with thousands of people breaking a stay-at-home order on Saturday to demonstrate against the restrictions in the country's largest such protest of the pandemic.
>
> The country's vaccination program has also been a source of consternation. The campaign began in earnest only last month, and fewer than half of people 12 and older have been fully vaccinated, leaving New Zealand far behind most developed countries.
>
> [Prime Minister Jacinda Ardern] began to acknowledge the public discontent two weeks ago, when she announced, after more than a month of a highly restrictive stay-at-home order, that some rules would be relaxed in Auckland even as much of the lockdown order remained in place. About 200,000 people were allowed to return to work, and restaurants and cafes could reopen for takeout orders.
>
> At the time, Ms. Ardern said the country was still trying to eliminate the virus. But to epidemiologists, who believed it was still possible to beat Delta and who were encouraging New Zealand to stick with the zero-Covid strategy, it was a gamble.
>
> Now, they say, it is clear that easing restrictions ended any chance of wiping out the virus again. New Zealand is still report-

ing dozens of new cases a day, almost all of them in Auckland, after the latest outbreak began in mid-August.[919]

The responses are at this point cultural archetypes. Philosopher Byung-Chul Han connects capitalism's death drive and the Valhalla consumer-citizens have been trained to seek beyond their hearth:

> Production increasingly resembles destruction. Humankind's self-alienation may have reached a point "where it can experience its own annihilation as a supreme aesthetic pleasure." What [Marxist critic Walter] Benjamin said of fascism is today true of capitalism. . . .
> Capital's logic of accumulation corresponds exactly to the archaic economy of violence. Capital behaves like a modern version of mana. Mana is the name of that powerful, mysterious substance that one acquires through the act of killing. One accumulates it in order to create a feeling of power and invulnerability.[920]

Han goes on in favor of reintroducing death as a cure to capitalism's celebration of the undead: "The mania for health is the biopolitical manifestation of capital itself." But he makes the mistake presuming capital isn't fully aware that—as we describe in our latest PReP dispatch on COVID in Los Angeles—foisting death upon the underclass allows the wealthier to live even as "botox zombies."[921]

The imbalance in mana explains in part President Biden's exhilaration at the May press conference announcing the CDC's recommendation that those vaccinated—still a deeply classist-imperialist condition stateside and globally—could go unmasked as if the pandemic were over. "A great day!" "The finish line." Birds chirping in the background.[922]

Now vaunted New Zealand bends back in that direction:

> The country's most at-risk communities are also its least vaccinated. While more than 95 percent of people of Asian descent and 80 percent of white people have received at least one dose,

the figure falls to about 73 percent for Pacific Islanders and less than 57 percent for Maori people.

Minimizing Auckland's outbreak has been complicated by a surge of cases among vulnerable people, including those living in emergency or transitional housing, said Dr. Michael Baker, an epidemiologist at the University of Otago.[923]

In a post on Twitter, the Maori writer and political commentator Morgan Godfery expressed concern about what abandoning the elimination strategy might mean for those in disadvantaged communities. "The PM says we must now live with the virus," he wrote.[924] "But the 'we' means these same lines of inequality. The virus will now burrow in gangs, the transitional housing community, and unvaccinated brown people. In 2020, Jacinda asked for shared sacrifice. In 2021, it's a particular sacrifice."

JOURNALIST BEN EHRENREICH GAVE *Dead Epidemiologists* a glowing blurb. If I returned the favor on Facebook in March, it was more out of sincere admiration than the cash he Venmoed me. Or the vaccine appointment he lined me up for, ahead of several thousand nursing home residents here in Minnesota.

Before the Delta variant proved Biden's CDC a lying, dog-faced pony epidemiologist, the path to pandemic "victory," atop the bodies of half-a-million Americans and rubbernecking past 130 countries without a single vaccine dose, had been such a grimly peppy march as to induce psychoseptic shock. We paraded right back into the normal that brought about the disaster (and which keeps the disaster in place). I felt my eventual stick might free me from my apartment, only to return me, as us all, into an epistemic prison.

Ehrenreich's own *Desert Notebooks* weaves the histories, imperial ecologies, and desert mirages that entrap us much the same way in climate change.[925]The book is no wonky scold, however. It's a triumph in the wandering essay. He's mastered Joan Didion's jump cut and W. G. Sebald's higher-order integration in topic, alongside the latter's use of photos. Clearly a big fan of the Barry Lopez we explored earlier in this book.[926]

Ehrenreich's inferences aren't positivist, they're visceral. They are grist for our anima, using the mill of long human understanding as far flung as the Popol Vuh, Walter Benjamin back again, Joshua Tree National Park, owl mythology, an expedient Lilith, nuclear testing in the desert, the messianic Ghost Dance, writing as cosmology, Las Vegas and the desert of the real, against anarchist anthropologist James Scott, and, magnificently, the cultural origins of time itself. That's hardly a comprehensive index.

Ehrenreich lands all the raptors he launches in style. But if one feels unmoored at the end, it's because he articulates few explicit answers. The resolution may be more affective. It may be probiotic, with a sense of arrival only when we act upon the world out there. As we must. Incrementalism is that death drive we already touched on with a long stick. To appropriate Ehrenreich's trope, we must bend linear just-in-time back into Earth's cycles.

ANY ETHOS, HOWEVER, CAN be repossessed. Neoliberal NGOs, Democratic candidates, and woke capitalists are diversifying the wardrooms of expropriation not only to protect themselves from accusations of racism or sexism, but, in the name of Obama Drone Strikers-in-Chief and Elizabeth Holmes girl bosses everywhere, to counterattack legitimate threats to such a system.[927]

Historian, commentator, and fellow CCNY radical Keeanga-Yamahtta Taylor commented in a recent interview:

> In the United States, the median income is what, $70,000? And that's skewed! That's white people! Black people? $47,000. The idea that this is the richest, most powerful country on the planet—and people are trying to live on $47,000? Or even $70,000?
> That's what's crazy with the white-privilege claim. They've

arranged it so that you have these millionaires and billionaires running the government, and then everyone's talking about how privileged these people making $70,000 a year are!

Is there racism? Absolutely. Does it mean that all these white people have advantages over Black people? Sure. No doubt. But if you think that is the extent of the fucking problem, then get a clue. These clowns in Congress are laughing all the way to the bank as they do the bidding for, to be crass, the capitalist class that is running things![928]

Ehrenreich notes that much as Christianity itself, a religion born out of poverty only to be weaponized by multiple empires, a more holistic time can be recolonized. Jews persecuted everywhere they roamed first bent time linear to escape their cycle of oppression: prosper, be oppressed, migrate, repeat. There must be another way!

Christianity followed the Jewish example, and the ever-forward march of Promethean progress that is destroying Earth's ecologies and Indigenous groups worldwide seeped into our sense of the natural with capitalism's emergence.

But fair warning, the return to more circular modalities needn't be steeped in solidarity or justice.

The USDA National Institute of Food and Agriculture, for instance, awarded a $10 million grant to Purdue University for a new project, "#DiverseCornBelt: Resilient Intensification through Diversity in Midwestern Agriculture":

> "What's new is that market and environmental research tailored to this part of the U.S. will inform our next moves, and individual farmers and stakeholders will be involved in every step of the process," [professor and project leader Linda Prokopy] says. "Growing only a rotation of corn and soybeans is not necessarily sustainable economically, environmentally or socially. We will be working with farmers in Indiana, Illinois and Iowa to evaluate alternative cropping systems that can be used in

the Midwest—we will be evaluating small grains and/or forage crops in rotations, perennial forage or bioenergy crops, agroforestry, horticultural food crops, and grazed livestock."[929]

The project mimics much of the work carried out by a decidedly less-funded Midwest Healthy Ag project I am a part of, integrating ecological analysis and farmer interviews, but apparently with little of the critical political economy MHA is pursuing.[930] The Purdue project's proposal included letters of support from General Mills, Smithfield, Kellogg's, Red Gold, and the Iowa Soybean Association.

Prokopy is spoken well of, her team well appointed, but this is likely less about persona than structurally neutralizing alternatives outside the control of the system's bigshots.

In the more technical treatment of our statistical test of the metabolic rift in agriculture across twenty-five U.S. states, evolutionary biologist Kenichi Okamoto, agrarian geographer Alex Liebman, and I warned:

Many of the growing number of agro-circular economic models aim at reconnecting nature to the neoliberal economy. The economies typically proposed in the stead of disembedded production presume linear biophysical cascades can be recoupled by recycling product and waste alike. As is the case in much of green capitalism, production efficiencies are proposed to minimize energy use and raw materials. . . .

Models in circular economy are often also presently framed in entrepreneurial terms, leaving out the contraindicative Jevons paradox against production efficiencies. Under the paradox, technological innovations cheapen production, helping open new markets for raw resources. As a result, more resources are used and more of the environment damaged. The issue extends beyond such perverse outcomes.

In promoting large-scale ecological change, many environmental modelers presume, even celebrate, continuing privatization of expropriated surplus value. The ethos is repeat-

edly operationalized as if the natural order of things. Entering
nature into the market, "selling nature to save it," is treated as
an unspoken social good. Irreplaceable "ecosystem services" are
proposed to be monetizable to the benefit of the very capital
destroying them.[931]

As anthropologist Maurice Godelier proposed against Marxist
cant, the base and superstructure we touched on above are in actuality
interrelated.[932] However irksome, returning to the vulgar distinction
might be required as green capitalists and their scientific apologists
are attempting to capture the language (and the power) of intervening
into the end of our epoch's ecologies. In the name of their moneybags.

Sometimes, we have to step the horses backwards out of the muck
to get around it.

FOR FAILING TO CONNECT strategy and tactics can be disastrous.
The United States, for one, lost the Afghan war the day it began.
Anthropologist Nancy Lindisfarne and clinic counselor Jonathan
Neale write:

The Pakistani military and intelligence services negotiated an
end to the stalemate. The United States would be allowed to take
power in Kabul and install a president of their choice. In return,
the Taliban leaders and rank-and-file would be allowed to go
home to their villages or into exile across the border in Pakistan.
This settlement was not widely publicized in the US and Europe
at the time, for obvious reasons, but we reported on it, and it was
widely understood in Afghanistan.

For best evidence for this negotiated settlement is what
happened next. For two years there was no resistance to the
American occupation. None, in any village. Many thousands of
former Taliban remained in those villages. . . .

The US and UK military occupied bases throughout the
villages and small towns of the Taliban heartland, the mainly

Pushtun areas of the south and east. These units were never told of the informal settlement negotiated between the Americans and the Taliban. They could not be told, because that would shame the government of President Bush. So the US units saw it as their mission to root out the remaining "bad guys," who were obviously still there.

Night raids crashed through doors, humiliating and terrifying families, taking men away to be tortured for info about the other bad guys. It was here, and in black sites all over the world, that the American military and intelligence developed the new styles of torture that the world would briefly glimpse from Abu Ghraib, the American prison in Iraq.[933]

Biden copped that the war never was about nation-building.[934] It was about crushing al Qaeda, which, he says, we accomplished ten years ago—eight years, according to Lindisfarne and Neale, too long. So, even by Biden's false account, a decade more to float the weapons sector and an imperial feminism impotent in the face of Texas's abortion ban until we rebuilt the enemy we were searching for.[935]

Not to be too flippant, but this is why some of us go to the shrink. We don't wish to act out our *Dasein*—our restless consciousness of our own human existence—through the task at hand, however much in this case it also led us, death drive first, to the graveyard of empires to begin with. The damage, as Byung-Chul Han describes it, was always going to be borne by the Afghans even to the imperial project's destruction.

We find a similar trap in our response to the pandemic or the Enbridge-bought counterinsurgency in Minnesota against environmentalists who opposed the Line 3 oil pipeline, flashes in the civil war at first approximation of rich upon poor, evoking the early 1980s graffiti I remembered spray-painted on 110th Street and Broadway in New York City: "U.S. Out of North America!"[936]

Where would we go? Anywhere but here, the Forever War, 230 out of 245 years fighting abroad, and everyday at home. "Some worlds are built on a fault line of pain," N. K. Jemison wrote, "held up by nightmares. Don't lament when those worlds fall. Rage that they were built doomed in the first place."[937]

IN THE DESERT, EHRENREICH describes he's learning how to track the constellations in the night sky. Until it all clicks in and he suddenly falls over dizzy with Earth's orbit through the solar system reflected in the movement of the stars.

My vertigo moment is the precipitation that we are lucky to walk the surface of a planet without a spacesuit (or a cowboy hat). That our air packs are built into our chests by four billion years of coevolution across the tree of life.

Both of us in these epiphanies are at best only lifting ourselves up off our knees onto the mind-land that Native Americans, and Indigenous the world over, have trod many thousands of years.

It isn't that modernity has nothing to offer. After a slow start and a determined public health campaign, American Indigenous groups are clocking in with some of the highest levels of COVID vaccination in the United States.[938] But positivism without the whys of mutual kindness, that's a barbarism best abandoned back on our feet at a standing sprint.

—PATREON, OCTOBER 15, 2021

Puzzled Patients

Jigsaw puzzle companies tend to use the same cut patterns for multiple puzzles. This makes the pieces interchangeable. As a result, I sometimes find that I can combine portions from two or more cool puzzles to make a surreal picture that the publisher never imagined.

—Tim Klein (2019)

IN MAY 2021, REPORTS from India identified a surge of "black fungus" in COVID patients.[939] Something of a misnomer, the fungus is a rare saprobic mucormycosis, the usual prevalence of which is seventy times higher in India than elsewhere.[940] The mold was subsequently found in COVID patients in lesser frequencies in Pakistan, Bangladesh, Nepal, Oman, Iran, Egypt, Chile, and Uruguay.[941]

These mucormycetes are typically in ecological balance with livestock and humans and, when inhaled as spores, cleared by the immune system.[942] But the mold can turn on a patient—in the immunocompromised, for instance, or by large exposure out in the field or in contaminated food, with a diabetes comorbidity, or following disturbance to gastric bacteria.[943] A bad infection can lead to discoloration, blurred vision, chest pain, difficulty breathing, and coughing up blood.

Like SARS-CoV-2 itself, the mold infection can grow in blood vessels, producing blood clots and tissue death and leading to oxygen deprivation and case fatality rates as high as 50 percent.[944] Also like COVID, at times it invades the central nervous system, although usually directly through the nose and eyes.

As an opportunistic infection in the immunocompromised and, in this case, in COVID patients taking immunosuppressant steroids, an India hit by the Delta strain mid-2021 proved a sudden epicenter, numbering 45,000 infections by July.[945]

Were doctors to blame for the new mucormycosis? Did overprescription of steroids and antibiotics drive one epidemic atop another? Jawaharlal Nehru University's Rajib Dasgupta argued "black fungus" in part originated in bad public health practice instead.[946]

After all, all the pieces to avoid the mold epidemic were already in place. Such COVID-related cases were detected in the first wave, as early as April 2020. They weren't entirely a surprise.

Antibiograms, Dasgupta continued, showing which infections are circulating locally and which antibiotics work on them, are usually routinely sent to hospitals. For severe infections, additional blood work is prescribed, to help identify the exact disease agent (and so the exact antibiotic needed). Both clinical steps aim to avoid prescriptions of broad-spectrum antibiotics that select for resistant pathogens as well, in this case, killing off good bacteria that block out fungal infections. Skipping the precautions is especially likely in hospitals under COVID siege.

Dasgupta also described Indian guidelines for key steroid methylprednisolone as recommending dosages as high as five times that recommended in other countries. If doctors were to blame, they were just following nationally set guidelines.

Causes for the dual epidemic may extend out beyond hospitals and public health systems. Agriculture is another sector where the mucormycosis finds its footing. An overapplication of antibiotics in livestock might select for a surge of fungal cases: "Mucormycotic ruminitis is therefore a well-known sequel to intensive antibiotic treatment of cattle."[947] Does such a pharmo-ecological interaction more directly connect farm to hospital? Do fungi adapt to antimicrobials beyond taking advantage of an opportunistic niche opening?

It wouldn't be the first time. The rapid spread of multidrug resistance in fungus *Candida auris* across human populations worldwide may be caused in part by a rise in antifungal application on farms.[948] We need ask whether an overapplication of antifungals in increasingly neoliberalized agriculture in India made it harder to treat fungal cases in human patients with amphotericin B, beyond the problem of shortages in the latter agent.[949] Inopportune juxtaposition may be more a systemic convergence.

If COVID is itself a difficult problem in part from its aerosolized mode of infection, transmission before symptoms appear, and a zoo of pathogenic pathways—from lung infection to multiple Long COVID syndromes—we see now the possibility that it can act in concert with other sources of disease to mutual amplification.

Sociopolitical Syndemics

The field of *syndemics* investigates the ways health problems intermesh.[950] At the molecular and clinical levels, sources of morbidity interact in webs of reciprocal activation often to synergistic effect.[951] Each disease amplifies the other. These inputs embody necessary but also insufficient explanations for health outcomes. From the field's start, the wider sociopolitical context from which these sources emerge were folded into models of syndemogenesis.[952]

A disease outbreak, for instance, represents more than a convergence of susceptibles, the exposed and infected, and those who have recovered from infection. Modeling far beyond the inveterate SEIR classes is required.

One recent series of socioecological models of Ebola and vector-borne diseases reversed perspective.[953] The series focused on the role systemic environmental stochasticity set by land use plays in driving epizootic outbreaks to extirpation or amplifying their propagation, including spillovers into humans. The broader landscapes through which pathogens circulate have definitional impact on the outcomes of outbreaks whatever the evolutionary state of the specific disease agent. Epidemiological causality is found as much in the etiological field as in the object of the pathogen or patient.

One pandemic can set the outcomes of another, in this case beyond the fungus. Virologist Nokukhanya Msomi and colleagues report that HIV patients were 30 to 50 percent more likely to die from COVID before the vaccine was introduced.[954] Patients with advanced HIV were even more likely to die. In the other direction, Long COVID appears associated with immune systems weakened by a variety of causes, including autoimmune diseases and cancer chemotherapy.

Such long infections may serve as incubators for the emergence of novel COVID variants, permitting quasispecies to accumulate multiple mutations in response to persistent immune attack.[955] We need keep in mind that such mechanistic explanations—entirely reasonable a possibility—shouldn't detract from the Global North's refusal to vaccinate the rest of the world.[956] In letting COVID spread and evolve, incubation can take place at the population level too. And, of course, HIV, diabetes, and all those other "preexisiting conditions" for a bad COVID outcome are themselves social in origin, with exposures foundationally tied to political economies of money and power.[957]

Opening each other new niches in the human body isn't the only way pathogens collaborate. Different viruses and bacteria can exchange genomic segments. Along with thirty substitution mutations and six deletions in its spike protein, the Omicron variant may have picked up insertion (ins214EPE) from another virus, including, perhaps, one of the viruses that together represent the common cold.[958] The receptors for SARS-2 (AEC2) and HCoV-229E (ANPEP) are expressed together in gastrointestinal and respiratory tissues, possible sites for a co-infection event. Other studies have shown co-infections of SARS-2 and non-SARS coronavirus.[959]

The immune system is itself such an open system. As our team modeled in the aughts, sociopolitical inputs can help set the parameter spaces over which the immune system chooses to respond to infectious and chronic diseases and the prophylaxes used to try to control them.[960] Similar boundary conditions are set at the level of epidemiological intervention, including vaccine effectiveness.[961]

Beyond the Body

Such effects across pathogens can be mediated by public health investment. Immunologist Pedro Reche's group hypothesized that children's comparative protection from COVID-19 may be cultural in origin.[962] The team hypothesized that general pediatric vaccination may offer cross-reactive protection against SARS-2. They found the diphtheria-tetanus-pertussis (DTP) vaccine offered significant potential cross-reactivity, particularly a variety of CD8 and CD4 T cell and neutralizing B cell epitopes in SARS-2's spike protein.

Sociocultural impacts can be felt in the other direction. General declines in hospital and public health services during a pandemic permit other pathologies to surge.[963] Epidemiologists Madhukar Pai and Ayoade Olatunbosun-Alakija noted that especially in the Global South, COVID lockdowns and demands upon personnel and supplies have sapped campaigns in routine immunization.[964] Treatment of TB, malaria, and HIV has also been disrupted, with as many as 1.3 million fewer cases of TB treated and 22 percent fewer HIV tests conducted.

The effects can be more distally felt. Wei Xia and colleagues proposed that the industrial African swine fever outbreak that cut into China's domestic hog supply the year before COVID-19's emergence —and which increased hog price and volatility—may have driven an increase in incursions upon bats.[965] The sudden gap in access to protein and the new freeway laid down may have led to a greater rate of spillover events, including in Yunnan, one possible SARS-2 point of origin. The hypothesis presumes, however, that SARS-2 arose in 2019, which much of the evolutionary genomics modeling doesn't support, placing the "new" coronavirus in human populations years before.[966]

But the team's key point stands. With multiple protopandemic pathogens emerging in parallel, the socioecological combinations driving disease emergence may be increasing, as much out of their economic impacts as from their reciprocal activation within potential hosts.[967]

For instance, a paper from a team led by disease ecologist Luis Chaves and geographer Luke Bergmann identifies where COVID and vector-borne infections—of seemingly incongruent etiologies— intertwine into sociospatial syndemics:

> Early COVID-19 rates rose syndemically in northeastern Chiapas and much of Panamá along with dengue infection rates; they also rose in northern and western Brazil with dengue and malaria. Although we found evidence for statistically significant spatial overlap of COVID-19 in the pandemic with vector-borne disease in northern Texas and coastal Chiapas, we did not find evidence of syndemic effects there; minimal overlap among diseases was observed in Costa Rica.[968]

The implications situate the interactions across SARS-2 and other diseases in their specific context:

> Our results suggest that synergies among diseases and socionatural processes are occurring, but they can be context-dependent in ways that identifying and understanding them requires a geographical data science in which processes may interact in different ways at different places, at different times, and at different scales.[969]

The travel and trade that bring about mind-boggling juxtapositions in the sciences and arts one side of the world to the other—the stuff of whole libraries—are as complex in their pathogenic manifestation. The increasing orders of interactions across diseases—across different places, times, scales, and domains—imply the illnesses must be met with public health responses of comparable dimensionality.[970]

Lucrative pharmaceuticals plied by the capitalist state individual-by-individual aren't sufficient by a long vaccine shot.

—PATREON, MARCH 25, 2022

Omicron Prime

Private property has made us so stupid and one-sided that an object is ours only when we have it, when it exists for us as capital or when we directly possess, eat, drink, inhabit it, etc., in short, when we use it. . . .

Therefore all the physical and intellectual senses have been replaced by the simple estrangement of all these senses—the sense of having.

— ANJA HEISLER WEISER FLOWER (2021)

One must imagine Sisyp . . . hey, the happy epidemiologist!

— JOSÉ HALLOY (2021)

READING IS A TYPE OF hallucination. Perhaps against the strictest Cartesian divides, deep thinking is a form of multiverse travel. Every world we think of may somewhere else exist.

Much attention is placed on the resulting gaps between theory and practice. Either hardheaded realists—just theorists of an expediently unselfconscious sort—dismiss theorists for missing a "real world" in large part of some theory's making. Or theorists themselves are shocked when any of their phantasmagoria prove dead right. What we dream about might suddenly matter. I wrote 50,000 words this summer recovering from my own projection last November that the Biden administration wouldn't wrap up COVID-19 by a long shot.[971] Only now, others more respectable are also beginning to mourn.[972]

Should any of us suffer a Cassandra complex, it is due in part to our refusal of the salacious advances of Apollo, the god of truth and prophecy and health and disease (and grants and tenure). Our unheard *warning* isn't merely the upshot of a society-wide superego, aiming, in psychoanalyst Melanie Klein's formulation, to crush what must be denied—if only as a matter of avoiding guilt—but also, I'll add here, serves as a convenient political target.[973] Power, in its negative form, is the capacity to avoid addressing counternarratives that suggest the present system produces its own dangers.

Even with the best data, such warnings are dismissed in Jungian Laurie Layton Schapira's articulation as nothing more than the occult.[974] The war and chaos that result from assiduously ignoring good advice are, ironically, more Ares than Apollo. We must burn down the immune village to save it, as only an imperial death cult would conclude.

So, in another example of information underload, epidemiologists, presenting a surprise already long reported on, announced the emergence of another SARS-2 variant of concern.[975] The B.1.1.529 or Omicron strain out of sub-Saharan Africa suddenly replaced the Delta strain in Gauteng province in South Africa.

Phylogeographer Trevor Bedford offered a preliminary analysis of the first 91 Omicron genomes uploaded to the GISAID database.[976] Bedford reported that Omicron represents no descendant of any of the previous variants labeled to that point, emerging out of SARS-2's phylogenetic tree mid-2020. The Omicron clade isn't a rubbish pile of loosey isolates collected together by long-branch attraction, an error in phylogenetic reconstruction whereby a few very different clades are grouped together. Omicron is a true-blue variant that emerged after quietly circulating for a whole year in areas of poor surveillance or by accelerated evolution in a chronic infection.

Tulio de Oliveira, the director of South Africa's Centre for Epidemic Response and Innovation, remarked on the wide array of mutations in the S1 domain of Omicron's spike protein, which may mark the kind of antigenic shift that promotes immune escape from natural immunity and vaccination:[977]

- Multiple mutations in the spike protein's receptor binding domain and amino-terminal domain associated with resisting neutralizing antibodies and monoclonal antibody therapies
- Mutations near the furin cleavage site promoting efficient cell entry and transmissibility
- Deletions associated with evading innate immunity and perhaps increased transmissibility
- Mutations in the nucleocapsid protein, enhancing infectivity

The new phenotype appears to accelerate transmission beyond that of the Delta variant, which in turn already had outpaced earlier pandemic strains.

Bedford circumvents the difficulties in using case frequencies to plot Omicron's transmission rate.[978] He uses a phylodynamic estimation that combines a branch-specific molecular clock and the branching patterns for 77 Omicron genomes from South Africa and Botswana to estimate a common ancestor dated to October 7, 2021 (95 percent confidence interval of September 19 and October 21) and a doubling in population of newly infected every 4.8 days.

Active research is underway to determine whether present vaccines control Omicron.[979] Either way, commentators have noted the way Omicron underscores the necessity of vaccinating the world. Epidemiologist Madhu Pai remarked:

Vaccine inequity (apartheid) is—Morally bankrupt—Ethically indefensible—Fiscally irresponsible—Epidemiologically foolish —Socially unjust.

If you are double or triple vaccinated and are worried about #Omicron, spare a thought for the 3+ billion people who are still waiting for their first dose. Do more than spare a thought. Advocate for vaccine equity![980]

In a *Science* commentary, Pai and Ayoade Olatunbosun-Alakija, Co-Chair of the Africa Vaccine Delivery Alliance, described the ongoing costs in lives and community well-being:

> Over 5 million people have died from COVID-19 so far, but the true death toll is probably threefold higher. As severe acute respiratory syndrome coronavirus 2 (SARS-CoV-2) continues to rapidly spread, vaccine inequity is the biggest threat to conquering the pandemic. Whereas 66% of the people in high-income countries are fully vaccinated, only 2.5% of the population in low-income countries are fully protected.[981]

Against the neoliberal notion that controlling the outbreak destroys the economy, Pai and Olatunbosun-Alakija note:

> Moreover, COVID-19 has rolled back most of the global gains in tackling poverty and disease. If the world does not tackle this inequity, all countries will face collateral damage of unimaginable proportions. The UN Sustainable Development Goals (SDGs) will remain unrealized.
>
> Consider the social and economic consequences of vaccine inequity. In 2020, the pandemic led to nearly 100 million more people in poverty, and the UN estimates that developing countries will suffer economic losses of $12 trillion through 2025. This will only get worse, as SARS-CoV-2 (Delta variant) is now primarily affecting countries with low vaccine coverage.
>
> Moreover, the pandemic has disrupted essential health services, especially in the Global South, where fragile health systems are falling apart. For example, routine immunization is suffering not just because of pandemic measures such as lockdowns, but also because personnel and supplies required for childhood immunization are now being utilized for COVID-19 vaccinations. Data suggest that global routine immunization rates in 2020 dropped to levels last seen in 2005. This could well derail global efforts to eliminate polio and result in a resurgence of measles.

Health services for the continuing threats of tuberculosis (TB), malaria, and HIV have been severely disrupted by the pandemic as well. According to a recent World Health Organization (WHO) TB report, 1.3 million fewer people with TB were treated in 2020 than in 2019. According to the Global Fund, HIV testing declined by 22% in 2020. Progress against malaria has stalled as there was no year-on-year growth in provision of malaria services.[982]

What to do?

The COVID-19 pandemic is the biggest test of humanity's ability to think and act as humankind. To pass the test, rich nations must stop vaccine hoarding, immediately redistribute surplus vaccines, meet their pledges to the COVID-19 Vaccines Global Access (COVAX) program, support the Trade-Related Aspects of Intellectual Property Rights (TRIPS) waiver, and mandate pharmaceutical companies to transfer know-how for diagnostics, vaccines, and therapeutics.[983]

Nothing about Omicron is a surprise. The repeated emergence of new variants in a world only lazily dedicated to controlling COVID was long expected.[984] Brutalist reality is spooling out of theory's playbook.

Even Gordon Brown, Tony Blair's follow-up prime minister, gets it, noting, perhaps only implicitly, what others have said out loud,[985] that those countries that so swiftly reported the Omicron emergence and that have been blocked from vaccine access are being punished with travel bans by the countries hoarding vaccines:

In the absence of mass vaccination, Covid is not only spreading uninhibited among unprotected people but is mutating, with new variants emerging out of the poorest countries and now threatening to unleash themselves on even fully vaccinated people in the richest countries of the world.

On Thursday, the UK's Department of Health, which has placed a travel ban on southern Africa, warned that the B.1.1.529 "Omicron" variant was the most "complex" and "worrying" seen so far. And yet with 9.1bn vaccines already manufactured and 12bn expected by the year's end—enough to vaccinate the whole world—this was the "arms race" that we could have won. No country should be facing yet another winter with the uncertainty of a new wave of Covid hanging over us. . . .

Only when we reject vaccine nationalism and medical protectionism will we stop outbreaks becoming pandemics.[986]

We might ask Brown, who now serves as WHO ambassador for global health financing, what his role was, if any, in turning over WHO's initial open medicine model to Bill Gates and the pharmaceutical sector. I noted in July 2021:

Noises early in the pandemic out of WHO, NIH, NIAID, and the *Financial Times,* among other surprising outlets, suggested all pharmaceuticals, vaccines included, would make open medicine available to all at no cost. Sentiments were turned into action or, to start, a platform—the WHO COVID-19 Technology Access Pool or C-TAP—to be made accessible to all private and public entities aiming to produce medicine.

Bill Gates, with overwhelming influence on public health up into UN executive offices, put a kibosh on the effort, getting the Covid-19 ACT-Accelerator launched under the WHO flag.

The Gates-run Accelerator—like the Vaccine Alliance Gates launched in 1999—organized R&D and distribution under the old model of intellectual property. That included COVAX, the WHO effort to distribute the vaccine to nations who couldn't afford the mad dash for vaccine access among the richer countries.[987]

The impacts upon the evolution of the virus and booster shots for the few were obvious:

What the variants win from a host system intent upon profitably denying itself herd immunity, the industry wins from the variants' proliferation.[988]

I more explicitly summarized the contrast a month later:

In other words, what should have been a race between the pathogen and a humanity aimed at vaccinating the world before vaccine escape set in was replaced by a race between the pathogen and booster shots for a fusillade of variants only a few countries can afford. Despite both involving the pathogen, vaccines, and people the world over, the two races are categorically different. The first would have made a real run at driving SARS-2 to extirpation. The second places profits (and the pathogen) before people.[989]

But more fundamentally what is necessary, even if the proverbial table wasn't tilted, isn't necessarily sufficient:

Vaccines are *not* the best bet in the race against new variants. Instead, it's keeping novel diseases from emerging in the first place. And keeping those that do emerge from spreading by organizing governance around public health and the public commons. Both interventions require replacing a mode of social reproduction organized around profit that sacrifices millions annually, including this year by COVID.[990]

Public health and well-being aren't found just in the object of medical innovations, but also in the field of relationships social and ecological upon which both virus and vaccine depend.[991]

If one relies on the news cycle or twitterverse or even our heroic epidemiologists alone, one might conclude from this repeat business of new variants that we're only getting faster at missing the point.

And what does the big picture of missing the point look like?

We're presently at 260 million documented COVID infections.

Even if this were an underestimate of ten times, meaning 2.6 billion have been infected really, and even if one-third of the human race is inherently immune, that would leave 2.59 billion people still fully susceptible, albeit omitting reinfections from one side of the ledger and vaccine jabs from the other.

Without a global Zero COVID campaign that many of our best and brightest have dismissed out of hand, the pandemic is likely far from over.[992] Again, not news. Early models projected COVID as far out as 2025.[993] The first European bout of the Black Death, killing at a much swifter pace at the individual level but perhaps slower at the population level, lasted from 1346 to 1353.[994]

Maybe COVID will attenuate as an infection, however long it reigns as a pandemic. Wishful thinking perhaps, with Omicron's emergence indicating we haven't reached an epidemiological ceiling in the virus's evolutionary ascent. Either way, long haul COVID is looking like more than just an individual patient's nightmare.[995]

That is, we're all likely to be stuck in COVID's grip for years. Such an outcome, marking us two years in as still at the start of the pandemic, is only partially a matter of the virus itself.

Biden spokesperson Jen Psaki's flippant dismissal of the suggestion that the United States might follow other countries and directly pay for every American's COVID test underscores the ongoing slog as much an outcome of neoliberal public health as any wily evolution on the virus's part.[996]

—PATREON, NOVEMBER 27, 2021

Corrupted Software

There's no point in designing software if researchers can't use it, and use it well for useful research. And there's no point in writing user guides and introductory texts to help them use it if it won't help them to do what they are trying to do . . .

But there is also no point in software developers telling researchers that they should be trying to do what this particular software supports. . . . The challenge of teaching research in the context of software is to resist all the time the pull of the software's tools.

—Lyn Richards (2019)

IN 2016, I WARNED of EcoHealth Alliance president Peter Daszak's compulsive lying.[997] However polite, such warnings often end careers. Not those of their objects, as many of New York Governor Andrew Cuomo's accusers sweated, but of their sources.[998]

Five years later, in what is shaping up as still the beginning of a pandemic, Daszak, a cornerstone of U.S. imperial epizoology, is now coming under increasing fire.[999] Whether or not EHA was in part responsible for COVID-19's lab escape, should that be a possibility, is still an open question, but the organization's repeated Nixonian response to the charge has only concentrated the dismay it sought to disperse.[1000]

Outside *Science Magazine*'s fawning portrayal of a reputable scientist under fire, the increasing skepticism of Daszak, and EHA more generally, has moved out from radical corners left and right and into the mainstream of the London *Sunday Times* and *Newsweek*.[1001] Indeed, warnings and skepticism have turned into outright denouncement.

Columbia University biologist Neil Harrison offers here perhaps the most scathing attack on a scientist this pandemic so far.[1002] And given *Dead Epidemiologists* on the one hand and Kentucky Senator Ron Paul on the other, that's saying a lot.[1003] "A graduate of the little known University College of North Wales," Harrison begins,

> Dr Daszak earned his PhD at the decidedly obscure University of East London, and then studied Crohn's Disease with research fraudster and anti-vaxxer Andrew Wakefield. After a series of unremarkable research positions in the United States, Daszak rose to prominence as "The Virus Hunter."
>
> Although less photogenic than [Elizabeth] Holmes, Daszak has nevertheless been widely profiled and photographed, often posed dramatically in khaki shorts—the scientist as outdoorsman—during a variety of daring field expeditions. He has been fêted by a variety of magazines, albeit of slightly lower profile than those that fawned over Holmes. Daszak has rarely been short of a quote for a decade or so, broadcasting the terrors of future pandemics, and he remains a favorite of many prestigious newspapers such as the *New York Times*, as well as the news sections of high-profile scientific outlets, including *Science* and *Nature*. . . .
>
> Success bred success for Daszak, as individuals and foundations were keen to support his organization and its One Health mission to save endangered animal species and prevent pandemics. Corporate punters were eager to join the action, unable to resist the combination of saving cute furry animals and battling nasty microorganisms. Daszak was able to partner with many universities around the U.S., including the University of North Carolina at Chapel Hill and the University of Texas Medical

Branch in Galveston. He also became an adjunct Professor at the prestigious Mailman Institute for Public Health at Columbia University.[1004]

The Bildungsroman takes an Oliver Twist:

Seasoned skeptics wondered how someone with no formal training in virology, and no actual laboratory (EcoHealth has offices, but no labs at its New York City HQ) was swinging such a large bag of research funding. Indeed, EcoHealth seems to function primarily as what is commonly known as a "pass-through" (this is funding agency speak for a kind of mailbox), gathering funding from a variety of sources and disbursing these research monies to its partners at a number of scientific institutions around the world, with the Wuhan Institute of Virology in China as its main partner. . . .

Their detailed and very expensive analyses (usually illustrated by maps of animal habitats, marked with colored blobs), had suggested that the "zoonotic" transfer of viruses from animals to humans would be observed in rural areas, where frontier activities of man encroach upon animal habitats, bringing farmers and animal traders into contact with bats and other animals likely to be harboring novel pathogens. This was certainly in keeping with the prevailing consensus, and was consistent with One Health principles. Doubling down on the EHA bloviation, Daszak recently claimed that such zoonotic events occur "up to 40,000 times a year."[1005]

Word about the damage Daszak is accruing finally started to circulate as much a matter of that iota of professional pride still promised at the end of Netflix's *The Chair* as professional jealousy:

Scientists are fond of dark humour, and while one colleague mused that EcoHealth has predicted and prevented "zero pandemics" in its history, another added "or perhaps minus one?"

If EcoHealth was a company, the stock and bond prices would have fallen precipitously. Markets like to get out ahead of bad news, and the market usually knows what's coming before you do. . . .

In fact, it would be more accurate to say that among scientists (even virologists) there is something of a silent "anti-Daszak" movement, albeit of modest proportions. It is worth noting that we rarely hear from Daszak about variants and vaccines, antivirals and other therapeutics, or about the ICU physicians and other clinicians who continue to save lives by treating critically ill COVID-19 patients. Instead, we hear a lot about the big Ps: pandemic prediction, prevention and, of course, Peter.

The problem for Daszak is that he invited undue attention with constant media appearances, and therefore brought suspicion on himself. His TV appearances on *60 Minutes*, and with Sanjay Gupta on CNN were at times excruciating, and rivaled the infamous Prince Andrew interview in terms of uncomfortable body language and credibility. . . .

Scientists are seriously spooked by Daszak and are unwilling to discuss EHA, which has become a kind of third rail, not only because of its extensive funding from NIH and DoD, but also due to the public relations offensive that has cast a dark spell over this field of biology. Daszak has repeatedly engaged in a PR campaign marked by disinformation, intimidation and distraction. These are not usually thought of as the tools of a scientist, but they are certainly central to the craft of a rather different trade, one that is coincidentally represented on the Advisory Board of EHA.[1006]

Elizabeth Holmes! Andrew Wakefield! Prince Andrew! And not too subtle implications of spycraft and hybrid war at home and abroad. Damn, Harrison wasn't playing around.

TO THIS CITY UNIVERSITY of New York boy, the notion Daszak came from the wrong school is so very British in its classism. So Columbia, down the hill from the City College of New York campus where, without a grant, I served as a doctoral student adjunct paying my bills teaching classes for nearly a decade.

And Harrison's withering critique—like Jeffrey Sachs's—has the smell of a ritual sacrifice.[1007] With only passing mention of the NIH's—and none of Anthony Fauci's—repeated defense of Daszak, not merely as a matter of rhetorical deflection, but of their out-and-out perjury before Congress.[1008]

Perhaps unbeknownst to Harrison, Daszak and EHA are far from sheep blackened by shame. They are at one and the same time on the cutting-edge of neoliberal science and ensconced deeply in the U.S. security state. It's a combo that speaks to the way fighting pandemics serves as a very means of protecting the systems of expropriation that produce those pandemics.

Sam Husseini reports that EHA took (and hid from the public) nearly $40 million from the Department of Defense.[1009] Most of it from the DoD's Defense Threat Reduction Agency, which aims to "counter and deter weapons of mass destruction and improvised threat networks." EHA received another $65 million from USAID, $20 million from Health and Human Services, $2.6 million from the National Science Foundation, another $2.3 million from the Department of Homeland Security, $1.2 million from the Department of Commerce, and smaller amounts from the Department of Agriculture and the Department of Interior.

Husseini identifies David Franz, former commander at Fort Detrick, the U.S.'s primary biowarfare facility, as an EHA policy adviser. Franz, Husseini continues, recently wrote an article in the neocon *City Journal* with disgraced former *New York Times* journalist Judith Miller of WMD infamy in favor of more funding for Fort Detrick.[1010]

About a decade ago, a One Health scientist queried me rhetorically, with a raised brow, what was virologist Nathan Wolfe doing in the Congo Basin on the DoD's dime?[1011] What some reporters were once in the thick of the Cold War—spies by another name—are now transmogrified into anthropologists, psychologists, and, at this historical juncture, disease scientists, who many expect can't be denied access to the far reaches of the world where the imperium's sword also thrusts.[1012]

To what aim? Against what targets? What food scholar and activist Raj Patel identified in a must-read as the anti-communist roots of the Green Revolution now appear shuttled along the epidemiological storylines of our era's gothic imaginarium.[1013] Blaming smallholders and Indigenous groups for the deforestation events that lead to spillover events weaponizes the absolute geographies of specific GPS coordinates that corporations can grab in the name of better protecting humanity from the next big outbreak.[1014]

To that objective, EHA follows the USAID model of soft and not-so-soft intervention in franchising out One Health labs across Latin America.[1015] Like Daszak himself, the efforts are hilariously shameless. I mean, one such lab in the Yucatán, Mexico, backed by French and German euros, is named "El Dorado"![1016] Among the objectives of the lab is to "provide scientific and integrative strategies that combine human health, biodiversity conservation and economic growth through sustainable development."[1017]

The lab's establishment goes hand in hand with the development agenda for the Yucatán Peninsula under President Andrés Manuel López Obrador. Yes, the objective is to build out the Yucatán as a tourist beach attraction on the coasts, a new Cancún, but also by way of Tren Maya, the lucrative megaproject train line to circle through Chiapas and the Yucatán, including through Mérida, where El Dorado is located.[1018]

The train system and new development towns along the 1,525-km route would destroy ecological reserves and spring possible pathogens against which the lab ostensibly aims to protect.

AMLO claims the development is an effort at ending the abandonment of the southeast region of the country. But few Mayans were queried whether they even wanted the duplicitly named train, on ramshackle target for sped-up, pre-election completion by 2024.[1019] The players that actually consulted for the megaproject included the likes of Woodhouse Lorente Ludlow, PricewaterhouseCoopers, Steer Davies & Gleve, and Goldman Sachs.[1020] The Regional Indigenous and Popular Council of Xpujil, among other Indigenous groups harking back to nineteenth-century uprisings against previous expropriation-ist regimes, is working to block the project as a threat to their very way of life.[1021]

Three million new tourists a year are planned for transport through the destroyed remnants of one of the last prime forest regions in the Western Hemisphere. "Nature will not be affected," AMLO, elected on a leftist platform, claimed. Is that true? The one study produced by Conacyt—Mexico's National Science Foundation and an El Dorado co-sponsor—describing the detrimental impacts of the project on local biodiversity was suppressed.[1022]

In 2022, Obrador again iterated "we are not going to destroy nature," admitting the area ecologically fragile, but that engineers were build-ing the line in such a way that the cenotes and underground rivers were protected.[1023] Four million trees, AMLO claimed, were being planted across the five states through which the train would run.

Construction refuted the assurances. Segment 5—running between Cancún and Tulum—was to run along a highway.[1024] Hotelier com-plaints sent planners rerouting the segment snaking through primary jungle—mere "shrub" ALMO waved his hand—atop porous bedrock over the underground rivers and one of the world's largest chains of caves and home to ancient Mayan ruins and artifacts.[1025] "It will col-lapse," said a former consultant to the project.[1026]

AMLO deployed a leftist attack that the protests were being led by "a number of interests," including unnamed businessmen and even the U.S. government, that were aiming to block the rail line:

There are interests here, where there is more money, to put it clearly here. And what doesn't sound logical sounds metallic.[1027]

Cancún's development thirty years ago left a wake of poverty and environmental degradation for local residents, outcomes many Indigenous workers and farmers in the planned Tren Maya region note.[1028] The farmers also observed that the announcement of the project set off regional land speculation, with foreign capital buying land out from underneath locals, a trajectory, agroecologist Peter Rosset comments, that was unachievable under the more conservative PAN and PRI governments.

The train would accelerate land grabs already long underway as oil palm, soybean, sugarcane, and pork and chicken production replace local Mayan production, promoted by both multinationals and the corporate conservation group Nature Conservancy in the name of a "green economy."[1029] The train project would now serve to anchor new agricultural industrial parks for "meat, fruit, forest products, organic food, and oil palm processing" as part of a "special economic zone."[1030]

Cargo trains on the new rail would also import food commodities to the added detriment of local producers, while acting also at larger scales of circuits of capital, alleviating the pressure on the Panama Canal in transporting international goods to the United States and Asia. Turning the Yucatan into Los Angeles.[1031] Another "factory without walls." The government has twisted opponents' characterization of this new scope of the project into the very grounds for justifying tagging the train as a matter of "national security."[1032] Such a tag, the government argues, sets the train beyond the purview of the lawsuits that environmental and Indigenous groups have brought to stay the project.

The fight continues, even at this late date with train cars on order. El Dorado, in contrast, has no plans to study the ecohealth impacts of the train. The gold it seeks apparently is to be found in ignoring the very subject of its study program.

Indeed, in a joint statement out of a July 2021 meeting, Mexico's Secretary of Foreign Affairs Marcelo Ebrard and France's Minister for Europe and Foreign Affairs Jean-Yves Le Drain acknowledged the lab and train megaproject as parts of the same program in international development.[1033] The ministers, a summary of the bilateral meeting reports,

- Welcomed the confidence that French companies have

shown for investing in Mexico, as seen by their partici-
pation in infrastructure projects, especially the Mayan
Train, the Azteca vaccine plant project and the Mayakan
gas pipeline.

- Confirmed the importance of swiftly signing and rati-
fying the modernized Mexico-European Union Global
Agreement, just as it was negotiated. They highlighted
the contribution its entry into force would make to both
countries' post-pandemic recovery and to the definition
of rules-based trade respectful of the collective pref-
erences of both parties that would allow us to increase
our ambitions and commitments regarding sustainable
development. . . .

- Expressed their satisfaction for the health cooperation
between our two countries as part of the fight against the
pandemic and highlighted their shared efforts to prevent
the emergence of zoonoses, especially Mexico's joining
the Prezode initiative and the creation of El Dorado, a
regional laboratory in Merida.[1034]

The way all the gold pieces appear to fall in place across extrac-
tivist rationale from 1517 on—from Jesus Christ's healing touch to
modern-day disease control—insinuates a deterministic inevitability.[1035] "*¡Qué elegancia!*" one Tren Maya puff piece put the $20 billion
project, as engineering and ethos both.[1036] But people and pathogens
in whose names this mining is pursued rarely cooperate with such
salesmanship.

STILL, HARRISON MAY REPRESENT one claque of a fracturing
establishment trying to come to terms with mainstream science's role
in bringing on the distrust of science it denounces outward, if not also
its possible role in starting the pandemic itself. That this is all out in
the open now speaks to a decline in class discipline one sees at any
local Chamber of Commerce.

The growing incoherence is now embedded in the very institutional cognition of a system in decline.[1037] For there's also no mention of the nature of the Biden response to the outbreak that only some in the mainstream—so very afraid of a Trumpist return on the heels of Weimar incompetence built in from day one—are beginning to acknowledge.[1038]

Along with the near-absence of real-world applications of the viral phylogeography U.S. science helped build as a field, the country is at best offering an empty gesture of a response to the Omicron variant.[1039] As what little phylogeography is conducted in the United States showed last year—excellent work—we're repeatedly six weeks behind any identified index case.[1040] We should expect no different from Omicron, now discovered to have been circulating in Europe at least a week before South Africa.[1041]

We're left with slack suggestions from the podium that the American people are to be left with vaccine boosters, Trumpist travel bans (even as Omicron is already stateside), and these numbers for a national public health response:

> Biden will also pledge to deploy more than 60 emergency response teams throughout the country to help combat the spread of Omicron this winter, including more than 20 "monoclonal antibody strike teams" to help administer these treatments, which can help prevent serious illness and death from Covid-19, and more than 15 "CDC expert deployments" to help state and local health officials track Covid-19 outbreaks.[1042]

Sixty, twenty, and fifteen, for the entirety of the country? In comparison to efforts elsewhere, what a joke.[1043]

Meanwhile, the eviction moratoriums are long lapsed.[1044] They were so 2020. Corporate profit margins are at their widest since 1950, up 37 percent in a year, with labor's share back down to near-postwar lows.[1045] One hundred new billionaires were certified this pandemic and 3.3 million Americans newly fallen into poverty.[1046] Hospital ERs and ICUs are widespread in their functional collapse.[1047]

All markers that the social fabric that sets the exposure matrix at the front end of infection continues to unravel, while a few Seal Team Six nerds doomed to fail to clean up the back end are presented as enough.[1048] Exactly the kind of strike forces Daszak proposed and implemented for epizootic interventions abroad.[1049]

Corruption isn't just about official lying or envelopes of cash.

—PATREON, DECEMBER 2, 2021

Station Ten

"Aches and pains. A sudden high fever. Difficulty breathing. Look,"
the epidemiologist said, "it's a fast incubation period. If you're
exposed, you're sick in three or four hours and dead in a day or
two."
"We're going to take a quick commercial break," the newscaster
said.

— Emily St. John Mandel (2014)

NEARLY TWO YEARS LATER and my August 2020 summary of
the various hypotheses about the origins of COVID-19 still rings true
enough to me.[1050]

I said then we should remain open to exploring a variety of possible explanations, even as I still lean to the long-haul field hypothesis:
SARS-CoV-2 emerged across a wending capital-led ecotone from
southwest China's encroached-upon forests up through wild food and
industrial livestock supply lines extending thousands of kilometers
east and north.

The main contenders, however, have since been updated.

Lab Leak 1

The Bioscience Resource Project has focused on both debunking the possibility of a field origins and marshalling more evidence in favor of the lab leak.

Jonathan Latham and Allison Wilson claim only southern China as home to an "exotic" palate that may have served as a COVID-19 source, even as the Wuhan Huanan Seafood Wholesale Market hosted a variety of wild foods species.[1051] Few bat species and circulating coronavirus have been documented in Hubei, Wuhan's province, if one assumes the spillover event that led to the Wuhan outbreak must have been local.[1052]

Latham and Wilson promised to put numbers on the unlikelihood of such a local emergence.[1053] But they skipped past niche modeling of local conditions that might promote or block spillover. They skipped the combinatorials of emergent molecular adaptations. Their back-of-the-envelope calculation appears more a rudimentary appeal to incredulity.

With bats inhabiting locales around the world and given the world's population (7 billion), the Bioscience Resource Project team offers that the chance a Wuhan resident (11 million) would serve as patient zero is 1 in 630 (11 million/7 billion). The same unlikelihood could be calculated for any spillover event, as all pathogens emerge in the specific places at specific times under specific conditions that Latham and Wilson dismiss:

> It truly is very, very, unlikely that a natural zoonotic pandemic would start in Wuhan. Yet no commentator on the outbreak seems to have properly acknowledged the true scale of this improbability.[1054]

The team argues the improbabilities extend to the SARS strains that happen to be under study at the Wuhan Institute of Virology. Of the twenty-eight documented coronaviruses, the one that WIV studied is also closely related to the SARS-CoV-2 that emerged.

The counterargument is that Zheng-Li Shi's lab at WIV studied this coronavirus pre- and post-pandemic because the strain showed itself previously capable of setting off an epidemic of deadly SARS.[1055] Latham and Wilson claim Zheng-Li Shi presumed no such focus, as several different strains of alpha and betacoronaviruses have spilled over into humans. The difference, however, is that WIV was studying strains associated with SARS-1. Except MERS—which emerged in the Middle East—none of the other spillover coronaviruses proved deadly or infectious enough to set off a detectable regional epidemic.

So, that SARS-2 emerged out of the same clade as the SARS-1-related strains WIV was studying represents to the BRP team a marker of a lab leak. But given SARS-1's deadliness and track record as a near-pandemic strain, that might be exactly the strain to study. It explains the long list of publications about SARS-like coronaviruses Latham and Wilson listed the WIV lab was studying. So, the notion that such a second trip to the pandemic well came out of a pathogen with attributes, and out of conditions, that might be spillover-ready doesn't read as the "surprising coincidence" Latham and Wilson claim. It's not a 17,640–1 chance—1/630 people multiplied by 1/28 SARS strains—the BRP team declares.

Latham and Wilson claim that critics will dismiss such geographic and phylogenetic evidence as merely circumstantial. The irony is that the BRP argument depends on abstracting out exactly such evidence by claiming every coronavirus strain (and every locale) equally likely to serve as a source to arrive at these 17,640–1 odds.

Lab Leak 2

In February 2022, a Hungarian team claimed it found traces of genetic signatures of what may be a lab leak strain.[1056] The team from Eötvös Loránd University performed a sweeping bioinformatic search across publicly available genetic sequences for early traces of the virus.[1057] The team reports it found an impossible complete SARS-2 genome, as well as mitochondrial DNA from humans, Chinese hamsters, and green monkeys in sequences from Antarctic soil samples collected December 2018–January 2019.

The soil samples were originally sampled from King George Island to test for the effects of sea animal activities on the nitrogen cycle microbial community.[1058] The samples had been sent to Sangon Biotech in Shanghai in December 2019 for DNA sequencing and may have been contaminated with samples Sangon sequenced for the Wuhan Institute of Virology. The signal for the soil SARS-2 genome proved strong (with reported average depth or unique reads reported first as 5.2x and then 17x).[1059] The mutations unique to the sequences were captured by multiple runs. Importantly, these SARS-2 sequences phylogenetically grouped with early pandemic isolates from the field.

How did this happen? The sequences may have been folded into the Antarctic reports from previous reads on the same flow cell at the Sangon facility in Shanghai.[1060] Flow cells are channels that adsorb mobile DNA fragments of 200–500 base pairs into random sequence libraries that are subsequently aligned together by high-power computing.[1061] The cells are large enough to take on billions of segments, increasing capacity, yes, but also increasing the likelihood of such barcode misalignment errors, including the kind of mix-and-match of a COVID-host sample and an environmental sample from Antarctica.

The mitochondrial DNA found may represent the host cells for the COVID sequences: decidedly non-Antarctic humans of a rare South Asian haplotype, as well as Chinese hamsters (*Cricetulus griseus*) and green monkeys (*Chlorocebus sabeus*).[1062] In vitro work on SARS receptors and vaccine development has been conducted on CHO lines made from Chinese hamster cells and Vero E6 and COS-7 cell lines from green monkeys. Combinations of hamster and green monkey lines have also been used in COVID-19 research. In something of an unintended positive control, the pouched lamprey, found widely in the Southern Hemisphere, was also found in the flow cell analysis.

I find this possibility intriguing. Others agree, including evolutionary geneticist Jesse Bloom:

My analysis confirmed main findings of first preprint: some samples did contain #SARSCoV2 reads, with most reads in 3 of

11 samples. In addition, some reads contained three key mutations: C8782T, C18060T, and T28144C, although there is clearly
a mixed viral population.

Those three mutations are intriguing because they are all
"ancestral" mutations that move the sequence *closer* to the
bat CoV relatives RaTG13 and BANAL-20-52 relative to first
reported Wuhan-Hu-1 sequence from the Huanan Seafood
Market.

A virus with those three mutations relative to Wuhan-Hu-1
is one of the two plausible progenitors for all currently known
human #SARSCoV2 (the other plausible progenitor has
C29095T rather than C18060T).[1063]

Although the stochastic recycling across mutations that RNA viruses
engage from one outbreak to the next makes Bloom walk back the
definitive "ancestral" nature of the mutations. That is, these mutations
subsequently emerged repeatedly, including in the Omicron variant.

As Bloom continues, there are also complications in the chro-
nology of the sequencing. The December 2019 submission of the
Antarctic soil doesn't mean the actual sequencing was conducted
(and the misalignment error introduced) before China's announced
start of the outbreak in late December. Against the *Wall Street
Journal's* editorial *j'accuse* that the Antarctica samples marked much
earlier COVID-19 in Wuhan, some of the first COVID samples
collected from already registered early Wuhan patients could have
been amplified in CHO and Vero E6 cells before arriving at Sangon's
facility for sequencing.[1064]

The Wuhan Market

In the early days of the pandemic, much focus was placed upon the
Huanan market. Subsequent environmental testing found uneven
support for a wild foods spillover there.[1065] Some of the first human
cases also were detected beyond the market itself, redirecting attention to alternate explanations.

Two years later and research returned the Wuhan market possibility front and center. Evolutionary geneticist Michael Worobey's team recently detected two different strains of SARS-2 in humans who visited the market in late 2019.[1066]

Here's the market story so far as the Worobey team (and the literature they collect) tell it. The two strains—lineages A and B—overlapped in time, with B starting a few weeks earlier, but not before early November 2019. Lineage A, on the other hand, retained two nucleotide substitutions found in coronavirus infecting *Rhinolophus*, the horseshoe bat genus, the likely ultimate source. All the SARS-2 isolates sequenced from humans associated with the market and all the environmental samples taken from the market are lineage B. The lineage A sequences were found in humans who lived near or visited close to the market. Lineage B's slightly earlier start, the Worobey team suggests, may account for B's predominance in China's early outbreak well beyond Wuhan.

The team published a second report on the geospatials of the December 2019 cases, finding all these early cases—both SARS-2 lineages—distributed in and around the market.[1067] Previous work had shown human cases (and positive environmental samples) in the market itself were most closely associated with the western end of the market where most of the live-mammal vendors were set up. The new analysis found the spatial connection strongest for patients who lived in the area *without* direct association with the market, indicating that community transmission had by this time already begun. The analysis ruled out an elderly population vulnerable to COVID near the market that would have biased case geographies. By January and February, the outbreak had spread to the rest of Wuhan (with no market-specific signal left).

Against the lab leak hypothesis, the Worobey team declared two putative index cases that had nothing to do with the market, and were first marked as getting infected in early December, in actuality took ill in late December. Those earlier dates were a clerical error. That leaves a Huanan market vendor the earliest case with a documented onset date. Against the Worobey group's argument, however, alluding to SARS-1's origins in a wild food market does not serve as evidence in favor of the same hypothesis for SARS-2, the kind of domain error members of this group have repeatedly made.[1068]

The second report also listed a series of SARS-susceptible live animals that were sold at the market November and December 2019. The team's Chris Newman had previously co-conducted an investigation of the market, and three others in Wuhan, May–November 2019, finding thirty-eight wild-caught and farmed wildlife species sold at the four markets.[1069] Among those observed at the Huanan market in November 2019 were animals previously documented to be susceptible to SARS at the family level of taxonomy, including some to SARS-2: raccoon dog, hog badger, Asian badger, Chinese hare, Chinese bamboo rat, Chinese muntjac, and red fox. The raccoon dogs, Chinese muntjacs, and red foxes were among caged animals photographed at the market in December 2019.

Setting aside "Huanan" refers to South China, the list puts to rest Latham and Wilson's overgeneralization that such sales are limited to southern provinces. But how does this translate to SARS-2's appearance? None of the PCR tests of the 457 samples taken from 188 animals across eighteen mammal species in and outside the market proved SARS-positive.[1070] Nor did nearly 80,000 samples taken across China. The Worobey team points out, however, that most of the 80,000 were sampled from species unlikely to be SARS-2-susceptible, including cattle and chickens, or from isolates collected long before SARS-2 arose or from regions of China unlikely to host possible ultimate and intermediate sources.

The 188 animals tested, the Worobey team further reported, included none of the species the group identified on-sale at the market November 2019. Instead, cats, dogs, snakes, rabbits, hedgehogs, pigs, chickens, salamanders, crocodiles, turtles, fish, and sheep were tested. Not a single raccoon dog. Nor any of the farms supplying these animals or the workers along the supply chain.

The first report investigated where genomics, phylogeny, and epidemic modeling meet. The report showed previously identified intermediate haplotypes between the A and B lineages—putatively connecting them by evolution—are in fact artifacts of contamination or bioinformatics.[1071] That the two lineages are indeed separate.

The team reconstructed an ancestral haplotype to both lineages that differs from previous attempts published in the literature.[1072] The maximum likelihood ancestral reconstruction of nonrecombinant regions of the early SARS-2 genome converged upon a combined sequence that is evolved further away from the closest bat ancestor but before the lineages diverged.[1073] The method offers a closer look at the likely line of evolution than an outgroup comparison with a bat sequence. The reconstruction differed by 381 nucleotide substitutions from the first reference human SARS-2 infection (Wuhan-Hu-1), including those two nucleotide substitutions lineage A retained, making lineage A closer to the reconstructed ancestor (even if lineage B *spread* first and farther in the early days).[1074]

The team insisted on noting, however, that evolutionary reversions were a common phenomenon even in samples isolated in the early days through February 2020.[1075] So an isolate further down the line, even early on in the pandemic, could seem as if closer to the recon-structed ancestor, but really isn't.

Worobey's group use the reconstructed ancestor in a novel Bayesian phylodynamic tree whose construction both reconstructed the coales-cent process for the tree and the genetic sequence of the most recent common ancestor. The reconstruction, the group declares, recapitu-lated documented substitution biases across the SARS-2 genome.

The team next modeled whether one or two introductions were most likely. They simulated epidemics with a small range of doubling times around 2.65 days given the rapid spread in the early days. How did these simulations jibe with the model of coalescent evolution?

Long story short, it was those simulations showing two introduc-tions matched up with the coalescent and sequence reconstructions that were best supported, in part because too many samples of both lineages were present in the early days to be accounted for by an ana-genetic event by which one lineage evolved from the other. The early outbreak was likely a polytomy, with different ancestral sequences at their origins. The team points out that many a Chinese city would subsequently be hit by such a combination, as both lineages spread to the same locales in the early pandemic.

Four additional implications follow, the team concluded. First, the most recent common ancestor of the two lineages was not in a human. Second, given the epidemic simulation showing so few cases at the most recent common ancestor, any cryptic circulation in Wuhan before December was so minimal as to be likely undetectable, an inference supported by thousands of SARS-2-negative samples from an influenza-like outbreak widely sampled in the months leading up to the pandemic.[1076]

Third, the two lineages were likely only the successful spillover events. The team simulated that it took five such events—perhaps as many as fifteen—to produce the two lineages, the others failing to infect enough susceptibles and burning out on their own. I'll add that the results raise the question of which is more likely: that two—or more—different SARS-2 lineages arose out of separate live animals at the market or that they emerged from two separate lab escapes? Thought experiments in probability can be played against each of the competing hypotheses.

For the fourth implication, the Worobey team concluded that two lineages running successfully one after the other means additional molecular adaptation was unlikely needed to spread the virus human-to-human. That capacity may have been in place even before entering whatever intermediate species set things off at the market. That grim possibility sparks the terrible thought of an airborne zoonotic RNA virus going epidemiologically radioactive once it reaches—or, given our two lineages, repeatedly reaches—an evolutionary threshold in a city of susceptibles.

The Worobey team published its results earlier than it intended because they were made aware of another surprise publication. Director of the Chinese Center for Disease Control and Prevention George Gao led a collaboration of Chinese scientists that posted results of the 923 environmental samples and 457 animal samples—corpses, strays, and feces—collected in the Huanan market early 2020.[1077]

Seventy-three of the environmental samples proved SARS-2-positive, most in the western zone of the market where live animals were sold. Forty-four positives were detected among twenty-one vendors, nineteen operating out of the western end. The Gao team suggested that the breadth of the positives indicates the virus had been circulating for some time in December.

Live viruses were isolated from three environmental samples and whole genome sequences were produced from three more. No samples from eighteen species tested were positive. The Gao team's table of animal samples includes some of the species the Worobey team claimed weren't sampled—hedgehog, muntjac, bamboo rat—although many were indeed missing, including the raccoon dog.

Does the question of whether any of the environmental samples included host cells other than human—which would help identify the source host—remain open? Jon Cohen reported in *Science*:

> The preprint by Gao and colleagues only notes that those samples contain DNA from many animals without specifying which one—other than humans. "The authors have already done the analysis, they have just not put all the results needed to interpret them in their paper," says evolutionary biologist Andrew Rambaut of the University of Edinburgh, a co-author of both [Worobey] studies. "This will undoubtedly be fixed if the paper gets through peer review."[1078]

On the one hand, the Gao team's Figure 4A implies exactly such unidentified species. Indeed, evolutionary geneticist Virginie Courtier-Orgogozo commented under the preprint: "Figure 4A: it would be nice to show also the list of species with significant correlation."[1079]

On the other hand, the Gao paper offers commentary that appears explicitly contradictory:

> To explore the potential origins of the SARS-COV-2, we conducted RNA-seq analysis using 27 SARS-CoV-2 positive environmental

samples collected on January 1st, 2020 from the [Huanan Seafood Market]. We analyzed the correlation of SARS-CoV-2 and the abundance of other species. The abundance of *Homo sapiens* showed the correlation to SARS-CoV-2, which highly suggests the SARS-CoV-2 might have derived from *Homo sapiens* in the [market]. No animals were included, implying that no animal host of SARS-CoV-2 can be deduced.[1080]

Lab leak proponents see the market as at best a superspreader event, an interpretation the Gao report champions, the authors declaring themselves unable to rule out an introduction from outside the market from animals and humans alike, as far as outside China itself—a position China's government supports—although not, it appears, from the Wuhan Institute of Virology.[1081] The Gao report repeats another governmental favorite that Zheng-Li Shi also floated in a talk in France: that SARS-2 could have been imported into China in frozen foods from abroad.[1082]

If the market is Wuhan's first epicenter, the Gao team explains it's all a matter of a busy day at the market: "The market might have acted as an amplifier due to the high number of visitors every day, causing many initially identified infection clusters in the early stage of the outbreak as indicated in the Report of WHO-convened global study of origins of SARS-CoV."[1083]

But didn't the team also identify the western end of the market with all those live animals the center of the positive environmental samples?

The Worobey group found the distribution of what were for them available positive environmental samples from the market was predicted independently by the distance to the closest vendor selling live animals and the distance to the nearest human case.[1084] By an implicit variography, the vendor distance supports the bigger spatial lag for positive environmental samples. That is, the vendors cast the bigger infection shadow.

A separate spatial relative risk analysis identified two vendors in the southwest region of the market—one selling live mammals, the other selling meat of unknown type—with the greatest risk density, controlling for the uneven sampling scheme. The human cases were centered elsewhere in the market, but the Worobey team declares humans in such a market more mobile than the animals. And not all the human infections that resulted were likely symptomatic.

Jesse Bloom weighed in again, this time that the three reports on the market here weren't the knife in the heart of the lab leak theory they implied.[1085] Bloom—in a running dispute with the likes of Worobey co-authors Kristian Andersen and Robert Garry—offered that he is especially skeptical that there were two zoonotic jumps at the market.[1086]

On the basis of fourteen partial sequences of early outpatient isolates collected by Wuhan University that against practice were deleted from the NIH's Sequence Read Archive and that Bloom cleverly recovered off of SRA's Google Cloud, Bloom concluded in 2021 that the samples collected from the Huanan market were *not* representative of the early Wuhan outbreak.[1087] "The progenitor of known SARS-CoV-2 sequences," Bloom wrote, "likely contained three mutations relative to the market viruses that made it more similar to SARS-CoV-2's bat coronavirus relatives."

The Worobey team pushed back that their modeling showed the likelihood one of the strains detected evolved from the other given the genetic sequences to be much less than two separate spillover events. Multiple zoonotic events characterized the launch of SARS-1 in 2002–2003 as well. If a SARS strain has arrived at an exact spillover combinatorial of evolution and circumstances, there's no reason that a wild food market can't serve as a superspreader conduit as any New York airport or Wisconsin supper club.

Worobey captures the frustration with putting a stake into the question of origins:

With the way that people have been able to just push aside any and all evidence that points away from a lab leak, I do fear that even if there were evidence from one of these samples that was full of red fox DNA and SARS-CoV-2 that people might say, "We still think it actually came from the handler of that red fox."[1088]

Field Hypotheses Farther Afield

But why the frustration? Does it emerge from beyond the matter of a lab leak as an unkillable and therefore unscientific hypothesis? Why does a stake need to be driven into the question as opposed to being answered as evidence and inference accumulate in the decade ahead? What are the origins of the compulsion to wrap up the matter in such short order, to the point of excluding even CDC director Robert Redfield from discussions?[1089]

An article by *Vanity Fair*'s Katherine Eban on Peter Daszak and the K Street machinations of the EcoHealth Alliance unpacks the financial and even emotional bonding many scientists enjoy with their imperial benefactors:

[Jesse] Bloom's paper was the product of detective work he'd undertaken after noticing that a number of early SARS-CoV-2 genomic sequences mentioned in a published paper from China had somehow vanished without a trace. The sequences, which map the nucleotides that give a virus its unique genetic identity, are key to tracking when the virus emerged and how it might have evolved. In Bloom's view, their disappearance raised the possibility that the Chinese government might be trying to hide evidence about the pandemic's early spread. . . .

[Then-NIH director Francis] Collins immediately organized a Zoom meeting for Sunday, June 20. He invited two outside scientists, evolutionary biologist Kristian Andersen and virologist Robert Garry, and allowed Bloom to do the same. Bloom chose [evolutionary biologist Sergei] Pond and Rasmus Nielsen, a genetic biologist. That it was shaping up like an old-fashioned duel with seconds in attendance did not cross Bloom's mind at the time. But six months after that meeting, he remained so troubled by what transpired that he wrote a detailed account, which *Vanity Fair* obtained.[1090]

Astonishingly, Andersen offers to purge Bloom for presidential medical adviser Anthony Fauci, also at the meeting:

> After Bloom described his research, the Zoom meeting became "extremely contentious," he wrote. Andersen leapt in, saying he found the preprint "deeply troubling." If the Chinese scientists wanted to delete their sequences from the database, which NIH policy entitled them to do, it was unethical for Bloom to analyze them further, he claimed. And there was nothing unusual about the early genomic sequences in Wuhan.
>
> Instantly, Nielsen and Andersen were "yelling at each other," Bloom wrote, with Nielsen insisting that the early Wuhan sequences were "extremely puzzling and unusual."
>
> Andersen—who'd had some of his emails with Fauci from early in the pandemic publicly released through FOIA requests—leveled a third objection. Andersen, Bloom wrote, "needed security outside his house, and my preprint would fuel conspiratorial notions that China was hiding data and thereby lead to more criticism of scientists such as himself."
>
> Fauci then weighed in, objecting to the preprint's description of Chinese scientists "surreptitiously" deleting the sequences. The word was loaded, said Fauci, and the reason they'd asked for the deletions was unknown.
>
> That's when Andersen made a suggestion that surprised Bloom. He said he was a screener at the preprint server, which gave him access to papers that weren't yet public. He then offered to either entirely delete the preprint or revise it "in a way that would leave no record that this had been done."[1091]

Fauci pivoted away when he got what he wanted:

At that point, both Fauci and Collins distanced themselves from Andersen's offer, with Fauci saying, as Bloom recalled it, "Just for the record, I want to be clear that I never suggested you delete or revise the preprint." They seemed to know that Andersen had gone too far.[1092]

Andersen had spoken what he should have only done. This is what happens when you hire a scientist for a hitman's job.

The science the Worobey team presents meanwhile supports other possibilities beyond lab and market the two sides here contend. I think the team's fourth inference that additional adaptations were unlikely needed to spread human-to-human in the market helps set the story of COVID-19's origins—as our group proposed in 2020—back through the live food supply line out of Wuhan.[1093]

The fourth inference also lends deductive support to evolutionary genomic work to the effect that the SARS-2 strain or precursors may have been circulating in humans for years, long before Wuhan.[1094] Weirdly, against its own premises and results, the Worobey group denies the possibility—despite its own discussion of multiple bouts of zoonosis and reverse-zoonosis—claiming instead that SARS-2 was unlikely circulating in humans before November 2019.

Medical and evolutionary geneticist Kostantinos Voskarides recently summarized the possibilities this way:

Taking into account the SARS-CoV-2 dating and its [most recent common ancestor] properties, three scenarios are most probable: (a) The SARS-CoV-2 ancestor has been incubating for years inside bats, accumulating mutations, and probably through a random event, e.g. in the Huanan wet market, the virus was transmitted in humans, (b) A less virulent SARS-CoV-2 ancestor was infecting humans for years, until accumulation of mutations increased its virulence, (c) The SARS-CoV-2 ancestor has been circulating in intermediate hosts until transmission to humans by a random event.[1095]

Detecting earlier SARS-2 spillover events before Wuhan is likely very difficult to test at this point, but the lack of present evidence doesn't refute the scenario as a *logical* possibility—exemplary of Worobey's nightmare of ever-permutating possibilities even as data accumulates.

I know that the Worobey group is attempting to cut off the notion SARS-2 arrived in Wuhan by train rather than by a truck of animals, but multiple skeins of infection across species and within are possible, with the Wuhan spillover the culmination of evolution and opportunity that punched through to pandemicity. Worobey himself, who helped pin the temporal origins of HIV, knows these epidemiological parallelisms well.[1096] It isn't just the Wuhan spillover, or the identity of the source species in a vendor's stall, it's the metapopulation of "natural" experiments across large tracts—in this case, as far south as Yunnan or Indochina—that serves as the origins of COVID-19.

On its face, then, it appears I share with the Peter Daszak team I've criticized on multiple accounts a sense of the scope of SARS-2 origins:

> We use probabilistic risk assessment and data on human-bat contact, human SARSr-CoV seroprevalence, and antibody duration to estimate that ~400,000 people (median: ~50,000) are infected with SARSr-CoVs annually in South and Southeast Asia.[1097]

The Daszak team, however, limits the implications and applications of such an expansive spatio-demographics to local communities breaching bat landscapes:

> Our approach may assist in better identifying regions for targeted surveillance of local communities at risk of spillover, for conducting viral discovery programs to identify novel bat-CoVs, for COVID-19 origins tracing, and for estimating human surveillance targets to identify spillover events earlier and more accurately. All of these are key goals for pandemic preparedness and prevention, and if used to target future surveillance and dis-

ease control, may help to reduce the risk of future COVID-like outbreaks. . . .

We estimated bat-human contact using data from previous human-animal contact surveys and ethnographic investigations, but contacts likely vary widely across the region due to different cultural practices and traditions. The type of contact may be critical to assessing the risk of transmission (e.g. hunting and butchering vs. living near a bat colony), and some types of contact may be unrecognized and therefore unreported (e.g. exposure to feces or urine on surfaces).[1098]

The Daszak team excises the circuits of capital out of New York, London, and Hong Kong, sources of capital that fund the worst deforestation and development driving disease emergence, as a matter of methodological operationalization.[1099]

It's these peculiar turns in the political economy of research that are monetized by Fauci's golden touch:

For more than a decade, EcoHealth Alliance hosted a series of cocktail parties at the Cosmos Club near DuPont Circle to discuss the prevention of viral outbreaks. There, expert biologists, virologists, and journalists mingled with the true guests of honor: federal government bureaucrats who were in the position to steer grants. . . .

Fauci signed on to give a presentation on the Zika virus at the Cosmos Club on March 30, and the RSVPs flowed in. The guests came from an array of deep-pocketed federal agencies: the Department of Homeland Security, the U.S. Agency for International Development, the Pentagon, even NASA. As Daszak would declare at a board meeting on December 15, the "Washington, DC cultivation events have been a great way to increase our visibility to federal funders," according to meeting minutes. A month earlier, Donald Trump had been elected president. One board member at the meeting asked what his incoming administration might mean for a conservation nonprofit dependent on federal grants. Daszak offered breezy reassurance: The organization's "apolitical mission" would help it adapt.[1100]

An EcoHealth Alliance wedded to such an ecologically abstracted set of GPS coordinates took first NIH money it schmoozed from Fauci, followed by agribusiness largesse, to pin blame on local small-holders for spillover events. As *Vanity Fair*'s Eban describes this "apolitical mission":

> One year, [EHA] proposed to honor at its annual benefit a mining company operating in Liberia that was paying it to assess the risks of Ebola virus. Another idea was to seek donations from palm-oil millionaires leveling rainforests who might be interested in "cleaning up" their image.[1101]

I described such EHA efforts in greenwashing the worst corporate offenders in 2016.[1102]

Beyond the possibility of a lab leak out of the Wuhan Institute of Virology that EHA helped fund, Alliance practices are helping select for the very pandemic strains out in the field from which it claims to be protecting us. The best way to control the future is to make it is one appalling epidemiological flex.

The gain-of-function studies EHA tried to hide represent a similar miscalculation.[1103] That line of research—selecting for dangerous SARS strains in the lab to see what made them dangerous—may have represented a Frankensteinian fascination with rewiring the SARS beast as operationalized by Department of Defense funding.[1104] But it also instantiated folding causality *down down down* into the objects of host and virus, rather than in their historical relationships with each other and the increasingly neoliberalized landscapes they share.

In that context, asking how many viruses dance on the head of a pin is as nonsensical as asking how many angels.

Other scientific approaches—based in statistical testing as any other—treat land, agriculture, disease, economics, and cultural premises in relational causalities far beyond singular coordinates or market stalls.[1105] These are foundationally different metaphysics than what most well-bred scientists trafficked into their work starting their very first day of university. "Science, in all its senses," dialectical biologists Richard Levins and Richard Lewontin put it,

> is a social process that both causes and is caused by social orga-
> nization. To do science is to be a social actor engaged, whether
> one likes it or not, in political activity. The denial of the inter-
> penetration of the scientific and the social is itself a political act,
> giving support to social structures that hide behind scientific
> objectivity to perpetuate dependency, exploitation, racism, elit-
> ism, colonialism.[1106]

An outcome the likes of Fauci and Daszak embody in decision after decision over long careers.

The Mojiang Mine

Jonathan Latham and Allison Wilson of the Bioscience Resource Project would continue their objections to hypotheses of a field emergence for SARS-2, referring to the 80,000 animals tested to total negative results.[1107] These negatives included eleven hundred bats in Hubei, Wuhan's province.

The lab leak proponents pivoted to some of the same literature that hypotheses of a field emergence far beyond Wuhan, as far south as Yunnan and into Indochina, focus on. In this direction, the team aimed for a rudimentary phylogeography that infers where SARS-2's direct ancestor emerged, based solely on percent genetic similarities and linear sample distances alone. No Markov chain, Monte Carlo Bayesian co-estimations of phylogeny, branch-specific molecu-lar clocks, ancestral spatial coordinates, or possible socioecological covariates.[1108] No accounting for variation in dispersal velocity.

The gaps aren't Latham and Wilson's fault. They instead beg why a more sophisticated analysis along these lines hasn't yet been pub-lished beyond mapping SARS-2's spread once within humans.[1109]

Latham and Wilson concluded the progenitor strain emerged out of, or nearby, the Mojiang, Yunnan, cave in which six men mining bat guano were apparently infected with coronavirus-like symptoms.[1110] Three of the miners died. Samples from the six were collected and analyzed at the Wuhan Institute of Virology, from which, incubated in a live model or cell line, Latham and Wilscon claim they likely escaped in late 2019.

Latham and Wilson declared their phylogeography refutes the frozen food, European origins, and bioweapon hypotheses of COVID-19's start. How, for instance, did a strain originating in Yunnan find its way into food shipped into China from abroad? In the other direction, what *does* this phylogeography show?

> Thus, if we knew nothing else about the origin of SARS-CoV-2 we would learn from this plot that, first, genetic variation among the bat viruses in this lineage is highly correlated with geographic location.
>
> Second, that the direct bat progenitor of SARS-CoV-2 came from a bat living at or near to the Mojiang mine in south-central Yunnan, China. In other words, the Mojiang area of Yunnan was the site of the key zoonotic leap where SARS-CoV-2's ancestor exited its bat reservoir.

Yunnan is certainly a favorite option for SARS-2's origins, however the virus ended up in Wuhan. Unfortunately, this phylogeography here, based on eight sequences alone separated by 40 to 100 years of evolution, offers no statistical test of the two assertions despite declarations of being "strongly correlated."

Hundreds of additional sequences along these evolutionary branches regularly and densely sampled by GPS coordinates—as work on other pathogens over much shorter time periods shows—could support a multitude of spatial origin stories: contiguous range expansion, restricted dispersal with isolation by distance, long-distance colonization followed by isolation by distance, multiple waves in multiple directions, expansion then collapse (among other possibilities).[1111] Especially with bat species swapping coronaviruses over habitat ranges stretching across the continent. A linear decay in great-circle distance and phylogenetic relatedness is hardly the only possible outcome.

Is this version of the lab leak theory best characterized as another version of the field hypotheses Latham and Wilson despise? The Daszak team, for instance, writes:

> Cave habitats were classified by the IUCN as suitable for nearly all species in our analyses, and carbonate rock outcrops (used here as a proxy for caves) made up a large proportion of species [areas of habitat]. Visiting caves, collecting guano, and using bat guano in crop production are likely particularly high-risk activities given these findings.[1112]

Latham and Wilson see the matter in the opposite direction: "The Chinese and international searches for SARS-CoV-2-related coronaviruses were supposed to reveal a zoonotic origin and refute a lab leak. Instead, they have achieved the almost direct opposite."[1113] How else but by transferring the mine samples up to the Wuhan Virology Institute did a SARS-2 of Yunnan origins end up in Hubei?

The Bioscience Resource Project team claims the decade it took researchers to find SARS-1 intermediaries doesn't excuse SARS-2's present field mystery given the much greater capacity for sampling and sequencing now available. The Worobey group, if you remember, claimed no such scope of sampling had *actually* been pursued, with sampling limited to cattle and chickens and the like, or samples collected long before SARS-2 emerged.[1114] Latham and Wilson pushed back that given Yunnan was long a SARS province of interest, sampling is more than merely adequate:

> Numerous different virology teams extensively sampled in Yunnan, especially at the Mojiang mine, even before the pandemic struck. For example, Zheng-Li Shi's colleagues alone visited the Mojiang mine seven times in the years following the

2012 outbreak. At least three other teams of virologists sampled the mine looking for coronaviruses prior to the pandemic. By their own accounts, WIV researchers alone took thousands of samples and found hundreds of coronaviruses. Post-pandemic, [the Associated Press] documented numerous wildlife sampling research projects in China as part of what it called a "hidden hunt for coronavirus origins" especially in bats, including in Yunnan.[1115]

As best practices suggest we test these hypotheses by attempting to refute them, similar sampling densities should also be pursued *elsewhere*. But, as Latham and Wilson describe, as of 2021, the publicly funded EHA refused to release even the Yunnan sequences to the public.

While the competing hypotheses alternately converge and clash, all three often miss the point. Proponents of the competing hypotheses willfully omit *why* coronaviruses are spilling over into human populations at a greater clip, whatever their ultimate delivery system outbreak-to-outbreak. The why, to which we will return, might matter to hypotheses of SARS-2's origins.

But, first, what of these Yunnan sources? Recent work on genomic recombination in SARS-2's inferred progenitor strains shows that bat genus *Rhinolophus*—the horseshoe bat—is "unambiguously" the source, perhaps directly out of one such cave, but also maybe through a wild food animal or traditional livestock intermediate.[1116] The work, led by molecular phylogeneticist Spyros Lytras, combines recombinant analysis, geographic distributions, and bat species hosting each sarbecovirus isolate to offer a next generation history of SARS-2's emergence.

Long story short, the most recent common ancestors shared by SARS-2 and the two evolutionarily closest bat isolates we have in hand are inferred forty and fifty years back in time, respectively. That offers a lot of time—eons in viral generations—over which many multiple SARS-like strains experimented across species. The Lytras team reports multiple recombinant events across multiple *Rhinolophus* species. Indeed, SARS-2's closest sister group includes Yunnan isolates found in *R. pusillus, R. malayanus,* and *R. spp,* with some recombinant segments originating in other provinces and in other kinds of coronaviruses nowhere near related to SARS-2:

> These relationships indicate ancestral movement of the nCoV viruses across large geographic ranges in China, spanning Yunnan in southwest China and Zhejiang on the east coast.
>
> As more countries initiate wildlife-infecting coronavirus sampling and sequencing efforts, the geographic range of the nCoV clade linked to bat host species will be further refined, evident from the recent reporting of bat sarbecoviruses closely related to SARS-CoV-2 from: 1) two samples collected in Cambodia from *Rhinolophusshameli* (RShSTT182 and RShSTT200) confirmed by whole-genome analysis, and 2) five bat samples from *Rhinolophusacuminatus* collected in Thailand with one fully sequenced genome of virus RacCS203.[1117]

The resulting dynamics in time and space—with closely related isolates recently found in Laos—batter the Bioscience Resource Project phylogeography of its easy-peasy conclusion.[1118] The Lytras team's results speak to a long history between bat and virus:

> Co-circulation and recombination between these viruses in the last few centuries is responsible for the observed patterns in their inferred evolutionary history, despite the current geographic range of at least 2,500km. This wide distribution of related viruses, including shared recombination breakpoints, highlights an important feature of bat species: Their frequently overlapping/sympatric ranges will provide ample opportunities for transmissions of viral variants from one bat species (or subspecies) to another.[1119]

It's a spatial scope that could also frame the human-specific sarbecoviruses that spill over into humans, some circulating for years, experimenting with our immune system, perhaps, as the Lytras team suggests for bats, using recombination as a mode of antigenic shift out from underneath host control.[1120] And perhaps it is all that evolutionary shadow work that helped inform one superstar strain about pandemicity upon being shipped to Wuhan in late 2019.

Indeed, that's exactly the supply-line scenario Latham and Wilson presented for SARS-1: "Presumably, civets being farmed in Kunming became infected via contact with bats. Subsequently, ones infected with the direct progenitor of SARS One were then transported to Guangdong [1200 km away]."[1121] We need ask then, other than as lab samples to the Wuhan lab, how else could a Yunnan SARS-2 end up in Hubei?

Certainly the virus was long well prepped for Wuhan, as the Worobey team itself admits. The work by Zheng-Li Shi's team we reviewed earlier in this volume offered a molecular mechanism by which SARS-like coronaviruses can splatter across human populations directly from bats.[1122]

Evolutionary phylogeneticist Oscar MacLean and colleagues identified the kind of natural selection underway at the base of the SARS-2 evolutionary branch.[1123] In bat lineages there, circulating hundreds of years ago, the team detected significant bouts of diversifying evolution in the Spike, ORF3a, and ORF nucleocapsid proteins likely associated with immune evasion. It also found depletion of dinucleotide CpG composition—cytosine followed by a guanine—associated with adaptation to bats' antiviral attack.

The branch also offered little evidence of additional selection special for humans. The virus appeared a born generalist, primed by combating the bat immune system to easily spill over into all kinds of other animals. That's a capacity we see in avian influenzas passed between migratory waterfowl gathering in the Arctic Circle every summer and that spill over into multiple poultry species farther south.[1124]

Additional sequences found in intermediate species before SARS-2's emergence might change that story. Maybe there *were* upticks of human-specific adaptations, but the MacLean team maintains its analysis here indicates probably not.

Either way, upon hitting the human jackpot, SARS-2 underwent little in the way of immune-driven corrections. Against early
phylogenetic work constrained by uneven sequence sampling, the
MacLean team found that once in humanity, SARS-2 evolved nearly
neutrally.[1125] Surges of positive selection, occurring only now and
then, survived being immediately purged out by traveling atop waves
of epidemic spread or upon evolution as new variants.

The team concludes with the kind of warning the Zheng-Li Shi
work implied. That the diversity of sarbecoviruses on the very edge
of human specificity, splattering across human populations and livestock, means a SARS-3 is just a recombination away. No lab leak
needed.

Is Solving the Mystery Even an Objective?

Whatever the ironies in the various hypotheses enriching each other,
are we in danger of producing a COVID industry aimed at reproducing itself in this high-stakes competition?

The eminent ecologist Charles Krebs recently described ecology's
own research mill:

> There is an extensive literature on hypothesis testing which can
> be crudely summarized by "Observations of X" which can be
> explained by hypothesis A, B, or C each of which have unique
> predictions associated with them. A series of experiments are
> carried out to test these predictions and the most strongly sup-
> ported hypothesis, call it B*, is accepted as current knowledge.
> Explanation B* is useful scientifically only if it leads to a new set
> of predictions D, E, and F which are then tested. This chain of
> explanation is never simple. There can be much disagreement
> which may mean sharpening the hypotheses following from
> Explanation B*. At the same time there will be some scientists
> who despite all the accumulated data still accept the Flat Earth
> Hypothesis. If you think this is nonsense, you have not been
> reading the news about the Covid epidemic.[1126]

While I agree with Krebs's warnings about misdirected efforts favoring mathematical modeling without enough data, the question remains, other than wacky conspiracy theories, which of the contending hypotheses for COVID's origins represents the "Flat Earth" hypothesis we should abandon bothering with?

"Reading the news" tells me that I'd like to see researchers continue to pursue all *four* classes of hypothesis: the saner lab leaks, the Huanan market, the field beyond Wuhan, and capitalism's regional production of new natures. Some explanations may fall by the wayside—Roger Frutos's group recently rejected the miners' symptoms were SARS—but several may serve as an answer in combination.[1127]

I'm betting with critical geographers Neil Brenner and Swarnabh Ghosh that the last of the list here, almost entirely omitted from the search of SARS-2's origins, isn't optional:

> The agro-ecological transformations of the neoliberal epoch are not only tightly intermeshed with processes of concentrated urbanization, but have been directly materialized within operational landscapes of extended urbanization through a range of large-scale infrastructure investments, financial speculations, and associated political-ecological transformations.
>
> The extensively capitalized and financialized spatial infrastructures of agro-industrial supply chains have not received systematic attention in food regime scholarship, but they represent the socio-metabolic circuitry within which primary commodities are cultivated, harvested, and circulated from the soil, the field, and the warehouse to the shipping container and the world market, and through which the manifold political-economic and biophysical contradictions of those processes are articulated.
>
> It is here, in the forests, fields, extractive hinterlands, and logistics matrices of the Global South, where new spatial strategies of land enclosure, infrastructure investment, landscape fragmentation, land-use simplification, and territorial management have been elaborated, that the [emerging infectious diseases] of the

neoliberal era have been engendered and from which they have been projected into the global metropolitan network.[1128]

For how—or why—do the new interfaces of so-called disease reservoirs and periurban landscapes emerge? Why at a quickening pace? And in response to exactly which contexts do repeatedly sprung pathogens evolve? "Deforestation" isn't enough. It boxes away in expedient abstraction both the historical moment and who's responsible. The why—as Frutos's group also converges on—sets the question of pathogen origins on its head.[1129]

But this is a body of work the Faucis of the world bury because it represents as much a structural forensics of the imperial program as an epidemiological investigation. And the expropriation that brought about the worst of the resulting damage mustn't be traced back to its causal source if this way of life is to be preserved even unto its imminent collapse.

—PATREON, APRIL 11, 2022

Don't Look Up...
COVID's Infectious Period

There is nothing to think in death, albeit the death of an empire, nothing but the intrinsic nullity of being.

—ALAIN BADIOU (1998)

Anyone who wants to defecate in the drinking water should be allowed to. One-way pooping works, & those arguing that clean water is important should simply not drink, cook, bathe, or clean with drinking water. Anything less makes you a clean water fanatic. #1854CholeraEpidemic

—NEOLIBERAL JOHN SNOW (2022)

THE OMICRON VARIANT IS everywhere in the United States at this point.[1130] Last Wednesday the country registered a world-record 484,377 COVID cases, topping it again with 512,500, 647,067, and, including reports from over the weekend, over a million the following Monday.[1131]

Many Americans who hadn't gotten COVID before are getting it now. And many previously infected or vaccinated (or both) are getting infected too. Three million new cases, or one in a hundred Americans, in just a week.

Omicron isn't the only variant in the mix. Delta and others still churn on. But Omicron's molecular biology—marked by multiple amino acid replacements in the spike protein's receptor binding domain and furin cleavage site, the nucleocapside protein's N-terminal domain and serine/arginine-rich linker region, and a deletion in the nonstructural protein 1—has evolved in such a way that the new variant is much more infectious.[1132] This virus largely attacks receptors in the upper airway and less in the chest, making the turnaround time in transmission much shorter.[1133]

Declarations we needn't worry as nose-and-throat Omicron isn't as deadly as previous variants miss the point, conflating, in what is now a pandemic staple, public health and individual outcomes.[1134] A variant with a lower case fatality rate can kill many more people if the virus's attack rate approaches the whole population and its doubling time speeds up. The Delta variant doubled in infections every two to three weeks. Omicron is doubling every two to three days.[1135]

The number of Americans hospitalized with COVID topped 103,000 Monday, the highest level in a year and rapidly approaching the record of 130,000 when vaccines weren't available. U.S. deaths are clocking in over a thousand a day, with weekly deaths no less than 5,000 since September.[1136] The Centers for Disease Control and Prevention is forecasting 85,000 deaths in the next month.[1137]

Treatment options have also narrowed. On the virus's end, Omicron has evolved around two monoclonal antibody therapies: bamlanivimab and casirivimab.[1138] Previous COVID infection offers little natural antibody protection against Omicron.[1139] All the variants together are slowly evolving vaccine resistance, even, as we will return, vaccines presently remain effective against hospitalization.[1140]

On our end, where humans control things, treatment effectiveness declines when ERs and ICUs are overloaded with new cases. That failure of capacity is a conscious decision. As one nurse put it, "Don't use euphemisms like 'hospital beds' when what you actually mean is nursing staff. The hospitals have not run out of furniture."[1141] Beyond hospitals, the early pandemic policies aimed at "flattening the curve" and preserving hospital capacity—postponing mass gatherings, mask mandates, and bar and restaurant closures—are now long abandoned.[1142]

Pandemic as Political Anima

At the sight of the new wave of patients flipped on their bellies and long bread lines at overpriced testing sites, one can't help but circle back with grim satisfaction to the deaths of right-wing talk show hosts killed by the COVID they denied.[1143] Their passings represent nigh on biblical rebukes of the denialist campaigns that continue to lead thousands of Americans to their COVID graves.

The nature of the resulting damage pivots us from righteous anger to gutting horror. Overworked nurses and doctors speak of the "talking dead," fully conscious patients whose lung capacities have been so destroyed that only machines are keeping them alive.[1144] Some use their final hours to continue to argue their health collapse was caused by something other than COVID.[1145] Even at this late moment before the Gates of St. Peter, they continue to organize their life force around fine-tuning a political etiology that cost them those very lives.

Other denialists have moved out of doubting COVID exists into dismissing its standard treatment, at times to brutally satirical lengths. One skeptic earlier this year queried about using livestock ivermectin, the antiparasitic, as a suppository, complaining about the taste of the paste at the front end.[1146]

A failure to act at the government level is far different than choosing to endanger oneself, albeit in doing so endangering others. "Ron DeSantis," Democratic organizer Thomas Kennedy tweeted,

> shut down all state-operated COVID testing sites [in May] and refuses to open them up despite cases in Florida increasing 1,000% and people waiting up to six hours for a test. He has not been seen in public since Dec 17th.[1147]

With data repeatedly showing the unvaccinated more likely to be infected (five times more) or killed (thirteen times) by COVID than the vaccinated, the meaning of our moment clearly matters.[1148] Materialism extends into the social and semiotic and, by their impacts on our behavior and beliefs, on back to who lives and who dies.[1149]

But surviving isn't confirmation enough.

The deaths of denialists do not ratify the decisions those still living made as good calls. The deceased, even those radically opposed to standard public health, aren't worthy of a Darwin Award, to reference a tongue-in-cheek competition of real-life stories about people killing themselves accidentally in spectacularly dumb ways. Against the bumper sticker, reality does not have a liberal bias, in the sense that the nature of things doesn't just embody the operative presumptions of Manhattan's gentrified Upper West Side.

There are thousands of working people who got infected with COVID commuting to and working in brick-and-mortar businesses, servicing those affluent enough to be able to shelter in place in West Sides across the country. From transit workers to meatpackers.[1150] Or these workers were infected living in overcrowded housing, with less ventilation and fewer options for self-isolation.[1151] The wealthy have little cause for patting themselves on the back for good citizenship. There was nothing inherently smart or responsible in being able to commute online without government support.

Like water follows cracks in ice, COVID flows through a social structure built long before the virus arrived. The contention isn't mere poetics, but a standard concept in social epidemiology.[1152]

Occupational health scientist Marissa Baker connected computer use at work, interaction with public at work, and median annual wage by occupational sector before the pandemic.[1153] She showed that workers largely in management, business, and science were able to stay home and get paid comparatively well. Workers in other sectors—construction, maintenance, production, transportation, shipping, sales, and the service economy—were likely to either work directly with the public or work on office computers. The information economy and its related sectors depend on the real economy it now helps structure, with the lowest-paid workers exposed to the epidemiological elements.

Manipulation imposed and self-induced appeared to accompany that divide. We need ask whether some of these blue and pink collars took on COVID skepticism or indifference as a form of traumatic bonding, if only to be able to help them get up to go to work under dangerous conditions daily for months on end and without the union protections that U.S. liberals and rightists together helped strip out.[1154] In a country with no federally mandated paid sick leave.[1155]

Meatpackers have described the pressure meat companies and state governments placed on workers to go to work at the height of outbreaks:

> Workers complain that many of the changes have been aimed at managing perceptions, while stubborn problems remain: not enough distance between people stationed at some parts of the assembly line, inadequate stocks of hand sanitizer, and subtle pressure to come to work even when they are ill.
>
> "It gets thrown in our faces if we're sick," said Mariel Pastrana, 23, who has worked at the plant for nearly three years, and whose wages jumped from about $18 an hour to more than $26 under the new contract. "They keep saying, 'Production is slow, demand is going up.'". . .
>
> The four largest meatpackers—including JBS—have collectively paid out more than $3 billion in dividends to shareholders since the beginning of the pandemic, according to a recent analysis from the White House.
>
> At the same time, many cattle ranchers are going broke. People who work in slaughterhouses—among them immigrants from Latin America, Asia and Africa—say they still face a grim choice between their safety and their livelihoods. . . .
>
> Signs throughout the plant direct people to stay home when they are sick. But workers say supervisors still sometimes urge them to continue showing up.[1156]

A second social psychology in play appears as a deeply tended nostalgia for a structural apartheid that delivered whites of all classes the race-specific protections increasingly not available to the poorest. The diseases of despair accumulating in rural counties long before COVID manifested in the largest switches in voting Obama 2012 to Trump 2016.[1157] Indeed, better to die than allow Black and Brown people access to health care whites also now lack.[1158]

A recent poll found that while unvaccinated whites (36 percent) were much less concerned about COVID than vaccinated whites (75 percent), Black people both unvaccinated (78 percent) and vaccinated (90 percent) remained concerned.[1159] For the latter, the failure to vaccinate was divorced from a denialism of the problem and more likely associated with either a distrust of the medical establishment or failure of vaccine access.

Go to Work Jack

The survivorship bias vaccinated-to-unvaccinated is now serving as the rationale for the public policy that bleeds back out to COVID outcomes. U.S. governance serves as a mirror by which to confirm those self-serving, if also ill-supported, presumptions that survival is a moralistic rite.

From the federal mask recommendations suspended in May to White House COVID coordinator Jeff Zients's December pronouncement that the unvaccinated are to blame for "the hospitals you may soon overwhelm," the Biden administration has organized its COVID response around an ethos of personal responsibility.[1160] COVID is spun as a pandemic of the unvaccinated even as the suddenly unmasked vaccinated can also spread the virus.[1161]

Many of the unvaccinated aren't ideologically motivated. Skepticism and hesitancy mark as much a failure of vaccine access, including the absence of a national door-to-door campaign to convince the 84 million Americans walking around without a single COVID shot to get vaccinated or to physically transport them to an appointment. Winning their trust is critical in controlling the outbreak stateside.

Zients's cheap shot smears the likes of Jesse Rouse, photographed in

November suffering his second bout of COVID here in Minneapolis.[1162] Rouse was reported to be unvaccinated after he previously underwent a double lung transplant. Researchers have proposed that lung transplantees are especially vulnerable to respiratory infection and should be vaccinated for COVID.[1163] Some people may refrain from vaccination for medical reasons specific to their situation, including out of conflicting data about how vaccination interacts with their health conditions or treatments. As it is, the celebrated booster shots appear to offer only ten weeks protection against Omicron.[1164]

Regardless of why particular people remain unvaccinated, thrusting culpability fully onto individuals is an act of political displacement. Like Ronald Reagan's campaign against "welfare queens," presuming public health problems emerge primarily from bad actors and individual decision-making obfuscates the systemic and structural roots of the failure of the U.S.'s response to the pandemic.

Much as Trump, Biden appears repeatedly intent on turning the COVID page, no matter the state of the pandemic itself. The May mask recommendations, which stated that vaccinated people could stop wearing masks in most indoor spaces, were textbook on that account. The administration ignored an October report from public health experts recommending free testing at a pace of 732 million tests per month in preparation for a holiday COVID surge:

> The plan, in effect, was a blueprint for how to avoid what is happening at this very moment—endless lines of desperate Americans clamoring for tests in order to safeguard holiday gatherings, just as COVID-19 is exploding again.
>
> Yesterday, President Biden told David Muir of ABC News, "I wish I had thought about ordering" 500 million at-home tests "two months ago." But the proposal shared at the meeting in October, disclosed here for the first time, included a "Bold Plan for Impact" and a provision for "Every American Household to Receive Free Rapid Tests for the Holidays/New Year."[1165]

Early in December, Biden spokesperson Jen Psaki scoffed at reporter

Mara Liasson's query why the United States doesn't just pay for home COVID tests for every American household like other countries do instead of making Americans submit for reimbursement from insurance companies that have routinely failed to pick up the bill.[1166] "How much is that going to cost?" Psaki asked.

Should a government that just voted $768 billion for the Pentagon, $24 billion more than Biden requested, just pay for COVID tests?[1167] Yes, April Wallace replied to Psaki for the *Washington Post*, yes, it should:

> I am a dual citizen of the United States and Britain, now living in Edinburgh, Scotland, and I am able get rapid antigen tests anytime I want to, at no cost and with no hoops to jump through. I know that Americans pay more than $20 for a package of two tests—if they're in stock. Here you can walk into your local pharmacy, and they will just hand you packs of seven tests at no charge. In my neighborhood I can also go to the local recreational center and collect packs of tests free for my family, or swing by a coronavirus testing center.[1168]

It turns out the U.S. reimbursement wasn't to start until mid-January anyway:

> The administration has already said that the plan will not provide retroactive reimbursement for tests that have already been purchased, which means that any tests you buy for the holidays will not be covered.[1169]

The Biden no-plan, expanded to a whole four rapid tests per household and three masks for each American, appeared to be phase one of a campaign of further eroding American expectations. As self-described shitposter @fingerblaster tweeted:

> Wild that the most unhinged republican president in history sent us $2000 checks back when we had like 12k cases a day and

now we have 300k cases a day and a dem president who's like "lol not my problem go to work jack"[1170]

The more august *New York Times* reported on the end of monthly child benefits millions of Americans were depending on:

> The end of the extra assistance for parents is the latest in a long line of benefits "cliffs" that Americans have encountered as pandemic aid programs have expired. The Paycheck Protection Program, which supported hundreds of thousands of small businesses, ended in March. Expanded unemployment benefits ended in September, and earlier in some states. The federal eviction moratorium expired last summer. The last round of stimulus payments landed in Americans' bank accounts last spring.[1171]

These benefit programs, as modest as they were, saved thousands of Americans from COVID deaths.

A March 2021 Families USA report summarized research showing a third of COVID deaths were tied to the lack of health insurance.[1172] The effect was multiplicative: "Each 10 percent increase in the proportion of a county's residents who lacked health insurance was associated with a 70 percent increase in COVID-19 cases and a 48 percent increase in COVID-19 deaths."

Controlling for stay-at-home orders, school closures, and mask mandates, another study, published November 2020, estimated that lifting eviction moratoriums state-to-state resulted in between 365,200 and 502,200 excess coronavirus cases and between 8,900 and 12,500 excess deaths.[1173]

Omicron's Delta Strain

So, public health clearly extends beyond necessary prophylaxes into necessary social interventions. But if to make sure there was no doubt as to which constituency the political class serves, in December, CDC cut down its recommendation for quarantine upon COVID exposure from ten days to five. The act was decidedly in response to pressure from employers, notoriously Delta Airlines's CEO Ed Bastian in a letter that Delta proudly posted.[1174]

The Delta letter summarized the scientific literature in favor of its request in two sentences. The science is in reality more nuanced, marked by a variety of definitional complications.

Omicron and other new variants are likely to modulate the vaccine effectiveness Delta Airlines cites as, full-stop, protection enough.[1175] Permitting COVID variants to circulate on Delta planes or elsewhere increases the chances they evolve enough to circumvent medical and nonpharmaceutical controls.[1176]

Other drawbacks refute such summary boosterism. Omicron is already associated with increased reinfection.[1177] The variant's other impacts are likely to be geographically specific, depending on a variety of local factors, including preexisting immunity and nonpharmaceutical interventions.[1178] What works as an intervention under one set of conditions does not necessarily hold under all.

More meta, the speed at which new variants evolve is outpacing even the frantic pace of the research conducted.[1179] "Flattening the curve" extends beyond our hospitals to research efforts aimed at discovering how to better control COVID.

In other words, under a more infectious Omicron, a variety of interventions, one layered atop another, is necessary, rather than stripping them back to serve criteria pretending to be scientific.

This isn't the first time the airline industry tried to bend basic COVID science to its financial advantage. JetBlue CEO and reopen proponent David Neeleman funded and helped coordinate a Stanford University study that whistleblower complaints showed used a testing kit that erred on the side of false positives.[1180] By these tests, the study concluded the COVID virus was more widespread in the public and therefore, given the underlying number of deaths in the study population, was less dangerous of a pathogen.

National Institute of Allergy and Infectious Diseases director Anthony Fauci, Lysenko on the Potomac, ran interference in the face of these obvious complications, parroting Bastian's arguments to the letter:

There is the danger that there will be so many people who are being isolated who are asymptomatic for the full ten days, that you could have a major negative impact on our ability to keep society running. So the decision was made of saying let's get that cut in half.

CDC director Rochelle Walensky once fought back tears over the likelihood of COVID mass deaths.[1181] Now, no better than a meat plant manager, she defends sending people back into the pandemic still infectious:

There are a lot of studies [from other variants] that show the maximum transmissibility is in those first five days. And [with Omicron] we are about to face hundreds of thousands more cases a day, and it was becoming very, very clear from the health care system that we would have people who were [positive but] asymptomatic and not able to work, and that was a harbinger of what was going to come in all other essential functions of society.[1182]

Washington had practiced cutting key epidemiological interventions in half only a few years ago:

With their loan payments still on the clock—outbreak or no— [Midwest] farmers are so desperate they've requested the second half of composting [poultry killed by bird flu H5N2] be allowed outside to free up their barns earlier.[1183]

In short, the combination of economic compulsion and traumatic bonding that sent Midwest farmers begging to put poultry back into production under the H5N2 outbreak and millions of workers into unprotected workplaces for COVID's first two years now represents state policy. The denialism for which liberals punch down on Trumpists is the labor law of the land. It is now a key part of the administration's public health campaign.

"I'm not letting COVID-19 take my shifts," one recent CDC ad declared. "My job puts me at high risk for COVID-19 exposure. I got vaccinated because it's better to be protected than to be out sick."[1184]

Another CDC post shamelessly used the U.S. privatized health care system as a cudgel of class discipline: "Hospital stays can be expensive, but COVID-19 vaccines are free. Help protect yourself from being hospitalized with #COVID19 by getting vaccinated."[1185]

In that spirit, Biden economic adviser Jared Bernstein waxed optimistic on the economy.[1186] The depletion of personal savings would drive low-paid workers back into the labor market during a pandemic, Bernstein cheered.

"We are intent," Zients declared mid-December, "on not letting Omicron disrupt work and school for the vaccinated. You've done the right thing, and we will get through this."[1187] The vaccinated are pure enough of soul to get back to working the gears of the economic machine. The unvaccinated are cast, to appropriate Hillary Clinton's characterization, as a basket of eschatological deplorables.

Zients, a Biden campaign donor, served as the CEO of the investment firm Cranemere before taking on the role as Biden's COVID czar, the position Deborah Birx filled under Trump. Zients served as the director of Obama's National Economic Council. His primary portfolio of priorities was always apparent.

The quarantine switcheroo follows CDC's changing recommendations for school distancing from six feet to three which it now pretends is the virus's limit.[1188] In reality, even six feet isn't enough for the airborne virus.[1189] But in changing it to three, CDC could legally accommodate efforts to stuff students back in brick-and-mortar school without changing day-to-day public health precautions.

Keeping kids out of school can have terrible impacts on learning outcomes and emotional well-being.[1190] Keeping kids in school, potentially leading to the deaths of other students or teachers in school, and older adults back home, can incur a different kind of emotional damage.[1191] Both risks serve as more the reason for bringing the outbreak under control with a full-spectrum intervention.

The CDC's position, sending students back to school without controlling the outbreak, is geared toward other aims. It's about putting the economic cart before the epidemiological horse. The kids need to go to school so that the parents can go to work.

Such misguided campaigns extend beyond the administration. Among the American Heart Association's new interim pandemic recommendations for medical staff is starting CPR without personal protective equipment.[1192]

Artist Rob Sheridan designed a series of counter-CDC posters:

- We Can Do It! We Can Sacrifice Grandma So Dave & Buster's Can Stay in Business!
- Quiet! Don't Cough! Pretend to Be OK! Your Boss's 8th Boat Depends on It!
- America's Youth is Ready to March Back to School! The Economy Demands Sacrifice![1193]

Across the internet—over a wide political expanse—other observers expressed as scathing an outrage:

- Comedian Zak Toscani: CDC recommends splitting up your quarantine over your two 15-min breaks.[1194]
- Sociologist Jenn Jennings: I guess I missed that rewrite of the Hippocratic Oath: first, do no harm to late capitalism.[1195]
- Comedian Roy Wood Jr: CDC just said you only need to quarantine if you are on a ventilator. But if ya ventilator got wheels and a battery pack you gotta take yo ass to work.[1196]
- Songwriter Certified Lover Girl: Y'all keep talking about the CDC, the CDC, the CDC . . . The CDC left you fa dead hoe![1197]
- Author Alexander Chee: If you have to deploy the military to support hospitals you may have spent your budget on the wrong part of the system, given the challenges we actually face.[1198]
- Designer Char: CDC okays pull-out method as "eh, good enough."[1199]

The administration is too full of itself to see it is losing the country.

Its caustic claims about "the science" aren't supported by the science, further undercutting research as a trusted source of both state strategy and public response.

The original ten-day quarantine that the CDC changed was grounded in the evidence-based realities of the virus itself, specifically its incubation time, generation time, and serial interval.[1200] At the same time, the ten days aren't a matter of an essentialist measure of *central tendency*—that is, a single value, like mean or median, that summarizes a dataset by reflecting the center of the data distribution.[1201]

Against CDC director Walensky's characterization, it's about the *variation* in patients' infectious periods.[1202] Some patients exit out of their infectiousness early, in the five days Walensky cited. Others can be infectious much longer. No one knows who's a late bloomer in transmission. As a matter of practical public health intervention, it's an unknown.

A public health campaign must therefore institute mask and quarantine policies that cover for the late transmissions, so that they don't serve as the means by which the outbreak rolls on—particularly as Omicron's infectiousness approaches measles and a 100 percent attack rate can still result from so small a population source.[1203]

Instead, we have slashed public assistance, shortened quarantines, offered no-to-little remote schooling, hired few community health workers, conducted little genomic sequencing of the virus, and let hospitals get overrun. The CDC gave in upon the subsequent furor around the shortened quarantine by adding only a recommendation—not a requirement—of a negative rapid antigen test before workers returned to work.[1204]

Beyond trying to circumvent the rancor of partisan criticism, why did Trump and Biden alike aim at pretending the pandemic away? Biden's trajectory is illustrative that capitalist realism has a way of eating away at even good faith efforts at addressing existential threats.

In October 2020, candidate Biden put the failings of his opposition in perspective: "We're eight months into this pandemic, and Donald Trump still doesn't have a plan to get this virus under control. I do."[1205]

"This crisis," President-elect Biden added, "demands a robust and immediate federal response."[1206]

A year later, President Biden pivoted: "There is no federal solution. This gets solved at a state level," months after state governors had lost or abandoned their emergency powers to impose mask mandates and shelter-at-home orders.[1207]

Other countries see federal jurisdiction differently, as if the very health of their ostensible constituencies has something to do with governance.

While the United States daily breaks record COVID caseloads, other countries appear of another world. COVID long-hauler Ravi Veriah Jacques reported these January 2 caseloads from abroad:

- New Zealand – 51
- China – 191
- Taiwan – 20
- Japan – 477
- Hong Kong – 18[1208]

China's reactions are both broader and triggered more quickly, with the public health results to show for it.[1209] Xi'an, a metropolis of 13 million people in Shaanxi Province, underwent an arguably arduous lockdown upon the emergence of 175 COVID cases.[1210] Western media has played on the difficulties in obtaining food in the city over the twelve days' quarantine, but not the campaigns to alleviate those problems.[1211]

Some may argue the Biden administration's reaction is better late than never, but that's not how controlling COVID's lightning strikes works. As epidemiologist Rodrick Wallace models, whatever the intervention, there's nothing worse than dithering.[1212] Given the insidious nature of the virus, we are routinely six weeks too late if spikes in cases, rather than anticipatory planning, are the trigger.[1213] Repeated delays mark U.S. COVID planning—among them, the spread of the original wave out of coastal cities to the rest of the country in spring 2020 and the arrivals of Delta and Omicron stateside since.

Rapid Confusion Test

It happens that the mass at-home testing the Biden administration passed over in October, setting up a program several months too late, is already a failure. Big picture, like vaccination, it represents yet another technicist intervention that, while necessary, is also insufficient. It's more a grand gesture that detracts from refusing to pursue multilevel systemic public health programming.[1214]

The specifics of such a rollout and the tests themselves also get in the way. It's much more than a matter of rapid tests permitting the deplorable unvaccinated an exit out of the shots, as the Biden administration feared.[1215] It's also not merely doctors defending their testing territory, as rapid test proponents argued.

Among several intrinsic errors that biotech consultant Dale Harrison explores around the rapid tests, there is the difficulty of self-administering them:

One important note is that at-home antigen tests will give VERY poor results (both high false-positives and high false-negatives) if you are sloppy or misuse them.

These are complex molecular assays and the EXACT usage is critical. You MUST read and follow every single detail in the instructions to get a reliable outcome. . . .

The difficulties extend beyond administering the tests. Interpreting is a difficult task, as much from being swayed by our hopes as a technical matter:

Now comes the tricky part . . .what happens if you get conflicting test results?

Let's say you get a positive result on an at-home antigen test (like the BinaxNow) and decide to take it again "just to be sure."

Then you get a negative result on the 2nd Binax test. Now you schedule an appointment to get a PCR test.

A couple of days later, it comes back negative.

ARE YOU INFECTED? Absolutely positively YES!

If you're non-symptomatic and get a [Binx+ Binax- PCR-] set of results. . . a positive and two negatives in any order.

In that case, it is 56-times MORE likely that you're infected than not infected . . . 5600% more likely!

And if you're FULLY symptomatic and get a [Binx+ Binax- PCR-] set of results, it is 20-times MORE likely that you're infected than not infected . . . 2000% more likely!

Even if you get ANOTHER PCR test and THAT test comes back negative as well [Binx+ Binax- PCR- PCR-] you are still 4-times more likely to be infected than not . . . 400 percent more likely!

And it does NOT matter the order of the test results . . . the math holds true regardless.[1216]

Even medical doctors conducting these tests in clinics stumble:

I know this seems VERY counter-intuitive and even most doctors who prescribe these tests (other than Infectious Disease specialists) tend to NOT understand this!

And when faced with multiple conflicting test results, most medical people will incorrectly select the LAST result as the "correct one."

This is a DANGEROUS mistake! Again, outside of certain specialties, few medical staff are trained to think in terms of Bayesian statistics.

Vanity Fair's palace intrigue set the COVID Collaborative of high-end epidemiologists recommending the holiday testing surge against the administration that ignored them.[1217] But that isn't quite right. Both sides agree on turning public health into an individualistic (and commoditized) option:

Once [ex-Harvard epidemiologist and now chief science officer at the eMed diagnostic company Michael] Mina began to advocate for rapid home tests, he encountered the same mindset: doctors "trying to guard their domain." Some doctors had long opposed home testing, even for pregnancy and HIV, arguing that patients who learned on their own about a given condition would not be able to act on the information effectively. Testing, in this view, should be used only by doctors as a diagnostic instrument, not by individuals as a public-health tool for influencing decisions.

The U.S. approach sticks the American people with the job of administering and then interpreting the conflicting results of multiple tests. The false positives might be low in part because nearly 100 percent specificity aligns with peak viral load. But, as Harrison describes, even should the test be administered correctly, the false negatives are legion and the results of one test do not necessarily change the implications of previous ones.

Techno-utopianism offers another iteration of blaming the victim if the outcome goes south: "It's your own fault you didn't do the test right." Don't let the easy lines on the lateral flow ag card confuse matters. Against Mina's insinuation, it's decidedly unlike a pregnancy test.

There is also the matter of what happens when organizing society's access to work and recreation around such tests collides with either a run on the tests at local stores already suffering supply chain problems or making the tests unavailable and priced beyond working people's budgets.

If, on the other hand, the Biden administration hired and *trained* a million community health workers to go door-to-door across the country administering these tests for free—like really free free—we wouldn't be in such a free-for-all, if you'll excuse the ironic phrasing.

If such teams had been put in place from the beginning, they may have been able to build the trust necessary to successfully introduce a variety of time- and place-specific public health interventions that would likely have minimized the duration and impact of each wave of the pandemic.

What's interesting about Harrison's direct and clearly written posts is that his recommendations are framed by the context of what the United States can, or is willing to, offer right now: not much.

Yes, everyone *should* be able to test themselves whenever they wish, all the time. But the United States chooses to position itself as unable to pursue such a public health program. Should the sensitivity and specificity reported on the test boxes match their actual outcomes?[1218] Yes, they should, however righteous the original testing went into bringing the products to market. Should the efficaciousness and effectiveness of vaccines match? Yes, that would be nice.

There are expectations individual American consumers hold about solutions—cheap and immediately effective—that the market repeatedly promises but can't deliver. In this case, the multifactorial virus doesn't cater to such an ideal of a single packet solution. And because the public health response we need, and the market treats as a rival, is starved to near-death.

Successful vaccination likewise depends on the same public health infrastructure that nonpharmaceutical interventions earlier in the pandemic needed but didn't get.[1219] Vaccine hesitancy isn't just a matter of occupational necessity for some, but, for others, also serves as a marker of a failure of vaccine access.

Privatizing Public Health

You see, no one knocked on people's doors to explain why a vaccine is a good idea.

As with testing, thousands of newly hired community health workers are needed to hit the streets to convince people that vaccines are safe and necessary. Daily conversations for weeks on end are needed to turn hundreds of thousands of skeptics or the disconnected into participants. It's the kind of program the Biden administration proposed to inadequate lengths for contact tracing before the inauguration and never pursued after.[1220]

That said, the resulting bloodbath—only inches deep but wide as a lake—isn't just a matter of any single administration. Trump's vindictive inaction killed half-a-million Americans the first year of the outbreak. Biden's smug insufficiency will likely help kill another half million by spring. But it's as much a matter of structural decline.[1221]

Beginning nearly fifty years ago, public health was increasingly abandoned or monetized under the neoliberal program.

Public health spending clearly saves lives. Ten years ago, healthy
policy analysts Glen Mays and Sharla Smith found that U.S. mortality
rates from preventable deaths—including infant mortality and cardiovascular disease, diabetes, and cancer—fell between 1.1 to 6.9 percent
for every 10 percent increase in local public health spending.[1222]

Yet this crucial spending has dropped. In 2018, Trust for America's
Health reported on the effective decline of such funding.[1223] CDC's
budget then was $7.15 billion, which, adjusting for inflation, was
flat for the previous decade. Most of the CDC's budget goes to states
and municipalities. There's also a CDC Prevention and Public Health
Fund, from which about $625 million a year also went directly to
states and municipalities.

The report described the Public Health Emergency Preparedness
(PHEP) Cooperative Agreement Program as the only federal program that supports state and local health departments to prepare
for and respond to emergencies. Except for one-time bumps for the
Ebola and Zika outbreaks, core emergency preparedness funding had
been cut by more than one-third (from $940 million in 2002 to $667
million in 2017).

The report went on to identify precipitous declines in public health
funding at the state level. Thirty-one states cut their public health
budgets 2015–16, with spending lower then than in 2008. The budget
cuts out of the Great Recession were never restored.

The impact was felt at the local level too. Local health departments
cut 55,000 staff the decade following the recession. By this system's
logic, an acute emergency is also grounds for such cuts. Thousands
of health staff were furloughed during the COVID outbreak due to
declines in more lucrative elective surgeries.[1224] One in five health
workers have left their jobs during the pandemic.[1225]

The Trust for America's Health report went on to describe incoming disasters for which the United States appeared unprepared in 2018.
These sound like headlines of the past year: weather disasters, flooding,
wildfires, extreme drought, hurricanes, infectious disease outbreaks,

deaths of despair, including out of racial disparities, opioids, and regional disparities that continue to drive governmental distrust.

Trust for America's Health placed particular focus on pandemics and the need to fully fund the Pandemic and All-Hazards Preparedness Act, the Hospital Preparedness Program, the Project BioShield Act, and PHEP.

The report recommended increasing funding for public health at all levels of jurisdiction—federal, state, and local. It called for preserving the Prevention and Public Health Fund, funding for preparing for public health emergencies and pandemics, establishing a standing public health emergency response fund, and surge funding upon an emergency to avoid the delays that were apparent in the Ebola outbreak, the swine flu pandemic, Hurricane Sandy, and the Zika outbreak.

Trust for America's Health concluded with a recommendation for a national resilience strategy to combat diseases of despair, for preventing chronic disease, and for expanding high-impact interventions across communities.

The recommendations were wrapped in the worst of language and precepts. Trust for America's Health accepted the class character of the state. Public health is a means of cleaning up messes that capitalist production produces. Public health outcomes were pitched in terms of Returns on Investment.

All terrible. And yet in the present context, the recommendations are radical, if only in pushing back against the damage of an empire at the end of its cycle of capital accumulation, organized around helping billionaires squeeze what's left of the commons and turning decades of social infrastructure back into bunker money.[1226]

Anti–Public Health—at Home and Abroad

We find an analog fallacy in U.S. COVID policy abroad. While the Biden administration has taken a stance in favor of waiving TRIPS rules against vaccine generics for COVID, tech billionaire and philanthrocapitalist Bill Gates, funding WHO efforts, effectively sets U.S. foreign policy on the matter.[1227]

Gates declared in April:

> There are only so many vaccine factories in the world and people are very serious about the safety of vaccines. And so moving something that had never been done, moving a vaccine from, say, a J&J factory into a factory in India, that, it's novel, it's only because of our grants and our expertise that can happen at all. The thing that's holding things back in this case is not intellectual property, there's not like some idle vaccine factory with regulatory approval that makes magically safe vaccines.[1228]

The reality is something different. Last month AccessIBSA and Médecins Sans Frontières identified 120 companies in Africa, Asia, and Latin America with the likely capacity to produce mRNA vaccines.[1229] Human Rights Watch reported:

> "Global vaccine production forecasts suggesting there will soon be enough Covid-19 vaccines for the world are misleading," said Aruna Kashyap, associate business and human rights director at Human Rights Watch. "The US and German governments should press for wider technology transfers and not let companies dictate where and how lifesaving vaccines and treatments reach much of the world as the virus mutates."[1230]

Two months earlier, the *New York Times* had investigated the possibility:

> "You cannot go hire people who know how to make mRNA: Those people don't exist," the chief executive of Moderna, Stéphane Bancel, told analysts.
>
> But public health experts in both rich and poor countries argue that expanding production to the regions most in need is not only possible, it is essential for safeguarding the world against dangerous variants of the virus and ending the pandemic.
>
> Setting up mRNA manufacturing operations in other coun-

tries should start immediately, said Tom Frieden, the former director of the Centers for Disease Control and Prevention in the United States, adding: "They are our insurance policy against variants and production failure" and "absolutely can be produced in a variety of settings."[1231]

Both home and abroad, pharm apologists propose nothing can be conceived, much less pursed, unless the largest companies make billions in profit. Our men of the year are to be treated as no less than gods with rocket wings. Few of the respectable establishment have described, much less denounced, the fallacy.

Others have been much more truculent in their commentary, connecting increasing wealth concentration with COVID failures:

- Economic historian Matthias Schmelzer started one thread early December: "The global concentration of capital is extreme: The richest 10% own around 60–80% of wealth, the poorest half less than 5%, according to just published World Inequality Report."[1232]
- Americans For Tax Fairness reported: "America's billionaires got $1 TRILLION richer in 2021, a 25% gain in collective wealth that will go largely untaxed."[1233]
- Union organizer Jack Califano encapsulated the externalized costs of such an arrangement: "COVID has been a perfect illustration of how our government now works. In a crisis, it will provide benefits, but only the absolute minimum it determines necessary to protect the system from political upheaval. And then, as soon as stability is restored, it will take them away."[1234]

The Pandemic Thinktank, whose members combine hundreds of years of epidemiology experience, has taken up the core matter in similarly direct terms. In a report it released in November, the ad hoc group—composed of a social psychiatrist, disease ecologist, medical anthropologist, epidemiologist, critical care physician, and county official—unpacked the origins of the COVID trap the United States had placed itself and offered a plan of escape other than "go to work."[1235]

The team described how social systems set the ways epidemics spread, the damage that accrued in the American system of disease control long before SARS-2 showed up, the history of successful public health efforts before that destruction, and what a working public health system looks like:

> Several lessons emerge from the COVID-19 pandemic and frame our approach to planning for the next pandemic.
>
> First, there are three "partners" in this enterprise: the government, the public health establishment, and the communities. Each partner has an important role to play in ensuring that we learn these lessons and can meet the next challenge with a better chance at survival. But there is an underlying issue of excess power held by the American oligopoly and the politicians allied with them. They profit in power and wealth from the array of policies David Harvey (2019) labeled "accumulation by dispossession."
>
> Any serious examination of pandemic threat must confront the danger contained in such one-sided power. Part of the way in which the oligopoly has gained and maintained power is by undermining communities and destroying their organizations. While this is good for short-term profit, it poses an enormous threat to long-term survival. Rebuilding community power is an essential part of epidemic control.

Rebellion as Intervention

So, there are minds stateside who understand both disease and the country in ways the establishment that rejects them does not. In contrast to Fauci and a CDC that repeatedly places commerce and empire before people, Pandemic Thinktank explicitly counsels a rebel alliance:

> Local health departments must, in many municipalities and counties, foment revolution.

This, like most revolutions, must occur in secret and with interactions with community groups in places like neighborhood bars, playgrounds, houses of worship, and barbershops/beauty salons.

In order to bring communities into condition for improved public health and for pandemic prevention and response, the health department must have the social and political muscle to pressure the elected executive into reforming the relevant agencies.

The health departments themselves must feel the pressure of empowered communities to establish egalitarian planning councils that will produce plans acceptable to and supportable by the various elements that form the local communities.

Unlike the COVID Collaborative of establishment epidemiologists who, like the CDC, push a more individualistic approach to public health, we can see why the Pandemic Thinktank holds no direct line to the president. Indeed, ultimately, it's going to take everyday people disconnected from the Beltway to help bend epidemiology back into a science for the people.

Younger epidemiologists are taking on that spirit, turning on Biden and their better-connected colleagues in confrontational terms for which most journeymen are punished:

- Perhaps with the COVID Collaborative and Michael Mina in mind, Columbia University's Seth Prins tweeted: "Turns out lots of blue check public health experts moonlight as pandemic profiteers."[1236]
- Ellie Murray, of Boston University's School of Public Health, tweeted: "Honestly baffled by people who claim the COVID plan put in place by the president of the united states, 'leader of the free world,' was so fragile that an assistant professor tweeting on her coffee breaks could undermine it, & that *isnt* somehow worse than the plan just failing?"[1237]
- Justin Feldman, a social epidemiologist at the Harvard FXB Center for Health & Human Rights, who wrote his own critique of Biden's

COVID year, followed up: "There's 'a lot to unpack' about how the only substantive criticism the media has been willing to pursue WRT Biden's pandemic response is failing to make a consumer product (rapid tests) available to individuals."[1238]

- Botswanan doctor Letlhogonolo Tlhabano, now based in North Carolina, weighed in: "I'm an intensivist and have been taking care of COVID patients since this pandemic began, and the new AHA guidelines are idiotic. We're not martyrs. The CDC guidelines are also motivated by the need to protect capital, and not necessarily by any science. We're on our own."[1239]

- Science organizer and biochemist Lucky Tran commented: "We are not 'learning to live with COVID.' When we give up on protecting our healthcare systems, workers, the immunocompromised, and the vulnerable, in reality we are 'surrendering to COVID.'" [1240]

- It really speaks to the tenor of our times when March for Science retweets Black radical Bree Newsome on the out-of-pocket costs of COVID testing.[1241]

I tried warning people about what was likely to come from Biden before the inauguration, twice, and wrote a book titled *Dead Epidemiologists,* underscoring the mortally wounded thinking of even some of the field's best and brightest practitioners.[1242]

The advocacy work of these younger scientists, however, may signal that our ugly future also offers hope. A more recent invitation to my millennial colleagues that we had a world to win reminded me of the generation-appropriate Marx T-shirt I'm getting my kid for his birthday: "You're a Wizard, Harry."[1243]

Of course, I don't have all the answers on how we'll get through this shit show—to use the technical term. I'm always learning alongside this new generation.

I experienced a bout of my own booster hesitancy, born out of the ethical quandary in which Gates trapped us all. Why a third inoculation for me when much of the world hasn't gotten stuck a single shot? The utter shame of it, with the appropriate symptoms of a red face and shortness of breath. I finally concluded that being alive allowed me to use what little power and platform I had to argue for a different public health order the world over.

For ending a pharmaceutical industry focused on commoditizing health and reinvesting in a public health organized around our shared commons here and abroad is the only way out of this pandemic in any short order. Otherwise, we are left to letting the virus burn out on its own by something like 2025, as early models projected.[1244] The Black Plague in Europe eventually ended after eight years. Unless we act now to restore an active, on-the-ground public health mobilization helping people block-by-block and farm-by-farm, we will be forced to assimilate the possibility that we are to suffer a pandemic of a similar duration.

My medical plan didn't have any boosters available. The Walgreens website was busted. I got an appointment at a CVS way out in West St Paul for ten days later. But a little corner pharmacy got me in earlier. The appointment online was easy to book. It pinged my phone a reminder the day before. The operation itself, although with only three people at the soda fountain counter, was a well-oiled machine, rotating multiple patients in and out every ten minutes.

And the personnel were kind and relaxed and had answers for every contingency. No vaccine card? No worries, we'll look up your shots. No medical card? No worries, homie, everyone showing up for a shot is leaving with one. You couldn't find N95 masks at Target? No worries, we got boxes of them. And plenty of rapid tests, however problematic their applicability. The Xmas bauble with the miniature vaccine card inside hanging over the fountain was a touch.

The lesson here isn't just the trouble I, or anyone else, has had getting a booster or a test on which the political class has placed the entirety of its fiasco of a COVID intervention, but the counterpoise of an American example that not everything public health need be run badly.

Excellent service is possible, even scaled up or out. We need extend it out from a few storefronts to millions of community health workers taking kind competence door-to-door across the country.

But that will depend on the kind of revolution Pandemic Thinktank counseled and Pandemic Research for the People champions—that the people demand that its better expectations be met. It's a possibility if, and only if, we step out of the desultory muck in which the billionaire class's representatives demand we wallow for our own good.

Otherwise, all that is left is to circle the proverbial drain, to use the medical colloquialism.

Philosopher Alain Badiou, writing in the pessimistic 1990s, described an end to another empire's truth of the state: "The USSR, the despotic gray totality, the reversal of October [1917] into its opposite."[1245]

One can't forget the associated collapse of public health that decade there, with declines in life expectancy the United States is now mimicking even before COVID.[1246] But for Badiou, the end of the USSR, embodying the loss of a counterpoise to rapacious global capitalism, also marked a serendipitous liberation, if only in separating communism from its antithetic representation.

Perhaps in this apparent collapse we ourselves can circle back to democracy. One need demand we make the journey without the apartheid and genocidal land grabs, the wealth from which—as this pandemic so blatantly demonstrates—continues to bloat on exsanguinating the public commons. As it took place under Trump and Biden both.

—PATREON, JANUARY 6, 2022
TRUTHOUT, JANUARY 21 AND 27, 2022

Governance Is Key

I co-authored the following draft commentary, first posted on the medRxiv server, with evolutionary biologist Kenichi Okamoto, disease ecologist Luis Fernando Chaves, and epidemiologist Rodrick Wallace.

CONSIDERABLE ATTENTION HAS BEEN paid to public health's impacts on the spread of SARS-CoV-2, the virus that causes COVID-19. Mask mandates, shelter-in-place orders, and broader interventions, including health care access and eviction moratoriums, mitigate SARS-2 transmission, albeit to varying degrees.[1247] Despite the striking emergence of multiple variants of concern, far less attention has been directed to policy's effects upon the evolution of the virus. Particularly troubling is how little modeling has been dedicated to policy's influence on the evolution of viral resistance to COVID-19 vaccines, for many policymakers our putative exit out of the pandemic.[1248]

Concerns about vaccine resistance may seem premature. Declines in vaccine effectiveness have indeed been documented across COVID variants, but the primary problem at hand still remains first getting millions around the world without vaccine access vaccinated, atop those skeptical and hesitant.[1249] The issues of vaccine access and the evolution of resistance are intertwined, however. Delays, gaps, or reversals in vaccination and other interventions pursued in various combinations since the start of the pandemic have already set the trajectory for the evolution of immune evasion.[1250]

Modeling Governance's Impacts

To evaluate the possible impacts of governance on the evolution in vaccine resistance, our group analyzed a stochastic model to quantify the risk that a mutant SARS-CoV-2 strain capable of evading immunity emerges 170 days following vaccine rollout. The novel strain evades both natural immunity and immunity acquired by vaccination, but in this model otherwise circulates similarly as the ancestral strain. We calibrated the model with publicly available data for four territories in the Western Hemisphere: Panama, Costa Rica, Texas, and Uruguay. The four represent societies of relatively high Human Development Index (HDI), but also substantively different modes of governance and public health policy as they relate to responding to COVID-19.

We assessed how readily such a novel strain spreads in an initially monomorphic, immune-susceptible viral population. We found that the ability of the strain to spread depends on the impacts of territorial policies on the ancestral strain's epidemiology at the time the mutant emerges. While some of these effects are likely to be relatively constant, others are time-varying. The transmission coefficients of the ancestral strain on each day in each location are estimated using an Ensemble Kalman Filter.[1251]

We then calculated the daily evolutionary invasibility of a mutant virus μ in each territory using a modified version of the basic reproductive number $R\mu$ for the novel strain, derived using the next-generation operator.[1252] We describe details of the modeling in the Supplementary Methods. All code is publicly available at github.com/kewok/immune_evasion and released under the GNU Public License (GPL 3).

The nearby figure shows SARS-CoV-2 exposure (and immunity)

steadily low in Panama and Costa Rica across the 170 days after vaccinations begin, low but slowly rising in Uruguay, and sharply rising in Texas. The results also show that as the vaccination campaign begins, public health policies in Texas readily select for an immune-evading strain over all infectivities (found above the invasibility threshold log $R_\mu = 0$). In Panama, only a high level of transmission (β_μ=5) permits immune evasion to evolve. No invasion appears likely in Costa Rica. Even with rising exposure, resistance appears highly unlikely to successfully emerge in Uruguay.

We see in the figure that the four territories differ substantively in their public health responses to the pandemic. The University of Oxford's COVID-19 Government Response Tracker combines containment and closure policies, measures of population economic support, health system policies, and vaccine policies into a government response index.[1253] The index shows Panama, Costa Rica, and Uruguay engaged in the kinds of combinations of control efforts that U.S. COVID science leaders recently publicly denounced.[1254] To be sure, these campaigns are in flux. Panama eventually converged upon a full-spectrum response: masks, vaccines, and household support. Costa Rica's nonpharmaceutical program pivoted to depending largely on vaccines alone beginning in 2021. Uruguay's startling early successes were subsequently mitigated by demands to reopen the economy.

The Oxford effort also compiles subnational control programs, including for U.S. states, which set their own control policy outside federal jurisdiction.[1255] Texas's responses were emblematic of an abandonment of COVID public health policies in the U.S. South, with minimal time under shelter-in-place, near-total reopening of businesses, and ending mask mandates despite new waves of COVID infection. Although Texas was among the first ten U.S. states to enact universal access to COVID vaccination (16 years and older), only 58 percent of Texans are fully vaccinated. That combination suggests SARS-CoV-2 populations there experience early and incomplete vaccine exposure and the granular geography of high- and low-vaccinated microhabitats to which resistance appears best able to evolve in response.[1256]

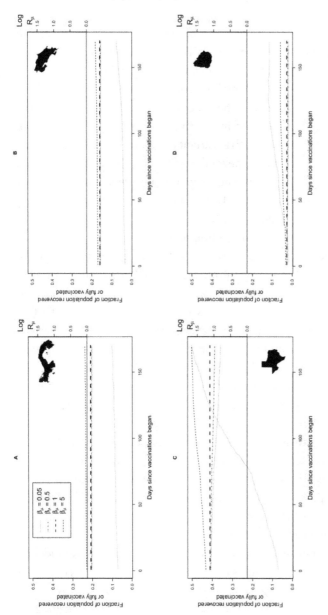

Exposure via infection or vaccination (solid line) and evolutionary invasibility (dashed lines) of an immune-evading mutant strain µ across 170 days in four Western Hemisphere territories with relatively high HDIs but qualitatively distinct public health strategies. (A) Panama, (B) Costa Rica, (C) Texas and (D) Uruguay. In all panels, the solid black lines represent the invasibility threshold (log $R\mu = 0$). The dotted lines represent invasibility of a mutant 5 percent as infectious as the resident strain, the heavy dashed lines represent the invasibility of mutants as infectious as the resident strain, and the light dashed lines represent a mutant 500 percent as infectious as the resident strain.

Rethinking Governance and Science

Such arrays of pandemic-specific health policies appear to capture only a part of the variation in COVID population burden. One control theory model showed that delays in responding alone degrade and destabilize governmental response capacity, whatever those interventions might be.[1257] The accumulating degradation promotes multiple infection waves of increasing severity, not unlike what we have seen across novel COVID variants. Dithering and denialism can amplify COVID's damage beyond any immediate wave. The control system itself tailspins into long-term, unstable dynamics of repeated crashes and overcorrections. Under this class of models, the disease endemicity many hoped for with the Omicron wave is replaced with explosive spikes of increasing amplitude.

The context of COVID-19 outcome can be expanded from public health responses to dominant modes of economic production. One study set epidemiological variables such as the exponential growth rate, and COVID cases and deaths 100 days after detection of a first case for clusters of countries against clusters based on uneven development variables, including HDI, the WHO Universal Health Coverage index, and several trade indicators.[1258] In Mesoamerica and the Caribbean, trade openness was associated with increases in COVID cases and deaths. Increases in concentration of imports, a marker of uneven development, correlated significantly with increases in early epidemic growth and deaths, even while accounting for COVID mitigation and prevention policies, and human travel across countries.

The implications of these lines of analysis extend beyond governance and public health practice and into research itself. A disease outbreak, for instance, represents more than a convergence of susceptibles, the exposed and infected, and those who have recovered from infection. Public health interventions and traditional SEIR modeling from which such campaigns often take direction must reach beyond cataloguing the emergent properties of populations of interacting individuals.[1259] The broader social landscapes in which pathogens evolve drive disease outbreaks.[1260] The causes for the evolution of diseases are found as much in the field of the social determinants of health as in the object of the pathogen or patient population.

We can take matters a step further. Modes of governance and production represent more than the ways a society impacts population health. They often embody a society's dominant principles and the institutional cognition—how groups think—by which such values are turned into policies.[1261] "Social determinants" of health in reality are *societal determinations* that are devised and acted upon by specific people.[1262] As our model suggests, statal and parastatal practices set many of the boundary conditions in time and space over which subsequent vaccine resistance in COVID-19 and any pandemics to follow likely emerge, long before any actual vaccination begins. More proactive and structural approaches to public health interventions must therefore be pursued to exit the rolling COVID trap and prevent novel pathogens from emerging out of the spillover queue.

Here are two strategic objectives to start. First, implement a program of integrated pharmaceutical and nonpharmaceutical interventions that removes the epidemiological space SARS-CoV-2 needs to evolve vaccine resistance and other adaptive life history changes.[1263] If not the Zero COVID programs some countries have instituted, governments and communities should implement timely, consistent, and collaborative programs across ministries or affinity groups that drive SARS-CoV-2 under its local rates of replacement.

Second, with the bigger picture in mind, governance must pivot back to supporting modes of production such as agroecology, community-controlled forestry, and open medicine that, on the front end of disease emergence, retard new pathogens from spilling over into human populations, and, on the back end, place public health and economic development on mutually supportive trajectories.[1264] Whatever the principles around which they organize themselves, societies across the globe are otherwise unlikely to flourish in the face of the epidemiological and climatic consequences of acting as if they are little more than a stock market with a country attached.

What Is "Land"?

In order to serve Progress, it's been necessary for us actively to refute the assertion of Indigenous . . . cultures that the land is sentient.
—BARRY LOPEZ (2006)

[In 1799] the American armies destroyed 40 Haudenosaunee (Iroquois) towns and burned their harvests while residents fled. At Chonodote, or Peach Town, the army burned 1,500 peach trees. The Haudenosaunee still call George Washington and all U.S. presidents Hanadahguyus. The name means town destroyer.
—"NATIVE NEW YORK" EXHIBIT, NATIONAL MUSEUM
OF THE AMERICAN INDIAN, NEW YORK CITY (2022)

The following dispatch was produced by the PReP Agroecologies working group for Pandemic Research for the People. I joined disease ecologist and lead author Luis Fernando Chaves, wildlife veterinarian Nicole Gottdenker, anthropologist Julie Velasquez Runk, agrarian geographer Alex Liebman, farmer and agroecologist Kim Williams-Guillén, anthropologist Lisa Kelley, agroecologist Ivette Perfecto, investment investigator Philip Seufert, farmer and anthropologist Tammi Jonas, geographer Luke Bergmann, and PReP interns Sophia Kruger and Katrina Anderson.

OVER THE PAST TWO DECADES, long before the COVID-19 pandemic, scientists increasingly attributed the emergence of new pathogens and reemergence of other diseases to land use change— the process of converting a specific area of land from one kind of use to another.

In the context of zoonotic disease emergence, shifts in land use from forest or other "wild" areas to agriculture or urban/suburban uses have received particular attention. But in talking about land use change, scientists may be racing past key assumptions, often taking fundamental concepts for granted. What, for instance, is "land," really?

Certainly land is a physical space where we and others live. But much is missed in so easy an answer. Cultures far and wide have long addressed such an oversimplification.

In his dialogue with the philosopher Huizi, the third century BC Daoist Zhuangzi observed:

> The earth is certainly vast and wide, but a man at any time uses only as much of it as his two feet can cover.
>
> But if you were to dig away all the earth around his feet, down to the Yellow Springs, would that little patch he stands on be of any use to him?[1265]

Huizi responds: "It would be useless." Yes, Zhuangzi says, "then the usefulness of the useless should be quite obvious." Paradoxically, carving away and isolating the "useful" turns it useless.

The lesson bears repeating today. Some of our brightest minds practice a way of understanding the world that is known as "reductionism."[1266] When trying to understand complex systems and concepts, many scientists reduce an inconceivable whole into more digestible bits, into conceptual fragments that are, taken in isolation, as representative of an elephant as its toenail. The approach has its place in the world. Sometimes the whole *is* the sum of its parts.

But in categorizing land use in terms of space, mode of production, or crop alone, many scientists appear to accept such reduced properties as the natural order of things for such a vast phenomenon. In doing so, the scientists tether the society that depends on their work to a rigid view of the human as both outside land and inherently unnatural.

This isn't the only path to understanding the world. Notions of land can take other forms. First Nations philosopher Leanne Betasamosake Simpson, for instance, offers that for many peoples, land is pedagogy.[1267] It is through the land and a compassionate web of interdependent relationships that we *know* people and place together.

In the terms of a modern radical political economy, it was through early capitalism and industrialization that we divorced ourselves from our relationships with land.[1268] What we see as our cultural instinct of a place without people is a historical hangover tied to turning land into an abstract commodity or financial instrument.

The impact on our understanding of disease follows. If we try to find the usefulness of "land use" as Huizi might have us, we can be easily swept away by the narrative of scientific research linking "land use change" and "disease emergence" or the process whereby deadly pathogens escape their previously limited ranges onto a wider stage.

The alienation of land and labor driving the new outbreaks echoes through the research itself. The ecology of years of intimate, locale-specific knowledge is replaced with a peculiar set of remote technologies and modeling. The two possibilities—intimate knowledge and modeling—needn't be mutually exclusive, but such a divide has been deployed by the powerful for their own benefit. As a result, humanity and nonhuman alike have been placed on the precipice of a series of globally felt environmental dangers.

Land as Pandemic Mirror

What we're saying is that it's a short step from thinking about land in a peculiarly utilitarian way to thinking about the pandemics that arise out of a land in much the same way. Many scientists appear to be able to recognize new infectious diseases and their treatment solely in the mirror of the ritual exploitation of the land from which the pathogens appear to originate.

The resulting paradigms are ugly. One particular narrative attracts media attention, funding support, and wide unconscious acceptance. It tells us that at the root of zoonotic disease spillover are "local" Indigenous populations and smallholders who are cutting down forests for agricultural plots as their population sizes grow out of control.[1269] This simplified narrative ignores settler colonialism and capitalism: a long and bloody history of grabbing lands and traditional knowledge out from underneath other peoples in imperialist and economic expansion.

Swidden-fallow agriculture that isn't tied to export schedules was long ago established as the most ecological means to cultivate in tropical forest regions.[1270] Recasting such rotational agriculture as destructive and coupling it with vilified wet markets and bushmeat reinforces the techno-scientific solutions of the reductionist, increasingly remote expertise of academic and intergovernmental science.

There is little new in this "blaming the victim" narrative. Karl Marx warned that "The ideas of the ruling class are in every epoch the ruling ideas, i.e., the class which is the ruling material force of society, is at the same time its ruling intellectual force."[1271] Brazilian geographer Milton Santos, one of the most important scholars from the Global South in the latter half of the twentieth century, described such modern fables as a fundamental component of the perversity that turns the most dangerous aspects of a society into the everyday normal.[1272] If we choose to be selectively blind to the real causes of our problems—to believe the fable—we can blame peasants and Indigenous populations for nature's destruction and the emergence of diseases, to the point of assigning their very existence as the major threat to nature's future.

In contrast, true radicalism always aims at getting to the root of the problem. Dialectical ecologist Richard Levins encouraged us to ask clarifying questions.[1273] Where is the rest of the world in any model? Can we see beyond what is expedient and in the now? What alternatives does history offer in its seed bank? Are alternate approaches already emerging into new futures?

The past is full of such possibilities. In ancient China, the Tang dynasty operated upon the *juntian* ("equal field") system that systematically redistributed agricultural land among people according to their capabilities to use that land and not their ability to extract value from it.[1274] Similarly, pre-Hispanic Mesoamerican societies saw land not as a good to be owned by individuals, but as a communal commons from where the community (*calpulli*) drew resources to reproduce itself.[1275]

By contrast, in ancient Europe, the Greeks, the society that would serve as a role model for the Western world, built its class structure around land tenure and private ownership. The contradiction underlying modern development appeared baked in from the start. So-called democratic principles were actualized within an economy sustained by shelving land aside and exploiting slaves, who were seen as the natural counterpart to free citizens.[1276]

The Romans, the intellectual children of the Greeks, followed this path in conquering territories. Land under Roman control was worked by those who were not citizens, creating and erasing borders along the way, and devising new means of expropriating others' resources as sources of energy sustaining the imperium.[1277] The provinces were stripped for a voracious core.

Today we can recognize the damage that followed. Pliny the Elder remarked that *latifundia perdidere italiam*—"the latifundia [or large landed estates and ranches] will destroy Italy." The social construct of "the land" as a good or commodity suggested to Pliny that the alienation of land from people was a swift step to societal self-destruction.

Centuries after Pliny reached this conclusion, Marx sketched the working dynamics of capitalism, finding that value extraction from nature accumulated when the means of production were concentrated and belonged to people different from those rendering the land useful.[1278]

The resulting runaway land grabs continue today, deep into the frontiers of the Amazon, the Congo, and Borneo. The push is propelled by crises of overaccumulation, governance narrowed to a politics around productivity, and the proliferation of farmland investment after the 2008 financial crisis.[1279] The paradox of abstracting land as a financial instrument and rendering land investible is that destroying land makes what little is left *more* valuable.[1280]

The global land rush and financialization over the past fifteen years has led to new levels of concentration. The Singapore-based agribusiness company Olam, for instance, owns and manages more than three million hectares of land and forests around the world, updating Pliny's prediction about latifundia's impacts to a chilling scope.

Latifundia, Disease, and Scientific Investigation

How does this shift in the notion of what land represents relate to emergent infectious diseases?

The late nineteenth-century physician Angelo Celli was among the first to propose a general theory of disease emergence linked to changes in land use and, importantly, ownership. Studying the history of malaria in the Agro Pontino Romano, he theorized that land accumulation was part of a vicious cycle fomenting the transmission of disease.[1281]

Celli suggested that disease could be a driver of latifundia, as much as disease is driven by land use. People who were protected from disease were more likely to keep their land or purchase land from the sick. Two mechanisms contributed to the vicious cycle: 1) the decreased utility of land exploitation by the reduced labor ability of sick landowners, and 2) the differences in the risk of acquiring infections, with the poorest more prone to getting sick.[1282]

Investigations in the decades to follow elaborated upon Celli's observation that how land was conceived and organized had a profound effect on the pathogens that emerged. The pioneering work of two research teams in the area of tropical medicine illustrates the broader approach which contemporary figures in the field appear to be avoiding as a matter of principle.

The late Karl Johnson was a global health scientist who conducted fieldwork and collaborated with scientists from many nations, mentoring peoples of different cultures and beliefs. He and his team discovered many new pathogens, including Ebola and Hantaan viruses.[1283] Closest to Johnson's heart, however, was the discovery of Machupo virus in the jungles of Bolivia.

In 1963, Johnson's team was tasked with investigating a novel hemorrhagic fever killing people around San Joaquin, Bolivia.[1284] The team embarked on a major study that combined exhaustive field studies and the best laboratory methods of the time. The study included sampling numerous bat, rodent, and insect species. The team was able to isolate the virus from the spleen of a deceased patient and establish that the large vesper mouse (*Calomys callosus*), a wild rodent native to South America, was the major reservoir of the pathogen.[1285]

Johnson concluded in much the way we find ourselves perplexed over COVID-19's origins: "The means of introduction is not clear. Infected rodents may have been imported with the baggage of humans, may have migrated directly into the town, or may have acquired the virus through contact with some other feral animal."[1286]

While studying the ecology of the system, Merle Kuns of the Middle America Research Unit found that the vesper mouse was abundant, and frequently infected with Machupo virus, in villages located in "elevated areas . . . known locally as 'alturas,'" where farmhouses were "usually located at the edge of the forest overlooking the grass covered marshlands or 'savannas.'" [1287] By contrast, more riparian villages, where the hemorrhagic fever was not observed, included both common rats (*Rattus rattus*) and common mice (*Mus musculus*), suggesting the presence of cosmopolitan rodents offered some protection against the Machupo virus.

Drawing upon his field experience, Johnson traced broader ecological connections. He proposed that DDT, the infamous pesticide with toxic neurological health effects on humans, might have had a role in impairing the ability of domestic cats to regulate rodent populations:

Cats were conspicuously scarce in San Joaquin. Residents of the town declared that these animals had been dying for several years of a peculiar neurological disease. Although we could not define its cause, oral administration of DDT reproduced the picture in cats imported for experimentation. Furthermore, subcutaneous and oral administration of Machupo virus to cats (the latter in the form of infected, sick, infant hamsters) did not result in illness. Neither were neutralizing antibodies found in response to these inoculations.[1288]

Later in life, Johnson hypothesized that rodent infestations were likely triggered by the plantains and cassava that farmers stored and on which the vesper mouse feasted and defecated, leaving Machupo virus in its wake.[1289]

Rather than blaming peasant farmers in San Joaquin for transforming the landscape in a way that promoted the emergence of the Machupo virus, we can better address the problem by asking, which and how many households store starchy vegetables? Disease causes become matters of conditional constellations of social practices tied to a mosaic landscape. The causes aren't essentialist in their racist, knee-jerk condemnation. Course corrections need not require removing populations that often represent the last resistance to multinational expropriation.

VHF and Structural Poverty

Another example. Epidemiologist Bob Tesh and his collaborators studied the Venezuelan Hemorrhagic Fever (VHF) caused by the Guanarito virus in the Portuguesa plains of western Venezuela.[1290]

Tesh and his team found that Alton's cotton rat and the short-tailed cane mouse, both common wild rodents at the study site, were the most likely reservoirs for the disease. Tesh suggested that private land ownership could have played a key role in the disease's transmission: "Property boundaries are often demarcated by tall grass or lines of trees, which serve as rodent habitats and refuges."[1291] Beyond that, however, Tesh and his team also asked a key question we should always keep in mind when studying emergent diseases:

One obvious question resulting from our study is why was VHF not recognized until 1989? We assume that Guanarito virus has existed in the local rodent population for a long time.

Also, people have lived in the VHF-endemic area for more than 200 years. There are a number of possible explanations. 1) The relatively small human population and the low prevalence of infection allowed sporadic cases to occur previously, without recognition as a distinct entity . . . ; 2) Increasing human migration into the region and the development of new agricultural lands have placed more people in contact with infected rodents; 3) Recent land-use changes in the region (i.e., deforestation and or large-scale cultivation of corn, sorghum, sun flowers, etc.) have provided more favorable habitats and food for granivorous species such as *S. alstoni* and *Z. brevicauda,* allowing populations of these rodents to increase significantly. This latter situation also would increase the risk of human contact with infected rodents.[1292]

In contrast, the reductionist fable insists that pathogen spillover and the emergence of disease need be attributed to land use change as driven by population growth, with the purpose of agriculture and urbanization. The compulsion is treated as internal to the locale. If we accept the fable, Milton Santos warned us, we assimilate a model of human nature that favors colonialist or neocolonialist objectives:

Growing unemployment is becoming chronic. Poverty is expanding and the quality of life of the middle classes is declining. Average salaries are tending to decrease. Famine and homelessness are spreading to all continents. New diseases such as AIDS are settling down, and old ones, supposedly extirpated, are returning triumphantly. Infant mortality remains in spite of medical developments and the dissemination of information. Good-quality education is increasingly difficult to access. Spiritual and moral disorders such as egoism, cynicism, and corruption are spreading and intensifying. The systemic perversity at the root of this negative evolution of humanity is related to a broad adherence to the competitive behaviours which presently characterize hegemonic actions.[1293]

The work of these Latin America-embedded researchers suggests that the complexity of the processes associated with the emergence of a disease is better encapsulated by a more comprehensive, holistic approach.

Celli's work, testing the hypothesis that low-quality housing was a major driver of malaria transmission, inspired more recent research that demonstrated that improving housing quality was associated with decreased malaria transmission in Costa Rica.[1294] The work also showed that more durable construction materials were associated with a reduction of sand flies, vectors of leishmaniasis, in rural Panamá.[1295]

So, if we are to blame "urbanization," we would better ask: What kind of urbanization? Is the problem urbanization or the massification of slums? Shall we worry about people living in suburbia and exurbia as it happens in the Global North? Or shall we worry about people living in the huge slums of Latin America, Africa, and Asia? From the perspective of rodents like the vesper mouse, is a house in the Dallas metroplex or in greater Los Angeles the same as informal housing in Iztapalapa, Paraisópolis, or Petare? In light of these more establishment analyses, it seems that living in Saitama or Riverside is the same as living in Tondo or Kibera. Land, after all, is just space. And by definition, land use is devoid of political economy.

There is another way. When we investigate the impacts of transforming natural ecosystems into agricultural land, mines, logged patches, or shopping malls, we should begin by taking into consideration the historical diversity and development of land covers past and present. Not all land was covered by forest before agriculture arose. Indeed, the African savanna and the Cerrado of South America have been savannas at least since the Pleistocene.[1296] As observed by Tesh's team, people have long been living where the Venezuelan Hemorrhagic Fever emerged, growing corn as a staple food, for hundreds, if not thousands, of years.[1297] It was, as we noted, only in 1989 that Guanarito virus became a problem.

Tesh and his team instead converged upon the new arrival of large-scale industrial agriculture, which had transformed the landscape before the outbreak. Coffee, for instance, can be grown under or without a forest canopy. In the shaded coffee agroforests, there is a richness of species and ecological interactions that regulate coffee pests.[1298] This doesn't happen in the sun coffee systems—monocultures under open skies—which, unlike the shaded ecosystem, bear little resemblance to a native forest in Mesoamerica.

Several studies of leishmaniasis from across Latin America have shown that shaded coffee agroecosystems have more diverse fauna, reducing the dominant vectors—those host species best at transmitting the parasite—in abundance.[1299] Sun coffee systems that host reduced biodiversity also host larger proportional and total abundances of the dominant vectors. The more ecologically exposed the dominant vector, the more cases of leishmaniasis.

All land conversion into agriculture is not the same. Generalizing terminology to the point where one speaks of "agricultural land transformation" ignores the heterogeneity of ecological processes involved and the foundational social, historical, and geographical relations underlying disease dynamics.[1300]

A Fistful of Dirt

Although not its explicit intention, establishment science helps to pave disease's way. Many research teams pursue sophisticated analytical methods—machine learning, artificial intelligence, and/or deep learning—using raster datasets or models that miss complex interactions across socioecologies.[1301] By omission or commission, the approaches reinforce the dangerous fables about the drivers of disease emergence.

What's missed? As detailed by ecological economist M. Graziano Ceddia, the big oversight is that increasing profits in commodity crops act as a major driver of deforestation.[1302] Depending on crop and locale, a 1 percent increase in investor wealth is associated with increases between 2.4 and 10 percent in commodity production at the expense of forests in Latin America and Southeast Asia.

Few disease ecologists address how these structural underpinnings of deforestation are repeatedly associated with the emergence and spillover of new pathogens, in spite of the evidence of the impacts that unequal ecological exchange impose.[1303] While agriculture and mining are increasingly addressed as the causes of the pandemic, the political economies driving these dynamics—the causes of the causes of the causes—are left on the side of the logging road.[1304]

Out in the world, they are felt in many directions. Uneven development and *horizontalities*—social impacts felt across contiguous tracts of land—have shaped, for instance, the emergence of two hemorrhagic arenaviruses, Machupo virus in Bolivia and the Junin virus in northern Argentina.[1305] Global *verticalities* raise borders against *some* people and *some* animals, while lowering them for other people and traded goods.[1306] By changing how land is used and *which* animals and people move around, migration policy and global trade disconnect long-standing disease ecologies and reconnect them in new ways that suddenly liberate pathogens that were previously boxed in by an earlier ecological regime.

Establishment science's penchant for abstractions devoid of such real-world complications helps enforce what is reimagined as "land"— what we see when we grasp a fistful of dirt—in favor of the powerful who are profiting from these new land use regimes. Across scales, from property lines to borders, this version of "land" is turned into the basis of governance and commodification. The scientific methods used to analyze the landscape reinforce these lucrative notions of land as a starting premise. It's not merely a matter of helping the logistics of extraction. Capital and science themselves are rationalized as a part of the natural order.

We are left with the spectacle of practitioners of the dominant paradigm in the field of ecology, its own disciplinary origins deeply embedded in white supremacist and colonialist thought, blaming people in slums and hinterlands from Colonia Azteca in Ciudad Juarez to Villa Fiorito in Buenos Aires, for the problem of emerging diseases.[1307] The impulse is an old one. A Calvinist discourse organizes a particularly Eurocentric civilizing mission around chastising and blaming the "other." Modern history—strewn with massacres,

slavery, and expropriation in the Global South—implies that the fable
ultimately acts as no more than a placeholder for supporting naked
imperialism and manifest destiny.

Such moralistic abuse has a long history. Slavery and conquest
are obvious examples, of course. Other instances serve as a bridge
to today's world order. Dutch colonialists, for one, appropriated
"unused" land to develop large-scale farms in Indonesia. The Javanese
were required to work for free on the new latifundia. As much as the
gun, administrative tactics were used to compel the labor. The Dutch
imposed taxes upon the Indonesian population both to fill colonial
coffers and increase productivity.[1308] The taxes maneuvered families
into serving up members as the cheapest option for fulfilling a village
or farm's labor quota.

The through line from one regime of exploitation to another is a
direct one. As political ecologist Nancy Peluso has shown, colonial
practices of asserting eminent domain over land perceived to be
"underutilized" or "unused" also formed the basis for the Government
of Indonesia's 1967 Basic Forestry Law.[1309] The law enabled the
Government of Indonesia to claim as property hundreds of thousands of lowland forests, grasslands, and croplands while recasting
customary practices as "criminal practices in huge chunks of the rural
landscape."

Massive state resource claims not only drove out local populations and propelled extensive deforestation from the 1960s onward,
today they form the basis for "green grabbing" projects throughout
the Indonesian archipelago.[1310] As was true historically, rather than
occupy "marginal," "idle," or "uninhabited" lands, such processes often
force local people who lose access to land-based entitlements, livelihoods, and existing ways of life into the capitalist labor market.[1311]

So what is spun in Global North terms as "overpopulation" or "too
many of them" still serves as a source of cheap labor. Maquilas and
other industrial operations that are headquartered abroad thrive
upon a standing army of labor that cannot be absorbed by otherwise
stripped-out and fenced-off local economies. Food sovereignty advocate Vandana Shiva has shown that at the other end of the rural-urban

circuit, the late twentieth-century's global connectivity and ease of movement (for some) renewed colonial style land monopolies and threatened seed sovereignty.[1312]

Racialism and imperialism are melded together.[1313] From Global South to North, the structural racism denounced by the Black Lives Matter movement has a long history rooted in labor needs for plantations, and, in a long continuation, in the perverse logic of redlining real estate and gentrification.[1314] Political scientist Samir Amin describes such impositions in uneven development in the Global South at larger scales, as brought on by the core-periphery economic dynamics of global capitalism.[1315] Even with the emergence of South-on-South exploitation, the capitalist core continues to appropriate land for commodities, driving people and pathogens across borders.[1316]

Next Imperial Greenwashing

The fate of the planet—with climate change and pandemics near-geological in their scale at this point—appears dependent on what we are to do with the next generation in such rationalization.

In February 2021, Peter Daszak, the president of EcoHealth Alliance, argued at a National Academy of Science webinar that the best way to bring about the appropriate interventions short-circuiting disease threats was to promote free trade. The very paradigm we saw Graziano Ceddia and others show is propelling the land grabs at the heart of the emergence of novel deadly pathogens.[1317]

EcoHealth Alliance, a New York-based NGO focused on the ecological origins of infectious diseases, has taken money from—and given awards to—the likes of Colgate-Palmolive and Johnson & Johnson, companies implicated in deforestation for oil palm.[1318] The Alliance is reported to have accepted (and tried to hide from the public) $40 million from the U.S. Department of Defense.[1319] The Alliance scored, lost, and scored back $7.5 million in funding from the National Institutes of Health to work, in part, on dangerous gain-of-function studies on pathogens, including coronaviruses, far beyond the scope of ecological research.[1320]

Such specifically sourced financing—corporations, military, and science—suggests the Alliance represents the modern-day equivalent of the Dutch East Indies Company, hopscotching from country to country rationalizing the neoliberal program in epizoology's name.[1321] Much as the technocratic Green Revolution aimed to box out communist insurgencies, the epidemiology-state nexus may represent a new mercantilized territorialism aimed at eradicating agroecological competition and subduing uncooperative farmers.[1322]

Case in point, Daszak has taken to retweeting missives on the ecological origins of outbreaks from the Capitals Coalition, an international NGO whose board includes representatives from Swiss pharmaceutical multinationals Novartis International and Roche, China-based real estate and manufacturing giant Giti Group, and, among others, the Director of the Enterprises Department at the International Labour Organization, who once served as the Chief Operations Officer of Business Unity South Africa.

One retweet linked to a plea from Patrice Matchaba, Group Head of Global Health & Corporate Responsibility for Novartis and Capitals Coalition board member, for capital-led interventions into pandemics and climate change:

> Responsibility falls on us all, and financial markets play a crucial role. Today, a growing body of Environmental, Social and Governance investors is looking at the financial rewards from sustainable practices. In his letter to CEOs, Larry Fink, BlackRock's Chairman and CEO, underlined climate risk as an existential threat to all companies and humanity. Companies that integrate the preservation and renewal of all forms of capital in their strategy will thrive, those that don't will not survive.
>
> I really hope the pandemic will force the world to shy away from the unilateral devotion to shareholder capitalism and short-term profits and move toward stakeholder capitalism, i.e. capitalism that promotes a capitals approach. Financial markets need to incentivize companies that are working on solutions for major global health challenges, particularly on cures for infec-

tious diseases that may not currently appear to have a financial return.[1323]

It doesn't take much to dwell on what Matchaba means. "Investing in governance" carries a variety of naughty connotations. Companies before humanity. Preserving labor and the environment, which are just different kinds of capital that capitalists get to control. Incentivizing pharmaceutical companies like Novartis by rewarding them with massive state subsidies to act in less sociopathic fashion.

As we forewarned near the top of this dispatch, Matchaba asks us to recognize and react to diseases in the mirror of the system that propagates them. Alongside characteristic opportunism, Matchaba's proposals—and Daszak's—exemplify the kind of conceptual incoherence that marks the present neoliberal order.[1324] Its incoherence and cruelty, however, do not serve as its refutation. It's going to take concerted political organization to defeat the new colonialism.

Radical Science with an Open Heart

A different kind of science is possible. Its origins aren't found in the latest statistical techniques, although eventually, with the right conceptual adjustments, such advances naturally follow. Disconnecting from the machinery of colonization is the first requisite.

In the face of such a daunting task, the world is awash in alternate ways of thinking and being upon which a resistance can draw. In Japan, despite a long history of assimilating technology from the world over, humans are seen as an essential part of the natural landscape. The sentiment is instilled early on. In the popular animated film *My Neighbor Totoro*, sisters Satsuki and Mei enjoy their time in their field house with Totoro and other Shintoist spirits. The grace of nature arrives as the children interact with beings of the forest: spirits, animals, and plants.[1325]

Beyond the aesthetic beauty of enjoying nature on its own terms, we are asked to understand that there is a struggle between humans and other species, but as a dialectical process with contradictions back

and forth. Against the Victorian Darwinism that was recruited to jus-
tify capitalism from the nineteenth century on, interactions between
different species aren't always matters of dog-eat-dog competition
and so need not serve as the basis of a voracious extractivism.[1326]
Ecological relationships are often also directly mutually beneficial
or in their emergent complexity more broadly enriching. Indeed,
humanity depends on these relationships, operating far beyond our
command and control, for its very existence.

The Japanese expression *kokoro no semai hito* translates as a "person
with a narrow heart" or a narrow mind, although the Japanese understand the mind and the heart as a unity. As we have argued up to this
point, having a narrow approach will unlikely help the world prevent
the emergence of new diseases. In fact, it may make matters worse
by imposing an opportunity cost: efforts to scientifically describe
disease emergence without reference to more sociopolitical circumstances *block* attempts to include them. Or worse, such well-funded
research programs may be supporting the new wave in corporatist
greenwashing.

Cultures beyond Japan object to such a colonialist science. But that's
only half the battle. Changing the world also requires action. Some of
that work includes scholarly research, yes. Ultimately, however, it'll
take the kind of political organization that rejects the expectation that
land is little but a source of commodities or, in the Capitals Coalition's
formation, just another form of capital.[1327]

We can take the stand of Ashitaka in *Princess Mononoke*, another
Hayao Miyazaki production. In the face of the destruction of the
forest and its spiritual poisoning, Ashitaka comes to terms helping
the forest spirit to rest in peace. He commits to helping Lady Eboshi
build a new human settlement that improves the lives of people, but
is also no longer a threat to the forest. Against any notion of the kind
of Half-Earth proposals of biologist E. O. Wilson and the like to clear
protected forests of the Indigenous and peasants, Ashitaka promises
to visit wild child San among the trees.[1328]

As Milton Santos and many others have proposed, another world
is possible. In fact, across many communities, it is already underway.

Indigenous, farmers, scientists, and many other people are working together on Richard Levins's question, "Where is the rest of the
world?" The answer for emerging diseases finds prophylaxes far
beyond vaccines and antivirals. They extend to housing improvement, land reform, public health for all, and ending the vicious cycle
of unequal development, commodification, and colonization driving
the worst of the new pathogens.

We can make better cities in the tradition of Lady Eboshi and
Ashitaka. We can visit San and the spirits in the forests upon which
we depend.

—PANDEMIC RESEARCH FOR THE PEOPLE
MARCH 28, 2021

Notes

Introduction

1. Wallace RG (2020). *Dead Epidemiologists: On the Origins of COVID-19*. Monthly Review Press, New York.
2. Wallace RG (2021). "Information underload." Patreon, November 13. https://www.patreon.com/posts/information-58647472
3. Tomšič S (2015). *The Capitalist Unconscious: Marx and Lacan*. Verso, New York.
4. Wallace R (2021). "How policy failure and power relations drive COVID-19 pandemic waves: A control theory perspective." https://hal.archives-ouvertes.fr/hal-03214718; Okamoto K, L Chaves, R Wallace, and RG Wallace. "Governance is key." This volume.
5. Žižek S (2021). *Pandemic! 2: Chronicles of a Time Lost*. Polity Press, Cambridge, UK.
6. Mitropoulos A (2020). *Pandemonium: Proliferating Borders of Capital and the Pandemic Swerve*. Pluto Press, London.
7. Wallace RG (2020). "Notes on a novel coronavirus." *MROnline*, 29 January. https://mronline.org/2020/01/29/notes-on-a-novel-coronavirus/.
8. Rogers A and M Raju (2022). "Democratic failures to pass Biden agenda force party to rethink 2022 strategy." CNN, 21 January. https://www.cnn.com/2022/01/21/politics/biden-agenda-2022-strategy/index.html.
9. Wilkie C (2022). "Biden says a Russian invasion of Ukraine 'would change the world." CNBC, 25 January. https://www.cnbc.com/2022/01/25/biden-says-a-russian-invasion-of-ukraine-would-change-the-world-.html; Anonymous (2021). "Biden-Xi talks: China warns US about 'playing with fire' on Taiwan." BBC News, 16 November. https://www.bbc.com/news/world-asia-china-59301167.

10. Emanuel E and M Osterholm (2022). "China's Zero-Covid policy is a pandemic waiting to happen." *New York Times*, 25 January. https://www.nytimes.com/2022/01/25/opinion/china-covid-19.html.

11. March E (2020). "A personality psychologist explains why some people can't admit when they lose—and how they spin failure to blame others." *The Conversation*, 12 November. https://www.businessinsider.com/personality-psychologist-explains-why-some-people-wont-accept-defeat-2020-11.

12. The People's CDC (2022). "The CDC's new guidelines are at odds with the fundamental tenets of equitable public health practice." Twitter, 4 March. https://twitter.com/PeoplesCDC/status/1499862495204454400.

13. Mina M (2022). "@CDCgov publishing its own results showing how POOR their own guidance is surrounding leaving isolation at 5 days w/out a negative rapid test." Twitter, 25 February. https://twitter.com/michaelmina_lab/status/1497312184480710662.

14. Pettypiece S and S Kapur (2022). "Biden's return-to-normal Covid strategy faces a new test as funding stalls." NBC News, 20 March. https://www.nbcnews.com/politics/politics-news/bidens-return-normal-covid-strategy-faces-new-test-funding-stalls-rcna20522.

15. Breslin M (2022). "Uninsured Americans now to be charged up to $195 per COVID test by some providers: report." *The Hill*, 26 March. https://thehill.com/policy/healthcare/medicaid/599898-uninsured-americans-now-to-be-charged-up-to-195-per-covid-test.

16. Pettypiece S (2022). "As Covid spreads through D.C., it's business as usual at the White House." NBC News, 8 April. https://www.nbcnews.com/politics/white-house/covid-spreads-dc-business-usual-white-house-rcna23492.

17. Wallace R and D Wallace (2022). "Concluding remarks." In R Wallace (ed), *Essays on Strategy and Public Health: The Systematic Reconfiguration of Power Relations*. Springer, Cham, pp 213–227.

18. Emanuel E and M Osterholm (2022). "China's Zero-Covid policy is a pandemic waiting to happen."; Feuer W (2020). "Biden Covid advisor says U.S. lockdown of 4 to 6 weeks could control pandemic and revive economy." CNBC, 11 November. https://www.cnbc.com/2020/11/11/biden-covid-advisor-says-us-lockdown-of-4-to-6-weeks-could-control-pandemic-and-revive-economy.html.

19. Wallace RG. "Biden's COVID plan isn't enough." This volume.

20. Stanway D (2022). "Shanghai eases lockdown in some areas despite record COVID infections." Reuters, 11 April. https://www.reuters.com/world/china/shanghais-covid-infections-rise-city-looks-get-moving-again-2022-04-11/.

21. Shear MD, SG Stolberg, S LaFraniere, and N Weiland (2022). "Biden's pandemic fight: Inside the setbacks of the first year." *New York Times*, 23 January. https://www.nytimes.com/2022/01/23/us/politics/biden-covid-strategy.html; Feldman J (2022). "A year in, how has Biden

done on pandemic response?" Medium, 4 January. https://jmfeldman. medium.com/a-year-in-how-has-biden-done-on-pandemic-response-88452c696f2.

22. Leonhardt D (2022). "A new COVID mystery: Why haven't cases started rising again in the U.S.?" *New York Times*, 6 April. https://www.nytimes.com/2022/04/06/briefing/covid-cases-us-omicron-subvariant.html; Leonhardt D (2022). "Covid and the 'very liberal.'" *New York Times*, 18 March. https://www.nytimes.com/2022/03/18/briefing/covid-risks-poll-americans.html; Leonhardt D (2022). "Do Covid precautions work?" *New York Times*, 9 March. https://www.nytimes.com/2022/03/09/briefing/covid-precautions-red-blue-states.html. Leonhardt D (2022). "COVID and race." *New York Times*, 9 June. https://www.nytimes.com/2022/06/09/briefing/covid-race-deaths-america.html

23. Yuan L (2022). "The army of millions who enforce China's Zero-Covid policy, at all costs." *New York Times*, 12 January. https://www.nytimes.com/2022/01/12/business/china-zero-covid-policy-xian.html; Yuan L (2022). "A coronavirus infection illuminates a migrant worker's tale of inequality in China." *New York Times*, 31 January. https://www.nytimes.com/2022/01/31/world/asia/covid-infection-illuminates-a-migrant-workers-tale-of-inequality-in-china.html; Yuan L (2002). "The 'China Model' is being tested by Covid, Russia and the economy. And it's coming up short." *New York Times*, 2 April. https://www.nytimes.com/2022/04/02/business/the-china-model-is-being-tested-by-covid-russia-and-the-economy-and-its-coming-up-short.html; Yuan L (2022). "Covid lockdowns revive the ghosts of a planned economy." *New York Times*, 25 April. https://www.nytimes.com/2022/04/25/business/china-covid-zero-economy.html; Yuan L (2022). "Has Shanghai been Xinjianged?" *New York Times*, 6 May. https://www.nytimes.com/2022/05/06/business/shanghai-xinjiang-china-covid-zero.html; Yuan L (2022). "Young Chinese feel suffocated." *New York Times*, 25 May. https://www.nytimes.com/2022/05/24/business/china-covid-zero.html; Yuan L (2022). "A solitary critic on 'Zero Covid'". 11 June. https://www.nytimes.com/2022/06/10/business/china-economy-covid-zero.html.

24. Yuan L (2022). "China's 'Zero Covid' strategy shows perils of autocracy." *New York Times*, 14 April. https://www.nytimes.com/2022/04/13/business/china-covid-zero-shanghai.html.

25. Harvey D (1982 [2006]). *Limits to Capital*. Verso, New York.

26. Tooze A (2021). *Shutdown: How Covid Shook the World's Economy*. Viking, New York.

27. Foster JB and I Sunwandi (2020). "COVID-19 and catastrophe capitalism: Commodity chains and ecological-epidemiological-economic crises." *Monthly Review* 72(2).

28. Harvey D (1982 [2006]). *Limits to Capital.*
29. Mandavilli A (2021). "The U.S. is getting a crash course in scientific uncertainty." *New York Times,* 22 August. https://www.nytimes.com/2021/08/22/health/coronavirus-covid-usa.html; Mandavilli A (2022). "The C.D.C.'s new challenge? Grappling with imperfect science." *New York Times,* 17 January. https://www.nytimes.com/2022/01/17/health/cdc-omicron-isolation-guidance.html;
30. LaFraniere S and N Weiland (2022). "Walensky, citing botched pandemic response, calls for C.D.C. reorganization." *New York Times,* 17 August. https://www.nytimes.com/2022/08/17/us/politics/cdc-rochelle-walensky-covid.html.
31. Anonymous (2022). "Some are winning - some are not: Which countries do best in beating covid-19?" Endcornavirus.org, 22 January. https://www.endcoronavirus.org/countries.
32. Harvey D (1982 [2006]). *Limits to Capital.*
33. Mitropoulos A (2022). "US likely 'dramatically undercounting' current COVID-19 resurgence, experts say." ABC News, 13 April. https://abcnews.go.com/Health/us-dramatically-undercounting-current-covid-19-resurgence-experts/story?id=84012793.
34. Trump D (2020). "Donald Trump speech transcript at PA distribution center for coronavirus relief supplies." Rev, 14 May. https://www.rev.com/blog/transcripts/donald-trump-speech-transcript-at-pennsylvania-distribution-center-for-coronavirus-relief-supplies.
35. LaFraniere S, MD Shear and SG Stolberg (2022). "Biden health officials warn of substantial increase in virus cases." *New York Times,* 19 May. https://www.nytimes.com/2022/05/18/us/politics/white-house-covid-briefing.html.
36. Ibid.
37. @CDCDirector (2022). "As of May 19th, over 45% of the U.S. population is in an area with a medium or high COVID-19 Community Level." Twitter, 20 May. https://twitter.com/CDCDirector/status/1527715083446636546.
38. Lopez G (2022). "Biden's unpopularity." Covid helps explain it." *New York Times,* 6 May. https://www.nytimes.com/2022/05/06/briefing/joe-biden-approval-rating-covid.html.
39. Lenton TM, CA Boulton, and M Scheffer (2022). "Resilience of countries to COVID-19 correlated with trust." *Scientific Reports* 12: 75; Qing Han Q, et al. (2021). "Trust in government regarding COVID-19 and its associations with preventive health behaviour and prosocial behaviour during the pandemic: a cross-sectional and longitudinal study." *Psychological Medicine* March 26: 1–11. doi: 10.1017/S0033291721001306; Covid-19 National Preparedness Collaborators (2022). "Pandemic preparedness and covid-19: an exploratory analysis of infection and fatality rates, and contextual factors associated with

preparedness in 177 countries, from Jan 1, 2020, to Sept 30, 2021." *Lancet* 399: 1489-51.

40. Lenton TM, CA Boulton, and M Scheffer (2022). "Resilience of countries to COVID-19 correlated with trust."

41. Galea S (2022). *The Contagion Next Time.* Oxford University Press, New York.

42. Albrecht DE (2022). "COVID-19 in rural America: Impacts of politics and disadvantage." Rural Sociology 87(1): 94-118; Jones B (2022). "The changing political geography of COVID-19 over the last two years." Pew Research Center, 3 March. https://www.pewresearch. org/politics/2022/03/03/the-changing-political-geography-of-covid-19-over-the-last-two-years/.

43. Van der Ploeg D (2009). *The New Peasantries: Struggles for Autonomy and Sustainability in an Era of Empire and Globalization.* Earthscan, London; Wallace RG (2018). "Vladimir Iowa Lenin, Part 2: On rural proletarianization and an alternate food future." *Capitalism Nature Socialism* 29(3): 21–35.

44. Kitchen C, et al. (2021). "Assessing the association between area deprivation index on COVID-19 prevalence: a contrast between rural and urban U.S. jurisdictions." *AIMS Public Health* 8(3): 519-530; Jackson SL, et al. (2021). "Spatial disparities of COVID-19 cases and fatalities in United States counties." *International Journal of Environmental Research and Public Health* 8(16): 8259; Monnat SM (2021). "Rural-urban variation in COVID-19 experiences and impacts among U.S. working-age adults." SocArXiv, 16 September. https://osf.io/preprints/socarxiv/tbhe2/.

45. Godelier M (2012). *The Mental and the Material.* Verso, New York; Tomšič S (2015). *The Capitalist Unconscious: Marx and Lacan.*

46. Han B-C (2021). "Capitalism and the death drive." In *Capitalism and the Death Drive.* Translated by Daniel Steuer. Polity Press, Cambridge, UK, pp 1–14. Han B-C (2021). *The Palliative Society: Pain Today.* Polity Press, Cambridge, UK.

47. Sitrin M and Colectiva Sembrar (eds) (2020). *Pandemic Solidarity: Mutual Aid during the COVID-19 Crisis.* Pluto Press, London.

48. Han B-C (2021). "Why revolution is impossible today." In *Capitalism and the Death Drive.* Translated by Daniel Steuer. Polity Press, Cambridge, UK, pp 15-20.

49. Han B-C (2021). "Capitalism and the death drive."

50. Dubos R (1959 [1996]) "The Gardens of Eden." In *Mirage of Health: Utopias, Progress, and Biological Change.* Rutgers University Press, New Brunswick.

51. Heti S (2022). *Pure Color.* Farrar, Straus and Giroux, New York.

52. Kapur S (2022). "Democrats turn against mask mandates as Covid landscape and voter attitudes shift." NBC News, 1 March. https://www.

nbcnews.com/politics/politics-news/democrats-turn-mask-mandates-covid-landscape-voter-attitudes-shift-rcna18043.

53. Cole D (2020). "White House chief of staff: 'We are not going to control the pandemic'." CNN, 25 October. https://www.cnn.com/2020/10/25/politics/mark-meadows-controlling-coronavirus-pandemic-cnntv/index.html.

54. LaFraniere S, MD Shear, SG Stolberg (2022). "Biden health officials warn of substantial increase in virus cases."

55. Peele A (2022). "The pandemic is waning. Anthony Fauci has a few more lessons to share." *Washington Post Magazine*, 29 June. https://www.washingtonpost.com/magazine/2022/06/27/anthony-fauci-post-pandemic-interview/.

56. The People's CDC (2022). "The CDC is beholden to corporations and lost our trust. We need to start our own." *The Guardian*, 3 April. https://www.theguardian.com/commentisfree/2022/apr/03/peoples-cdc-covid-guidelines; The People's CDC (2022). "What is the People's CDC?" https://peoplescdc.org/#about.

57. Diamond D (2022). "Transcript: Coronavirus: New variants with Rochelle Walensky." *Washington Post*, 22 July. https://www.washingtonpost.com/washington-post-live/2022/07/22/transcript-coronavirus-new-variants-with-rochelle-walensky/.

58. Weber L and C Cutter (2022). "Calling in sick or going on vacation, workers aren't showing up this summer." *Wall Street Journal*, 25 July. https://www.wsj.com/articles/calling-in-sick-or-going-on-vacation-workers-arent-showing-up-this-summer-11658741402.

59. LaFraniere S and N Weiland (2022). "Walensky, citing botched pandemic response, calls for C.D.C. reorganization."

60. Anthes E (2022). "C.D.C. eases Covid guidelines, noting virus is 'here to stay'." *New York Times*, 11 August. https://www.nytimes.com/2022/08/11/health/virus-cdc-guidelines.html.

61. Goodman B and E Cohen (2022). "CDC ends recommendations for social distancing and quarantine for Covid-19 control, no longer recommends test-to-stay in schools." CNN, 11 August. https://www.cnn.com/2022/08/11/health/cdc-covid-guidance-update/index.html.

62. Goodman B (2022). "Biden administration will stop buying Covid-19 vaccines, treatments and tests as early as this fall, Jha says." CNN, 16 August. https://www.cnn.com/2022/08/16/health/biden-administration-covid-19-vaccines-tests-treatments/index.html.

63. Anthes E (2022). "C.D.C. eases Covid guidelines, noting virus is 'here to stay'."

64. Yuko E (2022). "White House to establish office on Long Covid." *Rolling Stone*, 3 August. https://www.rollingstone.com/politics/politics-news/long-covid-white-house-department-1392205/.

65. Chengxi Zang C, et al. (2022). "Understanding post-acute sequelae of

SARS-CoV-2 infection through data-driven analysis with longitudinal electronic health records: Findings from the RECOVER Initiative." MedRxiv, 23 May. https://www.medrxiv.org/content/10.1101/2022.05.21.22275420v2.full.

66. Yong E (2022). "America is sliding into the long pandemic defeat." *The Atlantic*, 27 June. https://www.theatlantic.com/health/archive/2022/06/pandemic-protections/661378/.
67. Ibid.

Biden's COVID Plan Isn't Enough

68. Winck B (2020). "US weekly jobless claims rise to 898,000 as labor market recovery stumbles." *Business Insider*, 15 October. https://www.businessinsider.com/us-jobless-claims-weekly-unemployment-benefits-insurance-filings-rise-economy-2020-10.
69. Blow CM (2020). "Third term of the Obama presidency." *New York Times*, 8 November. https://www.nytimes.com/2020/11/08/opinion/biden-obama-presidency.html.
70. OECD (2020). "Income inequality (indicator)." OECD Data. https://data.oecd.org/inequality/income-inequality.htm.
71. Biden-Harris campaign (2020). "Joe and Kamala's plan to beat COVID-19." https://joebiden.com/covid19/.
72. Cole D (2020). "White House chief of staff: 'We are not going to control the pandemic." CNN, 25 October. https://www.cnn.com/2020/10/25/politics/mark-meadows-controlling-coronavirus-pandemic-cnntv/index.html.
73. Tankersley J and A Rappeport (2020). "Biden calls for stimulus ahead of a 'dark winter' for the country." *New York Times*, 16 November. https://www.nytimes.com/2020/11/16/business/economy/biden-speech-stimulus-economy.html.
74. Siegel B and L Bruggeman (2020). "Postal Service's plan to send 650M face masks to Americans allegedly nixed by White House." ABC News, 17 September. https://abcnews.go.com/Politics/postal-services-plan-send-650m-face-masks-americans/story?id=73081928.
75. Derysh I (2020) "Trump's decision to block coronavirus aid to hard-hit states will cost 4 million jobs." *Salon*, 15 August. https://www.salon.com/2020/08/15/trumps-decision-to-block-coronavirus-aid-to-hard-hit-states-will-cost-4-million-jobs-analysis/.
76. Kliff S (2020). "How to avoid a surprise bill for your coronavirus test." *New York Times*, 13 November. https://www.nytimes.com/2020/11/13/upshot/coronavirus-surprise-bills-guide.html.
77. Department of Health (2020). "COVID-19: Data". New York City. https://www1.nyc.gov/site/doh/covid/covid-19-data.page.
78. Ramos S and A Perez (2020). "U.S. tops 193,000 COVID-19 cases in 24 hours." ABC World News, 13 November. https://www.facebook.com/watch/?v=359826191972897.

79. KOTA Staff (2020). "Total cases surpass 50,000 in South Dakota, 22 new COVID-19 deaths Thursday." KOTA-TV, 5 November. https://www.kotatv.com/2020/11/05/total-cases-surpass-50000-in-south-dakota-22-new-covid-19-deaths-thursday/.

80. Stone W (2020). "COVID-19 hospitalizations hit record highs. Where are hospitals reaching capacity?" NPR, 10 November. https://www.npr.org/sections/health-shots/2020/11/10/933253317/covid-19-hospitalizations-are-surging-where-are-hospitals-reaching-capacity; Gates B (2020). "Austin hospitals taking overflow El Paso patients to make room for massive COVID-19 surge." KXAN, 17 November. https://www.kxan.com/news/coronavirus/austin-hospitals-taking-overflow-el-paso-patients-to-make-room-for-massive-covid-19-surge/.

81. Carlson J (2020). "Quarantined Minnesota health care workers feel pressure to return to work early." Star Tribune, 9 November. https://www.startribune.com/quarantined-minnesota-health-care-workers-feel-pressure-to-return-to-work-early/573011541/.

82. Luo E, N Chong, C Erikson, C Chen, S Westergaard, E Salsberg, and P Pittman (2020). "Contract tracing workforce estimator." Fitzhugh Mullan Institute for Health Workforce Equity. https://www.gwhwi.org/estimator-613404.html.

83. Grabell M, C Perlman, and B Yeung (2020). "Emails reveal chaos as meatpacking companies fought health agencies over COVID-19 outbreaks in their plants." ProPublica, 12 June. https://www.propublica.org/article/emails-reveal-chaos-as-meatpacking-companies-fought-health-agencies-over-covid-19-outbreaks-in-their-plants.

84. Brenner R (2020). "Escalating plunder." New Left Review, May/June. https://newleftreview.org/issues/ii123/articles/robert-brenner-escalating -plunder.

85. Corkery M and D Yaffe-Bellany (2020). "As meat plants stayed open to feed Americans, exports to China surged." New York Times, 16 June. https://www.nytimes.com/2020/06/16/business/meat-industry-china-pork.html.

86. LeBlanc P (2020). "Biden describes his phone call with Trump about coronavirus response." CNN, 7 April. https://www.cnn.com/2020/04/07/politics/biden-trump-phone-call-coronavirus-cnntv/index.html.

87. Tankersley J and A Rappeport (2020). "Biden calls for stimulus ahead of a 'dark winter' for the country."

88. Biden-Harris campaign (2020). "Joe and Kamala's plan to beat COVID-19."

89. Unwin HJT, et al. (2020). "State-level tracking of COVID-19 in the United States." Nature Communications 11: 6189. https://www.nature.com/articles/s41467-020-19652-6.

90. Planned Parenthood (2020). "What are pre-existing conditions?" https://www.plannedparenthoodaction.org/issues/health-care-equity/what-are-pre-existing-conditions.

91. Wallace RG, A Liebman, LF Chaves, and R Wallace (2020). "COVID-19 and circuits of capital." *Monthly Review* 72(1). https://monthlyreview. org/2020/05/01/covid-19-and-circuits-of-capital/.

92. Strobel WP and S Siddiqui (2020). "Biden aims to out-tough Trump on China while invoking his Obama experience." *Wall Street Journal,* 2 May. https://www.wsj.com/articles/biden-aims-to-out-tough-trump-on-china-while-invoking-his-obama-experience-11588420801.

93. Spinney L (2017). "Who names diseases?" *Aeon,* 23 May. https://aeon. co/essays/disease-naming-must-change-to-avoid-scapegoating-and-politics.

94. SCMP Reporter (2008). "Goldman Sachs pays US$300m for poultry farms." *South China Morning Post,* 4 August. https://www.scmp. com/article/647749/goldman-sachs-pays-us300m-poultry-farms; 5m Editor (2008). "Goldman Sachs invests in Chinese pig farming." *Pig Site,* 5 August. https://thepigsite.com/news/2008/08/goldman-sachs-invests-inchinese -pig-farming-1.

95. Wallace RG (2017). "Rogue resistance." *Farming Pathogens,* 29 March.   https://farmingpathogens.wordpress.com/2017/03/29/ rogue-resistance/.

96. Wallace RG (2016). "The Hillary Clinton boil." *Farming Pathogens,* 1   June.   https://farmingpathogens.wordpress.com/2016/06/01/ the-hillary-clinton-boil/.

97. McGirk T (2015). "How the bin Laden raid put vaccinators under the gun in Pakistan." *National Geographic,* 25 February. https:// www.nationalgeographic.com/news/2015/02/150225-polio-pakistan -vaccination-virus-health/.

98. Wallace RG. "The Alan Greenspan Strain." *Farming Pathogens,* 30   March.   https://farmingpathogens.wordpress.com/2010/03/30/ the-alan-greenspan-strain/.

99. Sifferlin A (2015). "Food illness outbreaks that cross state lines are the most deadly." *Time.* 3 November. https://time.com/4098438/ foodborne-illness-outbreaks/.

100. Wallace RG (2015). "Mickey the Measles." *Farming Pathogens,* 29 January. https://farmingpathogens.wordpress.com/2015/01/29/mickey -the-measles/.

101. Branswell H (2011). "Flu factories." *Scientific American.* January. https://www.scientificamerican.com/article/pandemic-flu-factories/.

102. Mena I, MI Nelson, F Quezada-Monroy, J Dutta, R Cortes-Fernández, JH Lara-Puente, F CastroPeralta, LF Cunha, NS Trovão, B Lozano-Dubernard, A Rambaut, H van Bakel, and A García-Sastre (2016). "Origins of the 2009 H1N1 influenza pandemic in swine in Mexico." *Elife.* 5.pii:e16777.

103. Wallace RG (2009). "The NAFTA flu." *Farming Pathogens.* 28 April. https://farmingpathogens.wordpress.com/2009/04/28/the-nafta-flu/.

104. Kissler SM, C Tedijanto, E Goldstein, YH Grad, and M Lipsitch (2020). "Projecting the transmission dynamics of SARS-CoV-2 through the postpandemic period." *Science* 368(6493):860-868.

105. Gilmore RW (2007). *Golden Gulag: Prisons, Surplus, Crisis, and Opposition in Globalizing California.* University of California Press, Berkeley, CA; Johnson W (2013). *River of Dark Dreams: Slavery and Empire in the Cotton Kingdom.* Harvard University Press, Cambridge, MA; Gisolfi MR (2017). *The Takeover: Chicken Farming and the Roots of American Agribusiness.* The University of Georgia Press, Athens, GA.

106. Taylor K-Y (2016). *From #BlackLivesMatter to Black Liberation.* Haymarket Books, Chicago, IL.

107. Bettez S (2013). *The Social Transformation of Health Inequities: Understanding the Discourse on Health Disparities in the United States.* Dissertation, Department of Sociology, University of New Mexico. https://digitalrepository.unm.edu/cgi/viewcontent.cgi?referer=&https redir=1&article=1005&context=soc_etds.

108. Wrigley-Field E (2020). "US racial inequality may be as deadly as COVID-19." *PNAS* 117(36):21854-21856.

109. Feuer W (2020). "Biden Covid advisor says U.S. lockdown of 4 to 6 weeks could control pandemic and revive economy." CNBC, 11 November. https://www.cnbc.com/2020/11/11/biden-covid-advisor-says-us-lock-down-of-4-to-6-weeks-could-control-pandemic-and-revive-economy.html.

110. Marcotty J (2015). "Scientists race to decode secrets of deadly bird flu." *Star Tribune*, 8 June. https://www.startribune.com/scientists-race-to-decode-secrets-of-deadly-avian-flu-strain/306436121/.

111. Relman DA, ER Choffnes, and A Mack (2010). *Infectious Disease Movement in a Borderless World: Workshop Summary.* Institute of Medicine (US) Forum on Microbial Threats. National Academies Press, Washington DC. https://www.ncbi.nlm.nih.gov/sites/books/NBK45719/.

112. Wallace RG (2015). "Made in Minnesota." *Farming Pathogens*, 10 June. https://farmingpathogens.wordpress.com/2015/06/10/made-in-minnesota; Wallace RG. "Industrial production of poultry gives rise to deadly strains of bird flu H5Nx." IATP blog, 24 January. https://www.iatp.org/blog/201703/industrial-production-poultry-gives-rise-deadly-strains-bird-flu-h5nx.

113. Cohen E (2020). "China says coronavirus can spread before symptoms show—calling into question US containment strategy." CNN, 26 January. https://www.cnn.com/2020/01/26/health/coronavirus-spread-symptomschinese-officials/index.html.

114. Emanuel EJ (2014). "Why I hope to die at 75." *The Atlantic*, October. https://www.theatlantic.com/magazine/archive/2014/10/why-i-hope - to-die-at-75/379329/.

115. Hall SS (2019). "A doctor and medical ethicist argues life after 75 is not worth living." *MIT Technology Review*, 21 August. https://www.technologyreview.com/2019/08/21/238642/a-doctor-and-medical-ethicist-argues-life-after-75-is-not worth-living/.

116. Ibid.

117. Goldsmith J (2017). "America's health and the 2016 election: An unexpected connection." *The Health Care Blog*, 4 January. https://thehealthcareblog.com/blog/2017/01/04/americas-health-and-the-2016-election-an-unexpected -connection/.

118. Madani D (2020). "Dan Patrick on coronavirus: 'More important things than living.'" NBC News, 21 April. https://www.nbcnews.com/news/us-news/texas-lt-gov-dan-patrick-reopening-economy-more-important-things-n1188911.

119. Klitzman R (2020). "How hospitals will decide who lives and who dies in the COVID-19 crisis." *The Hill*, 29 March. https://thehill.com/opinion/healthcare/490034-how-hospitals-will-decide-who-lives-and-who-dies-in-our-coronavirus-crisis.

120. Baker MG, N Wilson, and A Anglemyer (2020). "Successful elimination of Covid-19 transmission in New Zealand." *NEJM*, 7 August. https://www.nejm.or.g/doi/full/10.1056/NEJMc2025203.

121. Karlamanglas S and M Mason (2020). "Thousands of healthcare workers are laid off or furloughed as coronavirus spreads." *Los Angeles Times*, 2 May. https://www.latimes.com/california/story/2020-05-02/coronavirus-california-healthcare-workers-layoffs-furloughs.

Bidenfreude

122. Taylor A (2016). "Universities are becoming billion-dollar hedge funds with schools attached." *The Nation*, 8 March. https://www.thenation.com/article/archive/universities-are-becoming-billion-dollar-hedge-funds-with-schools-attached/.

123. Panitch L and S Gindin (2012). *The Making of Capitalism: The Political Economy of American Empire*. Verso, New York.

124. Bischoff E (ed) (2019). *Dimensions of Settler Colonialism in a Transnational Perspective*. Routledge, London.

125. Johnson W (2013). *River of Dark Dreams: Slavery and Empire in the Cotton Kingdom*. Harvard University Press, Cambridge, MA; Angus I (2016) *Facing the Anthropocene: Fossil Capitalism and the Crisis of the Earth System*. Monthly Review Press, New York.

126. Wallace RG, A Liebman, LF Chaves, and R Wallace (2020). "COVID-19 and ciruits of capital." *Monthly Review* 72(1).

127. Sheppard E (2020). "What's next? Trump, Johnson, and globalizing capitalism." *Environment and Planning A*, 22 April. https://doi.org/10.1177/0308518X20914461.

128. Neuburger T (2020). "To save the economy, Biden must first save

lives". *Naked Capitalism*, 24 November. https://www.nakedcapitalism. com/2020/11/to-save-the-economy-biden-must-first-save-lives.html.

129. Collins C (2020). "Updates: Billionaire wealth, U.S. job losses and pandemic profiteers". Inequality.org, 9 December. https://inequality.org/ great-divide/updates-billionaire-pandemic/.

130. The Decolonial Atlas (2020). "Do your part! Die for the market!" https://m.facebook.com/decolonialatlas/posts/1823790674454662.

131. Baek S, SK Mohanty, and M Glambosky (2020). "COVID-19 and stock market volatility: An industry level analysis". *Finance Research Letters* 37: 101748. https://www.ncbi.nlm.nih.gov/pmc/articles/ PMC7467874/.

132. Durand C (2017). *Fictitious Capital: How Finance Is Appropriating Our Future*. Translated by D Broder. Verso Books, New York.

133. Gibadullina A (2021). "Who owns the means of production? Uneven geographies of financialization." http://206.12.92.126:8838/ finance_geo/.

134. Foster JB, RJ Jonna, and B Clark (2021). "The contagion of capital: Financialized capitalism, COVID-19, and the great divide." *Monthly Review*, 72(8).

135. Paavola A (2020). "266 hospitals furloughing workers in response to COVID-19." *Becker's Hospital CFO Report*, 31 August. https:// www.beckershospitalreview.com/finance/49-hospitals-furloughing- workers-in-response-to-covid-19.html; Burlage R and M Anderson (2018). "The transformation of the medical-industrial complex: Financialization, the corporate sector, and monopoly capital." In H Waitzkin (ed), *Health Care Under the Knife: Moving Beyond Capitalism for Our Health*. Monthly Review Press, New York, pp 69-82.

136. Martin A (2021). "U.S. COVID-19 hospitalizations hit record." *Wall Street Journal*, 4 January. http://web.archive.org/web/20210107051236/ https://www.wsj.com/livecoverage/covid-2021-01-04.

137. Frankel TC, B Martin, A Van Dam, and A Flowers (2020). "A growing number of Americans are going hungry." *Washington Post*, 25 November. https://www.washingtonpost.com/graphics/2020/business/ hunger-coronavirus-economy/.

138. Tappe A (2020). "Another 787,000 Americans filed first-time claims for jobless benefits last week." CNN Business, December 31. https://www. cnn.com/2020/12/31/economy/unemployment-benefits-coronavirus/ index.html.

139. Bhattarai A and H Denham (2020). "Stealing to survive: More Americans are shoplifting food as aid runs out during the pandemic." *Washington Post*, 10 December. https://www.washingtonpost.com/ business/2020/12/10/pandemic-shoplifting-hunger/.

140. Kelly ML and M Pao (2020). "'These are deaths that could have been prevented,' says researcher studying evictions." NPR News, 2

December. https://www.npr.org/sections/coronavirus-live-updates
/2020/12/02/940720861/these-are-deaths-that-could-have-been-
prevented-says researcher-studying-evictio.

141. Brenner R (2020). "Escalating plunder." *New Left Review,* May/June.
https://newleftreview.org/issues/ii123/articles/robert-brenner-escalat-
ing-plunder; Ang C (2020). "The rich got richer during COVID-19.
Here's how American billionaires performed." Visual Capitalist, 30
December. https://www.visualcapitalist.com/the-rich-got-richer-dur-
ing-covid-19-heres-how-american-billionaires-performed/.

142. Kapur S and D Gregorian (2021). "Congress overrides Trump's veto
for the first time on major military bill." NBC News, 1 January. https://
www.nbcnews.com/politics/congress/congress-overrides-trump-
s-veto-first-time-major-military-bill-n1252652; Peter G. Peterson
Foundation (2021). "The United States spends more on defense than
the next 11 countries combined." 19 July. https://www.pgpf.org/
blog/2021/07/the-united-states-spends-more-on-defense-than-the-
next-11-countries-combined.

143. Tankersley J and M Crowley (2021). "Biden outlines $1.9 trillion
spending package to combat virus and downturn." *New York Times,*
14 January. https://www.nytimes.com/2021/01/14/business/economy/
biden-economy.html; Sarlin B and S Ruhle (2020). "As coronavirus
surges, countries spend more on economic aid. But not the U.S." NBC
News, 9 December. https://www.nbcnews.com/politics/politics-news/
coronavirus-surges-countries-spend-more-economic-aid-not-u-
s-n1250411.

144. Wallace R (2021) "Planet farm." *New Internationalist,* 6 January. https://
newint.org/immersive/2021/01/06/planet-fjf-farm.

145. Diamond D (2020). "'We want them infected': Trump appoin-
tee demanded 'herd immunity' strategy, emails reveal." *Politico,* 16
December. https://www.politico.com/news/2020/12/16/trump-appoin-
tee-demanded-herd-immunity-strategy-446408; Harrison DW (2020).
"Results from the AstraZeneca/Oxford Vaccine trials." https://dalewhar-
rison.substack.com/p/results-from-the-astrazenecaoxford.

146. Waitzkin H (ed) (2018). *Health Care Under the Knife: Moving Beyond
Capitalism for Our Health.* Monthly Review Press, New York; Kaufman
E, A Grayer, and S Murray (2020). "US officials promised 20 million
vaccinated against coronavirus by the end of the year. It's going slower
than that." CNN, 28 December. https://www.cnn.com/2020/12/23/
health/vaccine-rollout-slow-data-lags/index.html.

147. Szilagyi PG, K Thomas, and MD Shah (2020). "National trends in
the US public's likelihood of getting a COVID-19 vaccine—April 1 to
December 8, 2020." *Journal of the American Medical Association* 325(4):
396-398.

148. Sirota D (2020). "Joe Biden's love of austerity cut the stimulus bill in

half." *Jacobin,* 22 December. https://www.jacobinmag.com/2020/12/joe-biden-austerity-stimulus-bill-cut-in-half-covid-19.

149. Wallace R. "Biden's COVID plan isn't enough." This volume.
150. Marcetic B (2020). "Joe Biden said he'd 'follow the science' on the pandemic. He isn't." *Jacobin,* 10 December. https://jacobinmag.com/2020/12/biden-coronavirus-covid-lockdown-science.
151. Fisher M (2009). *Capitalist Realism: Is There No Alternative?* Zero Books, Hants, UK.
152. Ali T (2015). *The Extreme Centre: A Warning.* Verso, London; Foster JB, R York, and B Clark (2010). *The Ecological Rift: Capitalism's War on the Earth.* Monthly Review Press, New York.
153. Foster JB and I Suwandi (2020). "COVID-19 and catastrophe capitalism'" *Monthly Review,* 72(2); Twohey M, K Collins, and K Thomas (2020). "With first dibs on vaccines, rich countries have 'cleared the shelves.'" *New York Times,* 15 December. https://www.nytimes.com/2020/12/15/us/coronavirus-vaccine-doses-reserved.html.
154. Thrush G (2020). "'Accelerate the endgame': How Barack Obama nudged Bernie Sanders out of the race." *Chicago Tribune,* 14 April. https://www.chicagotribune.com/nation-world/ct-nw-nyt-barack-obama-bernie-sanders-democrats-20200414-tdpw52c46vgqjjevu54attf4yu-story.html; BBC News (2020). "Defund the Police: Obama says 'snappy slogan' risks alienating people." 3 December. https://www.bbc.com/news/world-us-canada-55169107; O'Donnell R (2020). "How Barack Obama helped convince NBA players to end their strike and return to play." *SB Nation,* 29 August. https://www.sbnation.com/nba/2020/8/29/21406770/barack-obama-nba-players-lebron-james-strike-chris-paul-meeting-call; Kashinsky L (2020). "Squad blasts Obama for 'critique' on 'defund the police' slogan." *Boston Herald,* 2 December. https://www.bostonherald.com/2020/12/02/obama-draws-progressive-ire-for-criticizing-snappy-slogans-like-defund-the-police/.
155. Goehl G (2020). "Biden's pick for agriculture secretary raises serious red flags." *The Guardian,* 21 December. https://www.theguardian.com/commentisfree/2020/dec/21/joe-biden-tom-vilsack-agriculture-secretary.
156. Edelman M (2021). "Hollowed out Heartland, USA: How capital sacrificed communities and paved the way for authoritarian populism." *Journal of Rural Studies* 82: 505-517.
157. Clinton Digital Library (1992). "The Man From Hope." Video. Clinton Presidential Library & Museum. https://clinton.presidentiallibraries.us/items/show/15890; Wikipedia. "Barak Obama 'Hope' poster." https://en.wikipedia.org/wiki/Barack_Obama_%22Hope%22_poster.
158. Alj M (2021). *A People's Green New Deal.* Pluto Press, London.

A Spray of Split Seconds

159. Flener M (2021). "Video provides new angle of fatal police shooting

of Malcolm Johnson in March." *KMBC 9 News*, 3 June. https://www.kmbc.com/article/video-provides-new-angle-of-fatal-police-shooting-of-malcolm-johnson-in-march/36623380#.

160. Crepeau M (2021). "Kim Foxx says her office's 'checks and balances' didn't work before faulty in-court statement on Adam Toledo shooting; her top assistant exits." *Chicago Tribune*, 5 May. https://www.chicagotribune.com/news/criminal-justice/ct-kim-foxx-adam-toledo-video-report-20210505-jfl4bwgf5feifaya6ih62lwtrm-story.html.

161. Bump P (2021). "How the first statement from Minneapolis police made George Floyd's murder seem like George Floyd's fault." *Washington Post*, 20 April. https://www.washingtonpost.com/politics/2021/04/20/how-first-statement-minneapolis-police-made-george-floyds-murder-seem-like-george-floyds-fault.

162. Star Tribune [@StarTribune] (2021). "We have removed this tweet because it falsely reported that the man who was shot and killed, later identified as Winston Boogie Smith, was a murder suspect. That information was initially sourced from law enforcement scanner audio. (1/2)." Twitter, 8 June. https://twitter.com/StarTribune/status/1402320864582934531.

163. Alec Karakatsanis [@equalityAlec] (2021). "Behind every cop who murders a 13-year-old child, there is a city lawyer working to keep the video secret, a prosecutor lying about it in court, a mayor giving cops more money and weapons, and a professor with a consulting firm deciding which 'reform' will make the most money." Twitter, 15 April. https://twitter.com/equalityAlec/status/1382827690382610434.

164. Goudie C, B Markoff, C Tressel, R Weidner, and J Fagg (2021). "No crimes reported by Chicago police after 86% of ShotSpotter gunfire alerts." *ABC 7 Eyewitness News*, 3 May. https://abc7chicago.com/chicago-police-cpd-shotspotter-news/10575861.

165. Richmond T and M Ibrahim (2021). "Brooklyn Center mayor blasts police tactics to control protesters." *Pioneer Press*, 17 April. https://www.twincities.com/2021/04/16/daunte-wright-brooklyn-center-minnesota-mayor-blasts-police-tactics-to-control-protesters.

166. Tucker E (2021). "States tackling 'qualified immunity' for police as Congress squabbles over the issue." CNN, 23 April. https://www.cnn.com/2021/04/23/politics/qualified-immunity-police-reform/index.html.

167. Kirkpatrick D (2021). "Split-second decisions: How a Supreme Court case shaped modern policing." *New York Times*, 25 April. https://www.nytimes.com/2021/04/25/us/police-use-of-force.html.

168. Dewan S and R Oppel Jr (2015). "In Tamir Rice case, many errors by Cleveland police, then a fatal one." *New York Times*, 22 January. https://www.nytimes.com/2015/01/23/us/in-tamir-rice-shooting-in-cleveland-many-errors-by-police-then-a-fatal-one.html.

169. Fry H (2021). "What data can't do." *New Yorker*, 22 March. https://www.newyorker.com/magazine/2021/03/29/what-data-cant-do.
170. Associated Press/WCCO (2015). "2 Minn. departments quit controversial police training." WCCO 4 CBS Minnesota, 15 May. https://minnesota.cbslocal.com/2018/05/15/bulletproof-mpd-rcs.
171. Cineas F (2021). "Why they're not saying Ma'Khia Bryant's name." *Vox*, 1 May. https://www.vox.com/22406055/makhia-bryant-police-shooting-columbus-ohio.
172. Kirkpatrick D (2021). "Split-second decisions: How a Supreme Court case shaped modern policing."
173. Rubright K and B Myszkowski (2021). "A call for justice: Community questions DA response in Hall case, mulls solutions for the future." *Pocono Record*, 9 April. https://www.poconorecord.com/story/news/local/2021/04/09/activists-plan-protest-christian-halls-death-police-shooting-treandous-cuthbertson/7156744002.
174. Ibid.
175. Jackman Y (2019). "Police chiefs propose ways to reduce 'suicide by cop.'" *The Washington Post*, 31 October. https://www.washingtonpost.com/crime-law/2019/10/31/police-chiefs-propose-ways-reduce-suicide-by-cop.
176. Ramos M (2021). "Medical examiner releases Adam Toledo autopsy details." *Chicago Sun-Times*, 6 May. https://chicago.suntimes.com/news/2021/5/6/22423497/adam-toledo-autopsy-fatal-police-shooting-medical-examiner-little-village.
177. Towers A (2021). "Sean Hannity blasted for calling Adam Toledo, child killed by Chicago police, a '13-year-old man.'" *The Wrap*, 15 April. https://www.thewrap.com/hannity-adam-toledo-13-year-old-man.
178. Goyal MK, N Kuppermann, SD Cleary, SJ Teach, and JM Chamberlain (2015). *JAMA Pediatrics* 169(11): 996-1002; Badreldin N, WA Grobman, and LM Yee (2019). "Racial disparities in postpartum pain management." *Obstetrics and Gynecology* 134(6): 1147-1153; Ly DP (2019). "Racial and ethnic disparities in the evaluation and management of pain in the outpatient setting, 2006-2015." *Pain Medicine* 20(2): 223-232.
179. Eligon J (2020). "Black doctor dies of Covid-19 after complaining of racist treatment." *New York Times*, 23 December. https://www.nytimes.com/2020/12/23/us/susan-moore-black-doctor-indiana.html .
180. Ibid.
181. Resnick B (2017). "Trump supporters know Trump lies. They just don't care." *Vox*, 10 July. https://www.vox.com/2017/7/10/15928438/fact-checks-political-psychology.
182. Wallace RG. "Biden's COVID plan isn't enough." This volume; Wallace RG. "Bidenfreude." This volume.
183. Lonas L (2021). "Powell cautions that US is reopening to a 'different

economy." *The Hill*, 8 April. https://thehill.com/policy/finance/547222-powell-cautions-that-us-is-reopening-to-a-different-economy; Brueck II and A Bendix (2021). "CDC director fights back tears as she warns of soaring COVID-19 cases: 'Right now I'm scared." *Yahoo! News*, 29 March. https://news.yahoo.com/cdc-director-fights-back-tears-172155352.html.

184. Weiland N and M Smith (2021). "Surging virus has Michigan's Democratic governor at loggerheads with Biden," *New York Times*, 12 April. https://www.nytimes.com/2021/04/12/us/politics/michigan-coronavirus-whitmer-biden.html.

185. Bogel-Burroughs N, S Dewan, and K Gray (2020). "F.B.I. says Michigan anti-government group plotted to kidnap Gov. Gretchen Whitmer." *New York Times*, 8 October. https://www.nytimes.com/2020/10/08/us/gretchen-whitmer-michigan-militia.html.

186. Knutson J (2020). "Trump blames 'blue states' for high coronavirus cases in U.S." *Axios*, 17 September. https://www.axios.com/trump-coronavirus-deaths-toll-blue-states-3bebf52a-d3ef-4ac0-91b0-7db96cd9f34a.html.

187. Institute for Health Metrics and Evaluation. "Covid-19 projections." Accessed May 22, 2021. https://covid19.healthdata.org/united-states-of-america?view=cumulative-deaths&tab=trend.

188. Institute for Health Metrics and Evaluation. "Estimation of excess mortality due to COVID-19." Accessed May 13, 2021. http://www.healthdata.org/special-analysis/estimation-excess-mortality-due-covid-19-and-scalars-reported-covid-19-deaths.

189. Defoe D (1772 [1995]). *A Journal of the Plague Year*. Project Gutenberg EBook. https://www.gutenberg.org/files/376/376-h/376-h.htm.

190. Galea S (2020). "The contagion next time: Underlying socioeconomic, racial divides, COVID risks and future pandemics." YouTube. Video, 39:46. https://www.youtube.com/watch?v=LHtbMebQw28.

191. Stobbe M (2021). "US deaths from heart disease and diabetes climbed amid COVID." *AP News*, 9 June. https://apnews.com/article/coronavirus-pandemic-diabetes-science-heart-disease-health-213fe132f33c9428ea39274ffb96aa01.

192. Waitzkin H (2021). "Re: [spiritof1848] COVID-19 mortality." The Spirit of 1848 listserv, 10 May.

193. Musgrove P, A Creese, A Preker, C Baeza, A Anell and T Prentice (2000). *The World Health Report 2000: Health Systems: Improving Performance*. World Health Organization, Geneva. https://www.who.int/publications/i/item/924156198X; Almeida C, P Braveman, M Gold, C Szwarcwald, JM Ribeiro, A Miglionico, et al. (2001). "Methodological concerns and recommendations on policy consequences of the World Health Report 2000." *The Lancet* 357(9269): 1692-1697.

194. Schwab T (2020). "Are Bill Gates' billions distorting public health

data?" *The Nation*, 3 December. https://www.thenation.com/article/society/gates-covid-data-ihme.

195. Ibid.

196. Lee S (2020). "JetBlue's founder helped fund a Stanford study that said the coronavirus wasn't that deadly." *Buzzfeed*, 15 May. https://www.buzzfeednews.com/article/stephaniemlee/stanford-coronavirus-neeleman-ioannidis-whistleblower.

197. Sanchez V (2021). "COVID long-haulers: What we know about the debilitating symptoms that last for months." *7News*, 8 June. https://wjla.com/news/coronavirus/covid-long-hauler-debilitating-symptoms-continue-months-after-diagnosis.

198. Wallace D and R Wallace (2017). "Benign neglect and planned shrinkage." Verso Books blog, 25 March. https://www.versobooks.com/blogs/3145-benign-neglect-and-planned-shrinkage; Complaint, Knight Institute v. CDC, (U.S.D.C. S.D.N.Y. 2020) (No. 20-2761).

199. BeMiller H (2020). "Fact check: Cosmetology training versus police training comparison lacks context." *USA Today*, 28 August. https://www.usatoday.com/story/news/factcheck/2020/08/28/fact-check-cosmetology-vs-police-training-comparison-lacks-context/5653808002.

200. Horton J (2021). "How US police training compares with the rest of the world." *BBC News*, 18 May https://www.bbc.com/news/world-us-canada -56834733.

201. ABC News (2000). "Court OKs barring high IQs for cops." ABC News, 8 September https://abcnews.go.com/US/court-oks-barring-high-iqs-cops/story?id=95836.

202. Cooper D and T Kroeger (2017). "Employers steal billions from workers' paychecks each year." Economic Policy Institute, 10 May. https://www.epi.org/publication/employers-steal-billions-from-workers-paychecks-each-year.

203. Watts M (2020). "Milwaukee PD criticized for old tweet congratulating cop who left Dahmer victim." *Newsweek*, 19 June. https://www.newsweek.com/milwaukee-pd-congratulate-retired-cop-who-laughed-off-teen-victim-dahmer-1512130.

204. Masters B (1993). *The Shrine of Jeffrey Dahmer*. Hodder and Stoughton, London.

205. Diski J (1993). "Good housekeeping." *London Review of Books*, 11 February. https://www.lrb.co.uk/the-paper/v15/n03/jenny-diski/good-house keeping.

206. Ibid.

207. Kravitz D (2021). "Bodies of hundreds of New York COVID victims still in trucks on Brooklyn pier." *The City*, 6 May. https://www.thecity.nyc/missing-them/2021/5/6/22423844/new-york-covid-victims-still-in-trucks-on-brooklyn-pier.

208. Audi A (2016). "Errol Morris on the time he filmed Donald Trump

missing the point." *Literary Hub*, 27 October. https://lithub.com/erroll-morris-on-the-time-he-filmed-donald-trump-missing-the-point.

209. Van Syckle K (2014). "'He's untouched by history': Errol Morris on Donald Rumsfeld." *Rolling Stone*, 1 April. https://www.rollingstone. com/politics/politics-news/hes-untouched-by-history-errol-morris-on-donald -rumsfeld-231576.

210. Holpuch A (2021). "US could have averted 40% of Covid deaths, says panel examining Trump's policies." *The Guardian*, 11 February. https:// www.theguardian.com/us-news/2021/feb/10/us-coronavirus-response -donald-trump-health-policy.

211. Galea S (2020). "The contagion next time: Underlying socioeconomic, racial divides, COVID risks and future pandemics."

212. Andrasfay T and N Goldman (2021). "Reductions in 2020 US life expectancy due to COVID-19 and the disproportionate impact on the Black and Latino populations." *Proceedings of the National Academy of Sciences* 118(5). https://www.pnas.org/content/118/5/e2014746118/ tab-article-info; Venkataramani A, R O'Brien, and A Tsai (2021). "Declining life expectancy in the United States: The need for social policy as health policy." *JAMA* 325(7): 621-622. https://jamanetwork. com/journals/jama/article-abstract/2776338.

213. Dorn S and R Gordon (2021). *The Catastrophic Costs of Uninsurance: Covid-19 Cases and Deaths Closely Tied to America's Health Coverage Gaps*. Families USA, 4 March. https://familiesusa.org/resources/ the-catastrophic-cost-of-uninsurance-covid-19-cases-and-deaths-closely-tied-to-americas-health-coverage-gaps; McLaughlin J, F Khan, S Pugh, F Angulo, H-J Schmidt, R Isturiz, L Jodar, and D Swerdlow (2020). "County-level predictors of COVID-19 cases and deaths in the United States: What happened, and where do we go from here?" *Clinical Infectious Diseases* 73(7): e1814-1821.

214. Leifheit K, S Linton, J Raifman, G Schwartz, E Benfer, F Zimmerman, and C E Pollack (2021). "Expiring eviction moratoriums and COVID-19 incidence and mortality." *American Journal of Epidemiology* 190(12): 2503-2510.

215. Block L (2021). "220,000 tenants on the brink and counting." Association for Housing and Neighborhood Development, 17 March. https://anhd.org/blog/220000-tenants-brink-and-counting.

216. Galea S (2020). "The contagion next time: Underlying socioeconomic, racial divides, COVID risks and future pandemics."

217. Qin A and C Buckley (2021). "A top virologist in China, at center of a pandemic storm, speaks out." *New York Times*, 14 June. https://www. nytimes.com/2021/06/14/world/asia/china-covid-wuhan-lab-leak. html.

218. Paul T (2021). "Distancing measures must continue during vaccine roll-out: study." Columbia School of Public Health website, 25 January.

https://www.publichealth.columbia.edu/public-health-now/news/distancing-measures-must-continue-during-vaccine-roll-out-study.

219. Freiman J (2021). "Texas Rangers allowing 100% capacity at stadium for opening day." *CBS News*, 11 March. https://www.cbsnews.com/news/texas-rangers-globe-life-field-100-capacity-opening-day; Carlsen A, P Huang, Z Levitt, and D Wood (2021). "How is the COVID-19 vaccination campaign going in your state?" National Public Radio/WNYC, accessed 15 July. https://www.npr.org/sections/health-shots/2021/01/28/960901166/how-is-the-covid-19-vaccination-campaign-going-in-your-state.

220. Tucker T (2021). "Braves expect crowd 'at or near sellout' for return to 100% capacity." *Atlanta Journal Constitution*, 6 May. https://www.ajc.com/sports/atlanta-braves/braves-expect-crowd-at-or-near-sellout-for-return-to-100-capacity/Y4OVVMK64FH5HG2OYOCHDU7GRE

221. Kurland J, A Piquero, W Leal, E Sorrell, and NL Piquero (2021). "COVID-19 incidence following fan attendance: A case study of the National Football League 2020-2021 season." *The Lancet*, 30 March. https://papers.ssrn.com/sol3/papers.cfm?abstract_id=3805754.

222. Peltier J (2021). "Crowds for European Championship soccer games are driving infections, the W.H.O. says." *New York Times*, 1 July. https://www.nytimes.com/2021/07/01/world/europe/euro-2020-covid-outbreak.html.

223. *The New York Times* (2021). "See reopening plans and mask mandates for all 50 States." *New York Times*, 1 July. https://www.nytimes.com/interactive/2020/us/states-reopen-map-coronavirus.html.

224. Jones S (2021). "De Blasio and Cuomo clash over reopening the city." *The Real Deal*, 29 April. https://therealdeal.com/2021/04/29/de-blasio-and-cuomo-clash-over-reopening-the-city.

225. Sexton J and Sapien J (2020). "How Andrew Cuomo and Bill de Blasio's failures made New York a Covid-19 epicentre." Scroll.in, 26 May. https://scroll.in/article/962891/how-andrew-cuomo-and-bill-de-blasios-failures-made-new-york-a-covid-19-epicentre.

226. Jewell B and N Jewell (2020). "The huge cost of waiting to contain the pandemic." *New York Times*, 14 April https://www.nytimes.com/2020/04/14/opinion/covid-social-distancing.html; Ramachandran S, L Kusisto, and K Honan (2020). "How New York's coronavirus response made the pandemic worse." *Wall Street Journal*, 11 June. https://www.wsj.com/articles/how-new-yorks-coronavirus-response-made-the-pandemic-worse-11591908426.

227. Wallace D (2020). "Firefighters and EMTs in this time of COVID-19." Pandemic Research for the People dispatch, https://drive.google.com/file/d/1fHOl8Mrrl-KnWUs6f4sLkI1p914yahXc/view; Gormley M (2020). "Virus exposes need for hospital beds after years of reductions." *Newsday*, 21 March. https://www.newsday.com/news/health/coronavirus/coronavirus-hospital-beds-1.43358677.

228. Gold M and E Shanahan (2021). "What we know about Cuomo's nursing home scandal." *New York Times*, 4 August. https://www.nytimes.com/article/andrew-cuomo-nursing-home-deaths.html.

229. Goodman, JD and D Hakim (2021). "Cuomo aides rewrote nursing home report to hide higher death toll." *New York Times*, 4 March. https://www.nytimes.com/2021/03/04/nyregion/cuomo-nursing-home-deaths.html.

230. Sirota D (2020). "Cuomo gave immunity to nursing home executives after big campaign donations." *The Guardian*, 26 May. https://www.theguardian.com/us-news/2020/may/26/andrew-cuomo-nursing-home-execs-immunity.

231. Goldberg B and S Gorman (2021). "New York Governor Cuomo hires defense lawyer in nursing home probe." *US News and World Report*, 1 March. https://www.usnews.com/news/top-news/articles/2021-03-01/new-york-governor-cuomo-hires-defense-lawyer-after-sexual-harassment-accusations.

232. Levine J (2021). "Families of female aides defending Cuomo rake in millions lobbying him." *New York Post*, 6 March. https://nypost.com/2021/03/06/families-of-female-aides-defending-cuomo-rake-in-millions-lobbying-him.

233. Zaveri, M (2021). "Vaccine czar asks county officials about loyalty to Cuomo." *New York Times*, 15 March. https://www.nytimes.com/2021/03/15/nyregion/larry-schwartz-cuomo.html.

234. Ibid.

235. Goodman JD, J Goldstein, and J McKinley (2021). "9 top N.Y. health officials have quit as Cuomo scorns expertise." *New York Times*, 1 February. https://www.nytimes.com/2021/02/01/nyregion/cuomo-health-department-officials-quit.html.

236. Goodman JD (2020). "N.Y.C. health commissioner resigns after clashes with mayor over virus." *New York Times*, 4 August. https://www.nytimes.com/2020/08/04/nyregion/oxiris-barbot-health-commissioner-resigns.html; Henning Santiago AL (2020). "The duel over NYC's contact tracing program." *City and State*, 15 May. https://www.cityandstateny.com/politics/2020/05/the-duel-over-nycs-contact-tracing-program/175999; Rashbaum W, J Goodman, J Mays, and J Goldstein (2020). "He saw 'no proof' closures would curb virus. Now he has de Blasio's trust." *New York Times*, 14 May. https://www.nytimes.com/2020/05/14/nyregion/coronavirus-de-blasio-mitchell-katz.html.

237. Smith G (2020). "Stringer sues de Blasio in the case of the missing pandemic preparation files." *The City*, 18 November. https://www.thecity.nyc/2020/11/18/21574299/stringer-sues-de-blasio-nyc-pandemic-preparation-investigation.

238. Lin SB (2020). "NYC now has 'functional immunity' from COVID." *Patch.com*, 10 June. https://patch.com/new-york/new-york-city/nyc-

now-has-functional -immunity-covid.

239. Zizek S (2008). "Rumsfeld and the bees." *The Guardian*, 27 June. https://www.theguardian.com/commentisfree/2008/jun/28/wild-life.conservation; Wallace R (2016). "Theory of conspiracy." *Farming Pathogens* blog entry, 29 January. https://farmingpathogens.wordpress.com/2016/01/29/theory-of-conspiracy.

240. Joseph A (2021). "5 pressing questions about the New York Yankees' breakthrough Covid-19 infections." *Stat*, 14 May. https://www.statnews.com/2021/05/14/5-questions-new-york-yankees-covid-19-infections.

241. Goldstein B (2001). "The precautionary principle also applies to public health actions." *American Journal of Public Health* 91(9): 1358-1361.

242. Simmons-Duffin, S (2021). "Confused by CDC's latest mask guidance? Here's what we've learned." National Public Radio/WNYC, 15 May. https://www.npr.org/sections/health-shots/2021/05/14/996879305/confused-by-cdcs-latest-mask-guidance-heres-what-weve-learned.

243. Holtgrave D and E Rosenberg (2021). "Public health experts: Why we're going to keep wearing our masks." CNN, 14 May. https://www.cnn.com/2021/05/14/opinions/cdc-new-mask-guidance-concerns-holtgrave-rosenberg/index.html.

244. Wolfson B (2021). Being vaccinated doesn't mean you must go without a mask. Here's why." *Los Angeles Times*, 15 June. https://www.latimes.com/science/story/2021-06-15/being-vaccinated-doesnt-mean-you-must-go-without-a-mask.

245. Yong E (2021). "The fundamental question of the pandemic is shifting." *The Atlantic*, 9 June https://www.theatlantic.com/health/archive/2021/06/individualism-still-spoiling-pandemic-response/619133.

246. Fottrell Q (2020). "Nurses are wearing garbage bags as they battle coronavirus: 'It's like something out of the Twlight Zone.'" *MarketWatch*, 13 April. https://www.marketwatch.com/story/nurse-at-brooklyn-hospital-on-coronavirus-protective-clothing-its-a-garbage-bag-its-like-something-out-of-the-twlight-zone-2020-04-07; National Nurses United (2021). "Nation's largest RN union condemns CDC rollback on Covid protection guidance." National Nurses United website, 14 May. https://www.nationalnursesunited.org/press/nurses-condemns-cdc -rollback-of-covid-protection-guidance.

247. National Nurses United (2021). "Nation's largest RN union condemns CDC rollback on Covid protection guidance."

248. Jewett C (2021). "'It's a little late': US orders healthcare worker protections after thousands die." *The Guardian*, 11 June. https://www.theguardian.com/us-news/2021/jun/11/us-orders-healthcare-worker-protections-coronavirus-covid.

249. Olson A (2021). "New federal COVID-19 safety rules exempt most employers." *ABC News*, 10 June. https://abcnews.go.com/Health/wireStory/federal-covid-19 -safety-rules-exempt-employers-78206118.

250. Wilson R (2021). "Line cooks, agriculture workers at highest risk of COVID-19 death: study." *The Hill*, 2 February. https://thehill.com/policy/healthcare/536948-line-cooks-agriculture-workers-at highest-risk-of-covid-19-death-study.

251. Defoe D (1772 [1995]). *A Journal of the Plague Year*.

252. Orrick D (2020). "Here's every Minnesota restaurant and bar that had a known COVID outbreak." *Pioneer Press*, 18 November. https://www.twincities.com/2020/11/18/here-is-every-minnesota-restaurant-and-bar-thats-had-a-covid-outbreak.

253. Watkins D, J Holder, J Glanz, W Cai, B Carey, and J White (2020). "How the virus won." *New York Times*, 24 June. https://www.nytimes.com/interactive/2020/us/coronavirus-spread.html.

254. Koenig D (2021). "Travel numbers climb as Americans hit the road for holiday." *APNews*, 28 May. https://apnews.com/article/ct-state-wire-travel-coronavirus-pandemic-holidays-government-and-politics-243d33f25a8 5766a83125490aead0644.

255. Thompson J (2021). "FAA seeks $124,500 in fines from travelers who agency says assaulted flight attendants, refused masks." *USA Today*, 23 June. https://www.usatoday.com/story/travel/airline-news/2021/06/23/southwest-allegiant-unruly-passengers-faa-124500-fines/5318546001.

256. Wallace RG. "Biden's COVID plan isn't enough." This volume.

257. Rabin RC (2021). "C.D.C. will not investigate mild infections in vaccinated Americans." *New York Times*, 25 May. https://www.nytimes.com/2021/05/25/health/cdc-coronavirus-infections-vaccine.html.

258. Weixel, N (2020). "Trump on coronavirus: 'If we stop testing right now, we'd have very few cases, if any.'" *The Hill*, 15 June. https://thehill.com/policy/healthcare/502819-trump-on-coronavirus-if-we-stop-testing-right-now-wed-have-very-few-cases.

259. Wen L (2022). "Yes, more variants may emerge in the future. That's why we should lift restrictions now." *Washington Post*, 1 Feburary. https://www.washingtonpost.com/opinions/2022/02/01/yes-more-variants-may-emerge-future-thats-why-we-should-lift-restrictions-now/; Wen L (2022). "CDC mask guidelines finally got it right." *Washington Post*, 25 Feburary. https://www.washingtonpost.com/opinions/2022/02/25/cdc-mask-guidelines-covid-pandemic-got-it-right/.

260. Goodman B and E Cohen (2022). "CDC ends recommendations for social distancing and quarantine for Covid-19 control, no longer recommends test-to-stay in schools." CNN, 11 August. https://www.cnn.com/2022/08/11/health/cdc-covid-guidance-update/index.html.

261. Yong E (2021). "The fundamental question of the pandemic is shifting."

262. Garneau M (2021). "I'm watching a press conference about that Miami building collapse…" Facebook post, 27 June. https://www.facebook.com/permalink.php?story_fbid=10157905327456128&id=530346127; Tolan C and C Devine (2021). "Surfside inspectors visited Champlain

Towers South dozens of times. Now its collapse is spurring calls for reform." CNN, 14 July. https://www.cnn.com/2021/07/14/us/florida-condo-collapse-building-inspections-invs/index.html.

263. Wallace RG (2019). "Review of Paul Richards' *Ebola: How a People's Science Ended an Epidemic*." *Antipode*, 13 May. https://antipodeonline. org/2019/05/13/ebola-how-a-peoples-science-helped-end-an-epidemic.

264. Wallace R, A Liebman, LF Chaves, and R Wallace (2020). "COVID-19 and circuits of capital." *Monthly Review* 72(1). https://monthlyreview. org/2020/05/01/covid-19-and-circuits-of-capital.

265. Jackson N (2021). "Sustaining 'hidden agency': Epistemic power across space and time." Paper presented at the American Association of Geographers Annual Meeting, 8 April. https://aag.secure-abstracts. com/AAG%20Annual%20Meeting%202021/abstracts-gallery/50027; Jackson N (2017). "'Social movement Theory' as a baseline legitimizing narrative: Corporate exploitation, anti-hegemonic opposition and the contested academy." *Human Geography* 10(1): 36-49.

266. Conrad J (2016). "Some reflections on the loss of the *Titanic*." *berfrois*, 25 July. https://www.berfrois.com/2016/07/joseph-conrad-titanic.

267. Wallace RG (2012). "Auld Lang Sine." *Farming Pathogens* blog entry, 24 December. https://farmingpathogens.wordpress.com/2012/12/24/ auld-lang-sine.

268. Patton D (2018). "China's multi-story hog hotels elevate industrial farms to new levels." Reuters, 10 May. https://www.reuters.com/ article/us-china-pigs-hotels-insight/chinas-multi-story-hog-hotels-elevate-industrial-farms-to-new-levels-idUSKBN1IB362;   Patton D (2020). "Flush with cash, Chinese hog producer builds world's largest pig farm." Reuters, 7 December. https://www.reuters.com/ article/us-china-swinefever-muyuanfoods-idUKKBN28H0CC; Patton D (2021). "African swine fever inflicts renewed toll on northern China's hog herd." *Agweek*, 1 April. https://www.agweek.com/ business/agriculture/6964350-African-swine-fever-inflicts-renewed-toll-on-northern-Chinas-hog-herd; Philpott T (2020). "Industrial hog farms are breeding the next pandemic." *Mother Jones*, 11 August. https://www.motherjones.com/food/2020/08/industrial-hog-farms -are-breeding-the-next-pandemic.

269. Gorman J (2021). "Some scientists question W.H.O. inquiry into the coronavirus pandemic's origins." *New York Times*, 4 March. https:// www.nytimes.com/2021/03/04/health/covid-virus-origins.html.

270. Joint WHO-China study (2021). "WHO-convened global study of origins of SARS-CoV-2: China Part." World Health Organization, 14 January-10 February. https://www.who.int/publications/i/item/ who-convened-global-study-of-origins-of-sars-cov-2-china-part.

271. Husseini S (2020). "Peter Daszak's EcoHealth Alliance has hidden almost $40 Million in Pentagon funding and militarized pandemic

science." *Independent Science News*, 16 December. https://www.independentsciencenews.org/news/peter-daszaks-ecohealth-alliance-has-hidden-almost-40-million-in-pentagon-funding.
272. Wallace RG. "The blind weaponmaker." This volume.
273. Gorman J (2021). "Some scientists question W.H.O. inquiry into the coronavirus pandemic's origins."
274. Ibid.
275. Wallace RG (2020). "Midvinter-19." In *Dead Epidemiologists: On the Origins of COVID-19*. Monthly Review Press, New York, pp 81-97.
276. Wallace RG. "The blind weaponmaker." This volume.
277. World Health Organization (2021). "WHO calls for further studies, data on origin of SARS-CoV-2 virus, reiterates that all hypotheses remain open." World Health Organization website, 30 March. https://www.who.int/news/item/30-03-2021-who-calls-for-further-studies-data-on-origin-of-sars-cov-2-virus-reiterates-that-all-hypotheses-remain-open.
278. Wang P, et al. (2021). "Antibody resistance of SARS-CoV-2 variants B.1.351 and B.1.1.7." bioRxiv, 12 February. https://www.biorxiv.org/content/10.1101/2021.01.25.428137v3; Wang P, et al. (2021). "Increased resistance of SARS-CoV-2 variant P.1 to antibody neutralization." *Cell Host and Microbe* 29(5): 747-751.
279. Wall E, et al. (2021). "Neutralising antibody activity against SARS-CoV-2 VOCs B.1.617.2 and B.1.351 by BNT162b2 vaccination." *The Lancet* 397(10292): 2331-2333.
280. Mukherjee S (2021). "Why does the pandemic seem to be hitting some countries harder than others?" *The New Yorker*, 22 February. https://www.newyorker.com/magazine/2021/03/01/why-does-the-pandemic-seem-to-be-hitting-some-countries-harder-than-others.
281. Wallace R (2021). "How policy failure and power relations drive COVID-19 pandemic waves: A control theory perspective." *HAL*, 2 May. https://hal.archives-ouvertes.fr/hal-03214718.
282. Okamoto K, V Ong, RG Wallace, R Wallace, and LF Chaves (2020). "When might host heterogeneity drive the evolution of asymptomatic, pandemic coronaviruses?" medRxiv, 22 December. https://www.medrxiv.org/content/10.1101/2020.12.19.20248566v1.
283. van Oosterhaut, N Hall, H Ly, and K Tyler (2021). "COVID-19 evolution during the pandemic—Implications of new SARS-CoV-2 variants on disease control and public health policies." *Virulence* 12(1): 507-508.
284. Hou C-Y (2020). "What is sterilizing immunity and do we need it for the coronavirus?" *Changing America*, 8 June https://thehill.com/changing-america/well-being/prevention-cures/501677-what-is-sterilizing-immunity-and-do-we-need-it .
285. The Nextstrain team (2021). "Genomic epidemiology of novel coronavirus—Global subsampling." Nextstrain.org web site, accessed 14 July. https://nextstrain.org/ncov/gisaid/global.

286. Buss L. et al. (2021). "Three-quarters attack rate of SARS-CoV-2 in the Brazilian Amazon during a largely unmitigated epidemic." *Science* 371(6526): 288-292.

287. Sridhar D and D Gurdasani (2021). "Herd immunity by infection is not an option." *Science* 371(6526): 230-231.

288. Mukherjee S (2021). "Why does the pandemic seem to be hitting some countries harder than others?"

289. Pandey G (2021). "Covid-19: India's holiest river is swollen with bodies." *BBC News*, 19 May. https://www.bbc.com/news/world-asia-india -57154564.

290. Taylor L (2021). "Why Uruguay lost control of COVID." *Nature*, 25 June. https://www.nature.com/articles/d41586-021-01714-4.

291. Jaffe S (2021). "The schools situation mirrors the global vaccination situation." Twitter, 26 April. https://twitter.com/sarahljaffe/status/1386686939454185475.

292. Boseley S (2021). "Campaign to waive Covid jab patent highlights $26bn shareholder payouts." *The Guardian*, 21 April. https://www.theguardian.com/world/2021/apr/22/campaign-to-waive-covid-jab-patent-highlights-26bn-shareholder-payouts.

293. Stolberg S G, C Hamby, and R Ruiz (2021). "Troubled vaccine maker and its founder gave $2 million in political donations." *New York Times*, 18 May. https://www.nytimes.com/2021/05/18/us/politics/emergent-vaccine.html.

294. LaFraniere S (2021). "F.D.A. details failures at a Baltimore plant that led to unusable vaccine doses." *New York Times*, 12 June. https://www.nytimes.com/2021/06/12/world/fda-baltimore-unusable-vaccine-doses-johnson.html.

295. Hamby C, S LaFraniere, and S G Stolberg (2021). "Baltimore vaccine plant's troubles ripple across 3 continents." *New York Times*, 6 May. https://www.nytimes.com/2021/05/06/world/baltimore-vaccine-countries.html.

296. LaFraniere S, C Hamby, and R Ruiz (2021). "Vaccine maker earned record profits but delivered disappointment in return." *New York Times*, 16 June. https://www.nytimes.com/2021/06/16/us/emergent-biosolutions-covid-vaccine.html.

297. Ibid.

298. Wallace R (2016). "Ghostface killahs." *Farming Pathogens* blog entry, 5 February. https://farmingpathogens.wordpress.com/2016/02/05/ghostface-killahs.

299. Chappell B (2020). "Florida agents raid home of Rebekah Jones, former state data scientist." National Public Radio/WNYC, 15 May. https://www.npr.org/2020/12/08/944200394/florida-agents-raid-home-of-rebekah-jones-former-state-data-scientist .

300. Zaitchik A (2012). "How Bill Gates impeded global access to Covid vac-

cines." *New Republic*, 12 April. https://newrepublic.com/article/162000/
bill-gates-impeded-global-access-covid-vaccines.

301. Latham J (2017). "Gates Foundation hired PR firm to manipulate UN
over gene drives." *Independent Science News*, 4 December. https://
www.independentsciencenews.org/news/gates-foundation-hired-pr
-firm-to-manipulate-un-over-gene-drives.

302. Liu C (2021). *Virtue Hoarders: The Case Against the Professional
Managerial Class*. University of Minnesota Press, Minneapolis.

303. Thiru (2021). "23 February 2021: South Africa's interventions at the
WTO TRIPS Council." Knowledge Ecology International website, 1
March. https://www.keionline.org/35453.

304. Dean H (2021). "India wants to copy American vaccines. Biden
shouldn't fall for it." *Barron's*, 11 March. https://www.barrons.com/
articles/india-wants-to-copy-american-vaccines-biden-shouldnt-fall-
for-it-51615511350.

305. Fang L (2021). "Howard Dean pushes Biden to oppose generic Covid-
19 vaccines for developing countries." *The Intercept*, 8 April. https://
theintercept.com/2021/04/08/howard-dean-biden-covid-vaccines.

306. Fang L (2021). "Pharmaceutical industry dispatches army of lobbyists
to block generic Covid-19 vaccines." *The Intercept*, 23 April. https://
theintercept.com/2021/04/23/covid-vaccine-ip-waiver-lobbying.

307. Fang L (2021). "Documents reveal pharma plot to stop generic
Covid-19 vaccine waiver." *The Intercept*, 14 May. https://theintercept.
com/2021/05/14/covid-vaccine-waiver-generic-phrma-lobby.

308. Fang L (2021). "Hollywood lobbyists intervene against proposal to
share vaccine technology." *The Intercept*, 27 April. https://theintercept.
com/2021/04/27/covid-vaccine-copyright-hollywood-lobbyists.

309. Ibid.

310. Koebler J (2020). "Hospitals need to repair ventilators. Manufacturers
are making that impossible." *Vice Magazine*, 18 March. https://www.
vice.com/en/article/wxekgx/hospitals-need-to-repair-ventilators-
manufacturers-are-making-that-impossible.

311. Singh P (2020). "Beyond the COVID-19 pandemic: Gauging neoliberal
capitalism and the unipolar world order." *International Critical Thought*
10(4): 635-654.

312. Pamuk H (2021). "U.S. to detail global distribution plan for 80
mln vaccine doses." Reuters, 2 June. https://www.reuters.com/
business/healthcare-pharmaceuticals/us-detail-plan-global-dis-
tribution-80-mln-vaccine-doses-2021-06-02; Bridge Consulting.
"China COVID-19 Vaccine Tracker." Accessed July 15, 2021.
https://bridgebeijing.com/our-publications/our-publications-1/
china-covid-19-vaccines-tracker.

313. Parker C, Schemm P, and Sullivan S (2021). "India sets another daily
coronavirus case record; U.S. pledges help." *Washington Post*, 25 April.

https://www.washingtonpost.com/world/asia_pacific/india-coronavi-
rus-deaths-pandemic/2021/04/25/ec0f208a-a51c-11eb-b314-2e993b
d83e31_story.html.

314. Ibid.
315. Alexandria Ocasio-Cortez [@AOC] (2021). "Let's do insulin next" *Twitter*,
    15 April. https://twitter.com/AOC/status/1390037473472942081.
316. Stoller M (2021). "Why Joe Biden punched Big Pharma in the nose
    over Covid vaccines." Matt Stoller Substack post, 9 May. https://matt-
    stoller.substack.com/p/why-joe-biden-punched-big-pharma.
317. Jones C (2021). "Civil rights leaders rally as services are planned for
    white officer-slain teen." National Public Radio/KUAR website, 2 July.
    https://www.ualrpublicradio.org/post/civil-rights-leaders-rally-ser-
    vices-are-planned-white-officer-slain-teen.
318. Carroll S (2021). "Arkansas deputy fired after fatally shooting teen;
    body camera wasn't on, sheriff says." KATV website, 1 July. https://katv.
    com/news/local/arkansas-deputy-fired-after-fatally-shooting-teen-
    didnt-turn-on-body-camera-sheriff-say.
319. Satterfield J (2021). "DA: We will not charge police officer who shot 17-year-
    old Anthony J. Thompson Jr. at Austin-East." *Knoxville News Sentinel*,
    21 April. https://www.knoxnews.com/story/news/crime/2021/04/21/
    austin-east-shooting-video-anthony-j-thompson-jr/7253027002.
320. Centers for Disease Control and Prevention. "Covid Data tracker
    weekly review". Accessed July 15, 2021. https://www.cdc.gov/
    coronavirus/2019-ncov/covid-data/covidview/index.html.
321. The COVKID Project. "COVID-19 hot spots in children and teens."
    Accessed July 15, 2021. https://www.covkidproject.org/hot-spots.
322. Stone W (2021). "Covid 'doesn't discriminate by age': Serious cases on the rise
    in younger adults." National Public Radio/KHN News, 4 May. https://khn.
    org/news/article/covid-cases-hospitalizations-rise-in-younger-adults.
323. Howatt G (2021). "Younger Minnesotans lead COVID-19 case growth."
    Star Tribune, 25 March. https://www.startribune.com/younger-min-
    nesotans-lead-covid-19-case-growth/600038488; Hotez P and A Ko
    (2021). "Why are so many children in Brazil dying from Covid-19?"
    New York Times, 4 June. https://www.nytimes.com/2021/06/04/opin-
    ion/Brazil-covid-children.html.
324. Vibhu P, K Booker, R Kalra, S Kuranz, L Berra, G Arora, and P Arora
    (2021). "A retrospective cohort study of 12,306 pediatric COVID-19
    patients in the United States." *Scientific Reports*, 13 May. https://www.
    nature.com/articles/s41598-021-89553-1.
325. Knutson J (2020). "CDC: Roughly 75% of children who die from COVID-
    19 are minorities." *Axios*, 15 September. https://www.axios.com/
    cdc-coronavirus-young-people-color-death-1c2edc2c-5d98-4d8d-
    9138-a51e193530a6.html.
326. ScienceDaily (2020). "Post-COVID syndrome severely damages chil-

dren's hearts." *ScienceDaily*, 4 September. https://www.sciencedaily.com/releases/2020/09/200904125111.htm.

327. Gandhi M and K Hunter (2021). "Opinion: Delta variant panic could cause more harm than good." *SFGATE*, 6 July. https://www.sfgate.com/california-politics/article/Delta-variant-California-COVID-19-masks-open-where-16296087.php.

328. Bullard J, et al. (2021). "Infectivity of severe acute respiratory syndrome coronavirus 2 in children compared with adults." *CMAJ* 193 (17): E601-E606.

329. Varma J, et al. (2021). "COVID-19 infections among students and staff in New York City public schools." *Pediatrics* 147(5): e2021050605.

330. Leonhardt D (2021). "Kids, COVID, and Delta." *New York Times*, 18 June. https://www.nytimes.com/2021/06/18/briefing/kids-covid-and-delta.html.

331. Lovelace B (2021). "WHO urges fully vaccinated people to continue to wear masks as delta Covid variant spreads." *CNBC* website, 25 June. https://www.cnbc.com/2021/06/25/delta-who-urges-fully-vaccinated-people-to-continue-to-wear-masks-as-variant-spreads.html.

332. Money L, R G Lin II, and M Hernandez (2021). "L.A. County will require masks indoors amid alarming rise in coronavirus cases." *Los Angeles Times*, 15 July. https://www.latimes.com/california/story/2021-07-15/l-a-county-will-require-masks-indoors-amid-covid-19-surge.

333. Gandhi M and K Hunter (2021). "Opinion: Delta variant panic could cause more harm than good."

334. Fox M (2021). "Pfizer says it's time for a Covid booster; FDA and CDC say not so fast." *CNN* website, 9 July. https://www.cnn.com/2021/07/08/health/pfizer-waning-immunity-bn/index.html.

335. Ibid.

336. Zimmer C (2021). "The world is worried about the Delta virus variant. Studies show vaccines are effective against it." *New York Times*, 6 July. https://www.nytimes.com/2021/07/06/science/Israel-Pfizer-covid-vaccine.html.

337. Speights K and B Orelli (2021). "Could Pfizer and Moderna be in trouble after the latest COVID vaccine findings?" *The Motley Fool*, 9 July. https://www.fool.com/investing/2021/07/09/could-pfizer-and-moderna-be-in-trouble-after-the-l.

338. Associated Press (2021). "Pfizer to discuss COVID-19 vaccine booster with US officials." *ABC7* website, 12 July. https://www.mysuncoast.com/2021/07/12/pfizer-discuss-covid-19-vaccine-booster-with-us-officials.

339. James C (2021). "Knoxville, Tennessee, is reeling after another Black high school student is killed—this time by police." *CNN* website, 1 May. https://www.cnn.com/2021/04/30/us/student-deaths-knoxville-reeling-go-there/index.html.

340. Totenberg N (2021). "Supreme Court rejects restrictions on life without parole for juveniles." National Public Radio/WNYC, 22 April.

https://www.npr.org/2021/04/22/989822872/supreme-court-rejects-restrictions-on-life-without-parole-for-juveniles.

341. Mullins L and MJ Stern (2018). "Some Kavanaugh supporters question his accountability for alleged assault as a teen." WBUR website, 19 September. https://www.wbur.org/hereandnow/2018/09/19/kavanaugh-assault-allegation -high-school.

342. Speri A (2019). "The NYPD kept an illegal database of juvenile fingerprints for years." *The Intercept*, 13 November. https://theintercept.com/2019/11/13/nypd-juvenile-illegal-fingerprint-database.

343. Goldstein J and A Watkins (2019). "She was arrested at 14. Then her photo went to a facial recognition database." *New York Times*, 1 August. https://www.nytimes.com/2019/08/01/nyregion/nypd-facial-recognition-children-teenagers.html.

344. Kimball W (2021). "NYPD's 'Shrek Bus' is fake, not a bus, and should be avoided at all costs." *Gizmodo*, 6 July. https://gizmodo.com/nypds-shrek-bus-is-fake-not-a-bus-and-should-be-avoid-1847237439.

345. Ibid.

346. Madhukar P (2020). "Police shouldn't tag students as potential criminals." Brennan Center for Justice, 22 December. https://www.brennancenter.org/our-work/analysis-opinion/police-shouldnt-tag-students -potential-criminals.

347. Ibid.

348. Martinez A (2018). "Investigation clears El Paso police officer who pulled gun on children; civil suit planned." *El Paso Times*, 30 August. https://www.elpasotimes.com/story/news/crime/2018/08/30/el-paso-police-officer-pointed-gun-children-cleared-wrongdoing-investigation/1144001002.

349. Burke G, J Linderman, and M Mendoza (2021). "Migrant children held in mass shelters with little oversight." *AP News*, 11 May. https://apnews.com/article/donald-trump-immigration-health-coronavirus-pandemic-government-and-politics-3b4e480c9021e6a8e02313f-4c73a497e.

350. Axford W (2018). "ICE's 'special prison bus for babies' causes online furor, but the truth is more nuanced." *Houston Chronicle*, 29 May. https://www.chron.com/national/article/immigration-ICE-bus-kids-detention-Texas-12951166.php.

351. Reuters (2021). "Kamala Harris tells migrants 'Do not come'." YouTube video. https://www.youtube.com/watch?v=c5dxMmfM2_4.

352. Price M (2019). "Harris in Vegas calls Trump immigration plan 'short-sighted'." *AP News*, 16 May. https://apnews.com/article/fd149f319e9c4cdebfa04fdd83ebb7ff.

353. Liptak A (2021). "Supreme Court limits human rights suits against corporations." *New York Times*, 17 June. https://www.nytimes.com/2021/06/17/us/supreme-court-human-rights-nestle.html.

354. Ibid.

355. Ibid.

356. Coghlan A (2014). "The reasons why Gaza's population is so young." *New Scientist*, 1 August. https://www.newscientist.com/article/dn25993-the-reasons-why-gazas-population-is-so-young.

357. Khoury J and Y Kubovich (2021). "Gaza authorities: 40 Percent of Palestinians killed in Israeli strikes are women and children." *Haaretz*, 14 May. https://www.haaretz.com/middle-east-news/palestinians/gaza-authorities-40-of-palestinians-killed-in-israeli-strikes-are-women-children-1.9808666.

358. Taylor A (2021). "With strikes targeting rockets and tunnels, the Israeli tactic of 'mowing the grass' returns to Gaza." *Washington Post*, 14 May. https://www.washingtonpost.com/world/2021/05/14/israel-gaza-history.

359. Butler C et al (2021). "Calls for further inquiries into coronavirus origins." *New York Times*, 7 April. https://www.nytimes.com/interactive/2021/04/07/science/virus-inquiries-pandemic-origins.html.

360. Personal communication.

361. Ginsberg J (2021). "Letter to the editor." *The New York Times*, 11 June. https://www.nytimes.com/2021/06/11/opinion/letters/climate-pay-legislation.html.

362. Wallace RG, et al (2016). "Did neoliberalizing West African forests produce a new niche for Ebola?" *International Journal of Health Services* 46(1): 149-165.

363. Baker M and K de Freytas-Tamura (2021). "Infighting and poor planning leave condo sites in disrepair." *New York Times*, 1 July. https://www.nytimes.com/2021/07/01/us/condo-associations-surfside-collapse.html.

364. Baker M, A Singhvi, and P Mazzei (2021). "Engineer warned of 'major structural damage' at Florida condo complex." *New York Times*, 26 June. https://www.nytimes.com/2021/06/26/us/miami-building-collapse-investigation.html.

365. Robles F (2021). "Collapse wasn't first for inspector who said tower seemed in 'good shape.'" *New York Times*, 1 July. https://www.nytimes.com/2021/07/01/us/ross-prieto-surfside.html.

366. chiara francesca [chiara.acu] (2021). "Capitalism will try and fool us into thinking that it didn't even happen..." Instagram, 22 May. https://www.instagram.com/p/CPLqEcdBm59.

367. Defoe D (1772 [1995]). *A Journal of the Plague Year.*

368. Mays G and S Smith (2011). "Evidence links increases in public health spending to declines in preventable deaths." *Health Affairs* 30(8): 1585-1593.

369. Lang A, M Warren, and L Kulman (2018). *A Funding Crisis for Public Health and Safety: State-by-State Public Health Funding and Key Health*

Facts. Trust for America's Health. https://www.tfah.org/wp-content/uploads/2019/03/InvestInAmericaRpt-FINAL.pdf.

370. Alfonso Y N, J Leider, B Resnick, J M McCullough, and D Bishai (2021). US Public Health Neglected: Flat or Declining Spending Left States Ill Equipped to Respond to COVID-19." *Health Affairs*, 40(4). https://www.healthaffairs.org/doi/full/10.1377/hlthaff.2020.01084.

371. Paavola D (2020). "266 hospitals furloughing workers in response to COVID-19." *Becker's Hospital CFO Report*, 31 August. https://www.beckershospitalreview.com/finance/49-hospitals-furloughing-workers-in-response-to-covid-19.html.

372. Meyer R (2021). "Congress is slashing a $30 billion plan to fight the next pandemic." *The Atlantic*, 2 August. https://www.theatlantic.com/science/archive/2021/08/congress-slashing-plan-end-pandemics/619640.

373. Salami J (2021). "The pandemic gets the Michael Lewis treatment, heroic technocrats and all." *New York Times*, 3 May. https://www.nytimes.com/2021/05/03/books/review-premonition-pandemic-michael-lewis.html; Lewis M (2021). *The Premonition: A Pandemic Story*. W.W. Norton, New York.

374. ChiVaxBot [@ChiVaxBot] (2021). "As of July 13, 2021, Chicago is reporting 1,369,775 people fully vaccinated: 49.6% of the population. Who is dying: Who is vaccinated." Twitter, 13 July. https://twitter.com/ChiVaxBot/status/1415114676963315717.

375. Tudor Hart J (1971). "The Inverse Care Law." *The Lancet* 297(7696): 405-412.

376. Kelley F (1892 [2005]). "The sweating system." *American Journal of Public Health* 95(1): 49-52.

377. Nugent W (2005). "Epidemics" entry. Encyclopedia of Chicago website. http://www.encyclopedia.chicagohistory.org/pages/432.html; Klinenberg E (2002). *Heat Wave: A Social Autopsy of Disaster in Chicago*. University of Chicago Press, Chicago.

378. Goodnough A and J Hoffman (2021). "The wealthy are getting more vaccinations, even in poorer neighborhoods." *New York Times*, 2 February. https://www.nytimes.com/2021/02/02/health/white-people-covid-vaccines-minorities.html; Ross, J (2021). "When a Texas county tried to ensure racial equity in COVID-19 caccinations, It didn't go as planned." *Time*, 2 March. https://time.com/5942884/covid-19-vaccine-racial-inequity-dallas; Ellis N (2021). "A vaccination site meant to serve a hard-hit Latino neighborhood in New York instead serviced more Whites from other areas." CNN website, 30 January. https://www.cnn.com/2021/01/30/us/new-york-vaccine-disparities/index.html; Goldhill O (2021). "In Palm Beach, Covid-19 vaccines intended for rural Black communities are instead going to wealthy white Floridians." *STAT*, 4 March. https://www.statnews.com/2021/03/04/covid19-vaccines-for-rural-black-communities-going-to-wealthy-white-floridians.

379. Nelson M (2021). "Report: Life expectancy gap widening between Black, non-Black Chicagoans." WTTW website, 23 June. https://news.wttw.com/2021/06/23/report-life-expectancy-gap-widening-between-black-non-black-chicagoans.

380. Dudek M (2021). "Critics slam Lightfoot's spending of $281 million of coronavirus relief money on police." Chicago Sun Times, 18 February. https://chicago.suntimes.com/city-hall/2021/2/18/22289859/chicago-mayor-lightfoot-cares-act-coronavirus-relief-money-police-department-costs-daniel-la-spata.

381. McGee C (2021). "Blue bailout: Covid-19 cash is militarizing cops across the country." Rolling Stone, 5 May. https://www.rollingstone.com/politics/politics-features/cares-act-covid-pandemic-funds-police-surveillance-1153439.

382. Strauss V (2018). "Chicago promised that closing nearly 50 schools would help kids in 2013. A new report says it didn't." Washington Post, 24 May. https://www.washingtonpost.com/news/answer-sheet/wp/2018/05/24/chicago-promised-that-closing-nearly-50-schools-would-help-kids-in-2013-a-new-report-says-it-didnt.

383. Esposito, S (2021). "Cook County Health nurses go on one-day strike." Chicago Sun Times, 24 June. https://chicago.suntimes.com/2021/6/24/22548496/cook-county-health-nurses-strike-staffing-stroger-hospital-provident; Schencker L (2021). "Nurses at Chicago's main safety-net hospital strike over staffing levels, say they're stretched to the limit. 'It's not fair to the patients at all.'" Chicago Tribune, 24 June. https://www.chicagotribune.com/business/ct-biz-cook-county-health-nurses-strike-20210624-d4f4lmgbnjaqrgynxpkht4kkg4-story.html.

384. Klein B (2021). "Biden administration urging state and local governments to use Covid relief funding to address uptick in violent crime." CNN website, 12 July. https://www.cnn.com/2021/07/12/politics/biden-administration-crime-covid-relief-funding/index.html.

385. Birn A E and R Kumar (2021). "Social determinants and determination of health." In Benatar S and G Brock (eds), Global Health: Ethical Challenges. Cambridge University Press, Cambridge; Chabon M (2005). "Inventing Sherlock Holmes." New York Review of Books, 10 February. https://www.nybooks.com/articles/2005/02/10/inventing-sherlock-holmes.

386. Thometz K (2021). "Have COVID-19 questions? The Nerdy Girls at 'Dear Pandemic' have answers." WTTW website, 2 March. https://news.wttw.com/2021/03/02/have-covid-19-questions-nerdy-girls-dear-pandemic-have-answers.

387. Varkony K (2021). "Anti-vaxxer tells Ohio lawmakers COVID-19 vaccine can leave people magnetized, interfaced with 5G towers." NBC4i website, 8 June. https://www.nbc4i.com/news/local-news/anti-vaxxer-tells-ohio-lawmakers-covid-19-vaccine-can-leave-people-magnetized-interfaced-with-5g-towers.

388. Spencer SH (2021). "Fact check: Evidence points to safety of COVID-19 vaccines for pregnant people." WCVB5 website, 11 June. https://www.wcvb.com/article/fact-check-evidence-points-to-safety-of-covid-19-vaccines-for-pregnant-people/36702883.

389. McEvoy J (2021). "Microchips, magnets and shedding: Here are 5 (debunked) Covid vaccine conspiracy theories spreading online." *Forbes*, 3 June. https://www.forbes.com/sites/jemimamcevoy/2021/06/03/microchips-and-shedding-here-are-5-debunked-covid-vaccine-conspiracy-theories-spreading-online/?sh=54c1115b26af.

390. Gurian-Sherman D and M Mellon (2015). "What Bill Nye got wrong in his about-face on GMOs." *CivilEats*, 3 June. https://civileats.com/2015/06/03/what-bill-nye-got-wrong-in-his-about-face-on-gmos/.

391. Those Nerdy Girls [dear_pandemic] (2021). "FALSEHOOD: A new occasional series..." Instagram, 11 June. https://www.instagram.com/p/CP_w8A4gFd0.

392. Bee KC (2021). "Sorry if this is hard to hear..." Facebook, 22 May. https://www.facebook.com/veronica.major.3158/videos/431140964720333.

393. Wallace RG, et al (2016). "Did neoliberalizing West African forests produce a new niche for Ebola?"

394. Wallace RG (2020). "Notes on a novel coronavirus." *MRonline*, 29 January. https://mronline.org/2020/01/29/notes-on-a-novel-coronavirus.

395. Wallace RG "The BoJo strain." This volume.

396. Wallace RG "Mo BoJo." This volume.

397. Lewontin R (1997). "Billions and billions of demons." *New York Review of Books*, 9 January. https://www.drjbloom.com/Public%20files/Lewontin_Review.htm.

398. Defoe D (1772 [1995]). *A Journal of the Plague Year*.

399. Saeed Jones [@theferocity] (2021). "In some ways, this side of the pandemic is lonelier than the early months." Twitter, 11 March. https://twitter.com/theferocity/status/1370124467410702341.

400. Stewart A (2021). "Zach Snyder's Justice League: a four hour Ayn Rand fantasia." *Counterpunch*, 26 March. https://www.counterpunch.org/2021/03/26/zach-snyders-justice-league-a-four-hour-ayn-rand-fantasia; MeMeLytics (2018). "What's your Superpowers again?? I'm RICH [HD]." YouTube video. https://www.youtube.com/watch?v=-2Z3rJMpCJY.

401. Wallace R (2016). "Caligula of Albany." *Farming Pathogens* blog entry, 24 March. https://farmingpathogens.wordpress.com/2016/03/24/caligula -of-albany.

402. Daraja Press (2021). "What conditions favour successful mutations of the COVID-19 virus?" Daraja Press website, 21 January. https://darajapress.com/2021/01/21/what-condition-favour-successful-mutations -of-the-covid-19-virus.

403. Stockholm Resilience Centre. "What is a regime shift?" Accessed July 15, 2021. https://regimeshifts.org/what-is-a-regime-shift.

404. Regeneration International. "Why Regenerative Agriculture?" Accessed July 15, 2021. https://regenerationinternational.org/why-regenerative -agriculture

405. Collins C (2021). "Update: U.S. billionaires pandemic wealth gains: $1.8 Trillion; Wealth gain could pay for President's family investment plan." Inequality.org, 14 July. https://inequality.org/great-divide/ updates-billionaire-pandemic.

406. Real Time with Bill Maher (2021). "Heather Heying & Bret Weinstein: The lab hypothesis." YouTube video. https://www.youtube.com/ watch?v=ZMGWLLDSA3c; Cressler C, D McLeod, C Rozins, J van den Hoogen, and T Day (2015). "The adaptive evolution of virulence: a review of theoretical predictions and empirical tests." *Parisitology* 143(7): 915-930.

407. Wallace RG. "The BoJo strain." This volume.

408. Chaw S, et al. (2020). "The origin and underlying driving forces of the SARS-CoV-2 outbreak." *Journal of Biomedical Science* 27: 73.

409. Wallace RG. "The blind weaponmaker." This volume.

410. Weinstein B (2021). "The day American justice died." *UnHerd*, 24 May. https://unherd.com/2021/05/the-day-american-justice-died.

411. Ibid.

412. Gorman J and C Zimmer (2021). "Scientist opens up about his early email to Fauci on virus origins." *New York Times*, 20 June. https://www.nytimes. com/2021/06/14/science/covid-lab-leak-fauci-kristian-andersen.html.

413. Andersen K, A Rambaut, W I Lipkin, E Holmes, and R Garry (2020). "The proximal origin of SARS-CoV-2." *Nature Medicine* 26: 450–452.

414. Prabhune M (2019). "Eradicating Malaria with CRISPR: Mosquito gene editing approach." *Synthego*, 9 October. https://www.synthego. com/blog/gene-drive-malaria.

415. Enzmann B (2018). "Gene drives explained: How to solve problems with CRISPR." *Synthego*, 4 December. https://www.synthego.com/ blog/gene-drive-crispr.

416. Thompson H (2015). "Could GM mosquitoes pave the way for a tropical virus to spread?" *Smithsonian*, 8 January. https://www. smithsonianmag.com/smithsonian-institution/could-gm-mosquitoes- pave-way-chikungunya-virus-panama-180953847/.

417. Hayden EC (2021). "Could editing the genomes of bats prevent future coronavirus pandemics? Two scientists think it's worth a try." *STAT*, 1 July. https://www.statnews.com/2021/07/01/ could-editing-genomes-of-bats-prevent-future-coronavirus-pandem- ics-two-scientists-think-its-worth-a-try.

418. Ibid.

419. Ibid.

420. Jonas T (2021). "Regenerative agriculture and agroecology—what's in a name?" *Food Ethics* blog entry, 23 June. http://www.tammi-

jonas.com/2021/06/23/regenerative-agriculture-and-agroecology-whats-in-a-name.

421. Wallace R (2017). "Prometheus rebound." *Farming Pathogens* blog entry, 31 October. https://farmingpathogens.wordpress.com/2017/10/31/prometheus-rebound.

422. BBC News (2021). "Berta Cáceres: Ex-dam company boss guilty of planning Honduran activist's murder." *BBC News*, 5 July. https://www.bbc.com/news/world-latin-america-57725007; Global Witness (2020). *Defending Tomorrow*. Global Witness, London. https://www.globalwitness.org/en/campaigns/environmental-activists/defending-tomorrow.

423. Liebman A, et al. (2020). "Can agriculture stop COVID-21, -22, and -23? Yes, but not by greenwashing agribusiness." Pandemic Research for the People dispatch, 10 December. https://drive.google.com/file/d/1M-yW7JakFwSV_ZFUNZdQLdYWhlbn_L6D/view.

424. Chaves L, et al. (2021). "Scientists say land use drives new pandemics. But what if 'land' isn't what they think it is?" Pandemic Research for the People dispatch, 28 March. https://drive.google.com/file/d/12cW-PkPU9Z5TtoEMqKuhPnUGsmOLVp16/view.

425. Wallace R, A Liebman, L Bergmann, and RG Wallace (2020). "Agribusiness vs. public health: Disease control in resource-asymmetric conflict." https://hal.archives-ouvertes.fr/hal-02513883.

426. Anonymous (2020). "Breonna Taylor: Police officer charged but not over death." *BBC News*, 23 September. https://www.bbc.com/news/world-us-canada-54273317.

427. Bailey P and T Duvall (2020). "Breonna Taylor warrant connected to Louisville gentrification plan, lawyers say." *Louisville Courier Journal*, 30 August. https://amp.courier-journal.com/amp/5381352002.

428. Fullilove M (2016). *Root Shock: How Tearing Up City Neighborhoods Hurts America, and What We Can Do About It.* NYU Press, New York.

429. Decolonial Atlas [@decolonialatlas] (2021). Instagram. https://www.instagram.com/decolonialatlas/?hl=en.

430. Ross C (2015). "A multi-level Bayesian analysis of racial bias in police shootings at the county-level in the United States, 2011–2014." *PLoS ONE* 10(11): e0141854.

431. Patience Zalanga [patiencezalanga] (2021). Instagram. https://www.instagram.com/patiencezalanga.

432. Almasy S, A Cooper and E Levenson (2022). "Ex-officer Brett Hankison was found not guilty of endangering Breonna Taylor's neighbors in a botched raid." CNN, 4 March. https://www.cnn.com/2022/03/03/us/brett-hankison-trial-closing/index.html.

433. Welsh-Huggins A (2022). "Ohio officer cleared in shooting of teenager Ma'Khia Bryant." Associated Press, 11 March. https://apnews.com/article/ohio-columbus-police-shootings-d42d225f2cea2cdf6a0d-6c7044fc941a.

434. Strozewski Z (2022). "Charges won't be filed in Amir Locke shooting involving 'no-knock' warrant." *Newsweek*, 6 April. https://www.newsweek.com/charges-wont-filed-amir-locke-shooting-no-knock-warrant-1695608.

435. Patel V (2022). "Prosecutors won't charge police officers in 2 high-profile killings in Chicago." *New York Times*, 15 March. https://www.nytimes.com/2022/03/15/us/adam-toledo-shooting-kim-foxx.html.

436. Peters L (2020). "Vaccinate the world against COVID-19 like we did with polio." *Crosscut*, 4 December. https://crosscut.com/opinion/2020/12/vaccinate-world-against-covid-19-we-did-polio.

437. Roush S and T Murphy (2007). "Historical comparisons of morbidity and mortality for vaccine-preventable diseases in the United States." *JAMA* 298(18): 2155-2163.

438. Antona D, et al. (2013). "Measles elimination efforts and 2008–2011 outbreak, France." *Emerging Infectious Diseases* 19(3): 357-64.

439. Aratani A (2021). "99.2% of US Covid deaths in June were unvaccinated, says Fauci." *The Guardian*, 8 July. https://www.theguardian.com/us-news/2021/jul/08/fears-of-new-us-covid-surge-as-delta-spreads-and-many-remain-unvaccinated.

440. Wallace RG. "Vic Berger's American public health." This volume.

441. Kelman B (2021). "Tennessee abandons vaccine outreach to minors—not just for COVID-19." *Nashville Tennessean*, 15 July. https://www.tennessean.com/story/news/health/2021/07/13/tennessee-halts-all-vaccine-outreach-minors-not-just-covid-19/7928701002.

442. Smith GJD, et al. (2006). "Emergence and predominance of an H5N1 influenza variant in China." *PNAS*, 103(45): 16936-16941.

443. Wallace RG. "The BoJo strain." This volume; Escorcia M, L Vazquez, S Mendez, A Rodriguez-Ropon, E Lucio, and G Nava (2008). "Avian influenza: genetic evolution under vaccination pressure." *Virology Journal* 5: 15.

444. Harrison D (2020). "Results from the AstraZeneca/Oxford vaccine trials." Dale Harrison Substack post, 15 December. https://dalewharrison.substack.com/p/results-from-the-astrazenecaoxford.

445. Medical News Today (2021). "Massachusetts outbreak demonstrates Delta variant's transmissibility." *Medical News Today*, 1 March. https://www.medicalnewstoday.com/articles/massachusetts-outbreak-demonstrates-delta-variants-transmissibility.

446. Gandon S, MJ Mackinnon, S Nee, and AF Read (2001). "Imperfect vaccines and the evolution of pathogen virulence." *Nature* 414(6865): 751-756.

447. O'Shea T, et al. (2014). "Bat flight and zoonotic viruses." *Emerging Infectious Diseases* 20(5): 741-745.

448. Saunders K, et al. (2021). "Neutralizing antibody vaccine for pandemic and pre-emergent coronaviruses." *Nature* 594: 553–559.

449. Baumler A, B Hargis, and R Tsolis (2000). "Tracing the origins of *Salmonella* outbreaks." *Science* 287(5450): 50–52.

450. Laland K and L Chiu (2020). "Niche construction." Niche Construction website, accessed 15 July. https://nicheconstruction.com/information.

451. Wallace RF, K Okamoto, and A Liebman (2021). "Gates ecologies." In DB Monk and M Sorkin (eds), *Between Catastrophe and Revolution: Essays in Honor of Mike Davis*. OR Books, New York, pp 307-319.

452. Wallace R (2017). "Prometheus rebound."

453. Marx K (1852 [1994]). *The Eighteenth Brumaire*. International Publishers Co., New York.

454. Badiou A (2019). *Can Politics Be Thought?* Duke University Press, Durham.

455. Bosteels B (2019). "Translator's introduction." In A Badiou, *Can Politics Be Thought?* Duke University Press, Durham.

456. Ball J (2018). "Australia doesn't exist! And other bizarre geographic conspiracies that won't go away." *The Guardian*, 15 April. https://www.theguardian.com/technology/shortcuts/2018/apr/15/australia-doesnt-exist-and-other-bizarre-geographic-conspiracies-that-wont-go-away.

457. Steinhauer J (2021). "What do women want? For men to get Covid vaccines." *New York Times*, 22 April. https://www.nytimes.com/2021/04/22/health/covid-vaccines-rates-men-and-women.html.

458. Wallace RG (2020). *Dead Epidemiologists: On the Origins of COVID-19*. Monthly Review Press, New York.

459. Macalester College (2021). "New study on efficacy of vaccine education reveals information, gender matter." Macalester College website, 13 April. https://www.macalester.edu/news/2021/04/new-study-on-efficacy-of-vaccine-education-reveals-information-gender-matter.

460. Smith S (2021). "Chauvin trial: Why didn't witnesses help George Floyd?" *USA Today*, 18 April. https://www.usatoday.com/in-depth/opinion/2021/04/18/george-floyd-witnesses-too-scared-to-stop-derek-chauvin-column/7186835002.

461. Berkow I (2020). "A baseball legend wrestles with removing his former boss's statue." *New York Times*, 30 June. https://www.nytimes.com/2020/06/30/sports/baseball/rod-carew-minneapolis-george-floyd-protests.html.

462. Ellis J (2021). "Minnesota values white comfort more than Black lives." *New York Times*, 16 April. https://www.nytimes.com/2021/04/16/opinion/sunday/george-floyd-daunte-wright-minnesota.html.

463. Bakst B (2021). "National Guard presence during Chauvin trial cost $25M." *MPR News*, 28 April. https://www.mprnews.org/story/2021/04/28/national-guard-presence-during-chauvin-trial-cost-25m; Schwartz ND (2015). "In the Twin Cities, local leaders wield influence behind the scenes." *New York Times*, 28 December. https://www.nytimes.com/2015/12/29/business/in-the-twin-cities-local-leaders-wield-influence-behind-the-scenes.html.

464. Lehman C (2017). "Slaveholder investment in territorial Minnesota."

Minnesota History. http://collections.mnhs.org/MNHistoryMagazine/
articles/65/v65i07p264-274.pdf.

465. Badiou A (2006). *Polemics.* Translated by S Corcoran. Verso, New York.

466. Althusser L (2001). *Lenin and Philosophy and Other Essays.* Monthly
     Review Press, New York.

467. Žižek S (2014). *Absolute Recoil: Towards a New Foundation of Dialectical
     Materialism.* Verso, New York.

468. Stevens G (2018). "What Fanon still teaches us about mental illness
     in post-colonial societies." *The Conversation,* September 4. https://
     theconversation.com/what-fanon-still-teaches-us-about-mental-ill-
     ness-in-post-colonial-societies-102426; Wallace RG (2016). "Strange
     cotton". In *Big Farms Make Big Flu: Dispatches on Infectious Disease,
     Agribusiness, and the Nature of Science.* Monthly Review Press, New
     York, pp 257-276.

469. Rahman K (2015). "'You're a disgusting human being': George
     Zimmerman provokes fury on Twitter AGAIN after posting image
     of Trayvon Martin's lifeless body." *Daily Mail,* 27 September. https://
     www.dailymail.co.uk/news/article-3251226/You-disgusting-human-
     George-Zimmerman-provokes-fury-Twitter-posting-image-Trayvon-
     Martin-s-lifeless-body.html.

470. Forliti A, S Karnowski, and T Webber (2022). "Kim Potter sentenced
     to 2 years in Daunte Wright's death." Associated Press, 18 February.
     https://apnews.com/article/death-of-daunte-wright-death-of-george-
     floyd-minnesota-george-floyd-minneapolis-a43a48970e37392ef-
     d85adfeae79ddf0; Li DK and D Silva (2022). "Legal experts question
     fairness of 2-year sentence for ex-cop who killed Daunte Wright."
     Yahoo! News, 18 February. https://www.yahoo.com/now/legal-experts-
     fairness-2-sentence-231629969.html.

471. Carlucci C (2021). "Wince Marie Peace Garden early morn-
     ing July 3, 2021." YouTube, 19 July. https://www.youtube.com/
     watch?v=sdLlxAC9lyc.

472. Georgiades N (2021). "Car attacker who killed Deona Marie charged
     with murder." Unicorn Riot, 16 June. https://unicornriot.ninja/2021/
     car-attacker-who-killed-deona-marie-charged-with-murder.

473. Du S (2021). "Minneapolis street outreach teams get caught between
     protestors, police." *Star Tribune,* 10 July. https://www.startribune.
     com/street-outreach-teams-come-under-fire-for-trying-to-curb-un-
     rest/600076888.

474. Hoban V (2021). "'Discredit, disrupt, and destroy': FBI records acquired
     by the Library reveal violent surveillance of Black leaders, civil rights
     organizations." *Berkeley Library News,* 18 January. https://news.lib.
     berkeley.edu/fbi; *FBI Strategy Guide FY2018-20 and Threat Guidance
     for Racial Extremists.* Documents uploaded by K Klippenstein. Scribd,
     accessed July 15, 2021. https://www.scribd.com/document/421166393/

FBI-Strategy-Guide-FY2018-20-and-Threat-Guidance-for-Racial-Extremists.

475. Murphy K (2020). "Prince's evolution as a race man took him from Minneapolis to 'Baltimore.'" *Andscape,* 9 June. https://andscape.com/features/princes-evolution-as-a-race-man-took-him-from-minneapolis-to-baltimore/.

476. Prince (1980). "Uptown." YouTube, accessed July 15, 2021. https://www.youtube.com/watch?v=ZiuSRQHLv88.

477. Mandavilli A (2021). "Immunity to the coronavirus may persist for years, scientists find." *New York Times,* 26 May. https://www.nytimes.com/2021/05/26/health/coronavirus-immunity-vaccines.html.

478. Center for Pathogen Evolution (2021). "What is antigenic cartography?" Center for Pathogen Evolution website, accessed 15 July. https://www.pathogenevolution.zoo.cam.ac.uk/antigeniccartography.

479. Speights K and B Orelli (2021). "Could Pfizer and Moderna be in trouble after the latest COVID vaccine findings?"

480. Turner J, et al. (2021). "SARS-CoV-2 infection induces long-lived bone marrow plasma cells in humans." *Nature* 595: 421-425.

481. Whitlow J (2018). "Anti-state statism and slumlord capitalism." *LPE Project,* 14 November. https://lpeproject.org/blog/anti-state-statism-and-slumlord-capitalism.

482. Wallace D and R Wallace (2017). "Benign neglect and planned shrinkage." Verso Books website. https://www.versobooks.com/blogs/3145-benign-neglect-and-planned-shrinkage; Bennington-Castro J (2020). "How AIDS remained an unspoken—but deadly—epidemic for years." History Channel website, 1 June. https://www.history.com/news/aids-epidemic-ronald -reagan.

483. Defoe D (1772 [1995]). *A Journal of the Plague Year.*

484. Callaway E (2021). "Had COVID? You'll probably make antibodies for a lifetime." *Nature,* 26 May. https://www.nature.com/articles/d41586-021-01442-9.

485. Starnes E (2017). "Silent evidence." Sigma Actuarial Consulting Group website, 13 December. https://www.sigmaactuary.com/2017/12/13/silent-evidence.

486. Duan Y, et al. (2020). "Deficiency of Tfh cells and germinal center in deceased COVID-19 patients." *Current Medical Science* 40: 618-624.

487. Makary M (2021). "Natural vs vaccine immunity for COVID: Is one more effective?" *Medpage Today,* 5 May. https://www.medpagetoday.com/opinion/marty-makary/92434.

488. InformedHealth.org (2020). "The innate and adaptive immune systems." National Center for Biotechnology Information website, accessed July 15, 2021. https://www.ncbi.nlm.nih.gov/books/NBK279396.

489. Vilar S and D Isom (2021). "One year of SARS-CoV-2: How much has the virus changed?" *Biology* 10(2): 91.

490. Ibid.
491. Ibid.
492. Wallace R (2002). "Immune cognition and vaccine strategy: Pathogenic challenge and ecological resilience." *Open Systems & Information Dynamics* 9: 51–83; Wallace R and RG Wallace (2002). "Immune cognition and vaccine strategy: beyond genomics." *Microbes and Infection* 4(4): 521-527; Cohen I (2000). *Tending Adam's Garden: Evolving the Cognitive Immune Self.* Academic Press, Cambridge.
493. Rimmelzwaan GF, EGM Berkhoff, NJ Nieuwkoop, DJ Smith, RAM Fouchier, and ADME Osterhaus (2005). "Full restoration of viral fitness by multiple compensatory co-mutations in the nucleoprotein of influenza A virus cytotoxic T-lymphocyte escape mutants." *Journal of General Virology.* 86(6): 1801-1805.
494. Kelley R (2017). "What did Cedric Robinson mean by racial capitalism?" *Boston Review,* 12 January. https://bostonreview.net/race/robin-d-g-kelley-what-did-cedric-robinson-mean-racial-capitalism.
495. Engel Di-Mauro S (2021). *Socialism, Socialist States and Environment: Lessons for Ecosocialist Futures.* Pluto Press, London.
496. Nowak MA (1992). "What is a quasispecies?" *Trends in Ecological Evolution* 7(4): 118-21.
497. World Health Organization (2021). "Antimicrobial resistance." World Health Organization website, accessed July 15. https://www.who.int/health-topics/antimicrobial-resistance.
498. Santora M and E Peltier (2021). "The variant first detected in India is forcing the U.K. to speed up delivery of second doses of vaccine." *New York Times,* 14 May. https://www.nytimes.com/2021/05/14/world/india-covid-second-doses-united-kingdom.html.
499. Capel C (2021). "U.K. virus cases surge even as 8 in 10 have received shots." *Bloomberg News,* 17 June. https://www.bloomberg.com/news/articles/2021-06-17/u-k-virus-cases-surge-even-as-vaccine-rollout-hits-milestone.
500. Winsor M (2021). "CDC director warns delta variant could soon become dominant coronavirus strain in US." *ABC News,* 18 June. https://abcnews.go.com/Health/cdc-director-warns-delta-variant-dominant-coronavirus-strain/story?id=78354918.
501. Emasculation Proclamation [@angryblkhoemo] (2021). "It's the fact that they knew about the delta variant before they released those premature recommendations for vaccinated individuals for me..." *Twitter,* 20 June. https://twitter.com/angryblkhoemo/status/1406802643918393347.
502. Anonymous (2021). "Delta variant of Covid-19 mutates into Delta Plus: All you need to know." *Times of India,* 24 June. https://timesofindia.indiatimes.com/india/delta-variant-of-covid-19-mutates-into-delta-plus-all-you-need-to-know/articleshow/83538387.cms; Khan A, et al. (2021). "Higher infectivity of the SARS-CoV-2 new variants is asso-

ciated with K417N/T, E484K, and N501Y mutants: An insight from structural data." *Journal of Cell Physiology* 236(10): 7045-7057.

503. Bradley J, S Gebrekidan, and A McCann (2020). "Waste, negligence and cronyism: Inside Britain's pandemic spending." *New York Times,* 17 December. https://www.nytimes.com/interactive/2020/12/17/world/europe/britain-covid-contracts.html; Kleinman M (2021). "Matt Hancock 'affair': Aide Gina Coladangelo's brother has top job at company with NHS contracts." *SkyNews,* 26 June. https://news.sky.com/story/matt-hancock-affair-aide-gina-coladangelos-relative-has-top-job-at-company-with-nhs-contracts-12341789; Ashton E and A Morales (2021). "U.K. lobbying scandal deepens as Hancock accused of cronyism." *Bloomberg News,* 15 April. https://www.bloomberg.com/news/articles/2021-04-15/second-u-k-official-gets-caught-up-in-greensill-lobbying-storm.

504. Javid S (2021). "The economic arguments for opening up Britain are well known. But, for me, the health case is equally compelling." *The Daily Mail,* 3 July. https://www.dailymail.co.uk/debate/article-9753313/SAJID-JAVID-health-arguments-opening-Britain-compelling.html.

505. Our World in Data (2021). "Daily new confirmed COVID-19 case per million people." Ourworldindata.org, accessed July 15. https://ourworldindata.org/explorers/coronavirus-data-explorer?zoomToSelection=true&time=2020-03-01..latest&facet=none&pickerSort=asc&pickerMetric=location&Metric=Confirmed+cases&Interval=7-day+rolling+average&Relative+to+Population=true&Align+outbreaks=false&country=USA~GBR~CAN~DEU~ITA~IND.

506. PA Media (2020). "There is such a thing as society, says Boris Johnson from bunker." *The Guardian,* 29 March. https://www.theguardian.com/politics/2020/mar/29/20000-nhs-staff-return-to-service-johnson-says-from-coronavirus-isolation; McLachlan H (2020). "Why 'there's no such thing as society' should not be regarded with moral revulsion." *The Conversation,* April 20. https://theconversation.com/why-theres-no-such-thing-as-society-should-not-be-regarded-with-moral-revulsion-136008.

507. Garrick LE (2004). "A historical context of municipal solid waste management in the United States." *Waste Management & Research* 22(4):306-322.

508. Wallace RG (2010). "Do pathogens time travel?" *Farming Pathogens* blog entry, 12 January. https://farmingpathogens.wordpress.com/2010/01/12/do-pathogens-time-travel.

509. Tomsic S (2015). *The Capitalist Unconscious: Marx and Lacan.* Verso Press, London.

510. Brown A (2021). "Local cops said pipeline company had influence over government appointment." *The Intercept,* 17 April. https://theintercept.com/2021/04/17/enbridge-line-3-minnesota-police-protest.

511. Hasson N and the Associated Press (2021). "Israel police release Al Jazeera reporter hours after arresting her in Sheikh Jarrah." *Haaretz*, 5 June. https://www.haaretz.com/israel-news/. premium-israel-police-arrest-al-Jazeera-reporter-at-protest-in-east-j-lem-s-sheikh-jarrah-1.9877327; Noor P (2020). "Teargassed, beaten up, arrested: what freedom of the press looks like in the US right now." *The Guardian*, 6 June. https://www.theguardian.com/us-news/2020/jun/06/george-floyd-protests-reporters-press-teargas-arrested; Committee to Protect Journalists (2021). "Journalist Alan Weisman arrested, strip-searched while covering anti-pipeline protest in Minnesota." Committee to Protect Journalists website, 11 June. https://cpj.org/2021/06/journalist-alan-weisman-arrested-strip-searched-while-covering-anti-pipeline-protest-in-minnesota.

512. Mannix A (2021). "Hennepin healthcare workers demand hospital reduce use of 'medical force' on patients." *Star Tribune*, 23 May. https://www.startribune.com/hennepin-healthcare-workers-demand-hospi-tal-reduce-use-of-medical-force-on-patients/600060524.

513. Mannix A (2018). "At urging of Minneapolis police, Hennepin EMS workers subdued dozens with a powerful sedative." *Star Tribune*, 15 June. https://www.startribune.com/at-urging-of-police-hennepin-emts-subdued-dozens-with-powerful-sedative/485607381.

514. Ibid.

515. Mannix A and Z Jackson (2022). "Hennepin Healthcare promised to address 'systemic racism.' Then came the blackface photos." *Star-Tribune*, 2 March. https://www.startribune.com/hennepin-health-care-promised-to-address-systemic-racism-then-came-the-blackface-photos/600152097/.

516. Collins B (2018). "Mayo issues an apology 156 years in the making." NewsCut blog, *MPR News*, 18 September. https://blogs.mprnews.org/newscut/2018/09/mayo-issues-an-apology-156-years-in-the-making/.

517. Nierenberg A (2020). "Gandhi Mahal restaurant burned in George Floyd riot, but owner still supports protest." *Pioneer Press*, 31 May. https://www.twincities.com/2020/05/31/gandhi-mahal-restaurant-burned-in-george-floyd-riot-but-owner-still-supports-protest.

518. Davis A and S Matsumoto (2021). "Talking farming with Minnesota farmers of color." *MPR News*, 8 June. https://www.mprnews.org/epi-sode/2021/06/07/talking-farming-with -minnesota-farmers-of-color.

519. Katchor B (2000). *Julius Knipl, Real Estate Photographer: The Beauty Supply District*. Pantheon Books, New York.

520. Ringgold F (1996). *Tar Beach*. Penguin Random House, New York.

521. Corman L (2021). "You are not a guest." *Tablet*, 28 April. https://www.tabletmag.com/sections/community/articles/you-are-not-a-guest -leela-corman

522. Ibid.

523. Ibid.
524. Graziosi G (2021). "Right-wing Oath Keepers are being trained by police, leader claims." *The Independent*, 19 April. https://www.independent.co.uk/news/world/americas/us-politics/oath-keepers-60-minutes-interview-b1834005.html.
525. Ben Crump [attorneycrump] (2021). Instagram. https://www.instagram.com/attorneycrump.
526. Benjamin W (2021). "Theses on the philosophy of history." In *Illuminations: Essays and Reflections*. Schocken Books, New York, pp 253-264; Berardi F (2019). *Futurability: The Age of Impotence and the Horizon of Possibility*. Verso Press, London and New York; Lazarus S (2015). *Anthropology of the Name*. Seagull Books, London and Calcutta.
527. Lopez B (2020). *Horizon*. Penguin Random House, New York.
528. Ibid.
529. Ibid.
530. Ibid.
531. Morton T (2013). *Hyperobjects: Philosophy and Ecology after the End of the World*. University of Minnesota Press, Minneapolis.
532. Thing Bad [@Merman_Melville] (2021). "kind of a bummer to have been born at the very end of the Fuck Around century just to live the rest of my life in the Find Out century" *Twitter*, 22 February. https://twitter.com/merman_melville/status/1364000670760669184.
533. Defoe D (1772 [1995]). *A Journal of the Plague Year*.
534. Global Social Theory (2021). "Zapatismo." Global Social Theory website, accessed July 15. https://globalsocialtheory.org/topics/zapatismo.
535. Srikanth A (2020). "What Angela Davis has to say about today's Black Lives Matter movement." *Changing America*, 20 October. https://thehill.com/changing-america/enrichment/arts-culture/521928-what-angela-davis-has-to-say-about-todays-black .
536. Gleeson J J and E O'Rourke (eds) (2021). *Transgender Marxism*. Pluto Press, London.
537. Kern S (2021). "No, billionaires won't 'escape' to space while the world burns." *Salon*, 7 July. https://www.salon.com/2021/07/07/no-billionaires-wont-escape -to-space-while-the-world-burns
538. Berardi F (2019). *Futurability: The Age of Impotence and the Horizon of Possibility*.
539. Shockman E (2021). "Minnesota students walk out of school to protest racial injustice." National Public Radio/ WNYC, 20 April. https://www.npr.org/2021/04/20/989074842/1-000s-of-minnesota-students-walk-out-of-school-to-protest-racial-injustice.
540. Stableford D (2019). "'How dare you': Greta Thunberg tears into world leaders over inaction at U.N. climate summit." *Yahoo! News*, 23 September. https://news.yahoo.com/greta-thunberg-un-climate-speech-how-dare-you-151148559.html.

The Blind Weaponmaker

541. Wallace RG (2016). "Homeland." In *Big Farms Make Big Flu: Dispatches on Infectious Disease, Agribusiness, and the Nature of Science*. Monthly Review Press, pp 295-296.
542. Wallace RG (2020). "Midvinter-19." In *Dead Epidemiologists: On the Origins of COVID-19*. Monthly Review Press, pp 81-97.
543. Latham J and A Wilson (2020). "The case is building that COVID-19 had a lab origin." *Independent Science News*, 2 June. https://www.independentsciencenews.org/health/the-case-is-building-that-covid-19-had-a-lab-origin/.
544. Latham J and A Wilson (2020). "A proposed origin for SARS-CoV-2 and the COVID-19 pandemic." *Independent Science News*, 15 July. https://www.independentsciencenews.org/commentaries/a-proposed-origin-for-sars-cov-2-and-the-covid-19-pandemic/.
545. Xu L (2013). "The analysis of six patients with severe pneumonia caused by unknown viruses." Master's thesis in Chinese (translated), School of Clinical Medicine, Kun Ming Medical University. https://www.documentcloud.org/documents/6981198-Analysis-of-Six-Patients-With-Unknown-Viruses.html.
546. Burki T (2018). "Ban on gain-of-function studies ends." *The Lancet Infectious Diseases* 18(2):148-149; Page J, B McKay, and D Hinshaw (2021). "The Wuhan lab leak question: A disused Chinese mine takes center stage." *Wall Street Journal*, 24 May. https://www.wsj.com/articles/wuhan-lab-leak-question-chinese-mine-covid-pandemic-11621871125.
547. Coulson D and C Upton (2010). "Viral bioinformatics: Recombination." *Viology Blog*, 8 September. https://www.virology.ws/2010/09/08/viral-bioinformatics-recombination/; Zhou H, et al. (2020). "A novel bat coronavirus closely related to SARS-CoV-2 contains natural insertions at the S1/S2 cleavage site of the spike protein." *Current Biology* 30: 2196-2203; Ge X-Y, et al. (2016). "Coexistence of multiple coronaviruses in several bat colonies in an abandoned mineshaft." *Virologica Sinica* 31: 31-40.
548. Xio K, et al. (2020). "Isolation of SARS-CoV-2-related coronavirus from Malayan pangolins." *Nature* 583(7815): 286-289.
549. Thomas L (2020). "Research sheds doubt on the Pangolin link to SARS-CoV-2." *Medical Life Sciences News*, 8 July. https://www.news-medical.net/news/20200708/Research-sheds-doubt-on-the-Pangolin-link-to-SARS-CoV-2.aspx.
550. Lee J, et al. (2020). "No evidence of coronaviruses or other potentially zoonotic viruses in Sunda pangolins (*Manis javanica*) entering the wildlife trade via Malaysia." *EcoHealth* 17:406-418.
551. Wallace RG (2020). "Midvinter-19."
552. Ibid.

553. Frutos R, J Serra-Cobo, T Chen, and CA Devaux (2020). "COVID-19: Time to exonerate the pangolin from the transmission of SARS-CoV-2 to humans." *Infection, Genetics and Evolution* 84:104493.
554. Boykin LM, LS Kubatko, and TK Lowrey (2010). "Comparison of methods for rooting phylogenetic trees: a case study using Orcuttieae (Poaceae: Chloridoideae)." *Molecular Phylogenetics and Evolution* 54(3):687-700.
555. Pipes L, H Wang, JP Huelsenbeck, and R Nielsen (2021). "Assessing uncertainty in the rooting of the SARS-CoV-2 phylogeny." *Molecular Biology and Evolution* 38(4):1537-1543.
556. Forster P, L Forster, C Renfrew, and M Forster (2020). "Phylogenetic analysis of SARS-CoV-2 genomes." *Proceedings of the National Academy of the Sciences* 117(17): 9241-9243.
557. Bloom J (2021). "Recovery of deleted deep sequencing data sheds more light on the early Wuhan SARS-CoV-2 epidemic." bioRxiv, 22 June. https://www.biorxiv.org/content/10.1101/2021.06.18.449051v1.full.pdf; Chan JF-W, et al. (2020). A familial cluster of pneumonia associated with the 2019 novel coronavirus indicating person-to-person transmission: A study of a family cluster. *Lancet* 395: 514–523.
558. Chookajorn T (2020). "Evolving COVID-19 conundrum and its impact." *Proceedings of the National Academy of the Sciences* 117(23): 12520-12521; Sánchez-Pacheco SJ, S Kong, P Pulido-Santacruz, RW Murphy, and L Kubatko (2020). "Median-joining network analysis of SARS-CoV-2 genomes is neither phylogenetic nor evolutionary." *Proceedings of the National Academy of the Sciences* 117(23): 12518–12519; Mavian C, et al. (2020). "Sampling bias and incorrect rooting make phylogenetic network tracing of SARS-COV-2 infections unreliable." *Proceedings of the National Academy of the Sciences* 117(23): 12522-12523.
559. Chaw S-M, J-H Tai, S-L Chen, C-H Hsieh, S-Y Chang, et al. (2020). "The origin and underlying driving forces of the SARS-CoV-2 outbreak." *Journal of Biomedical Science* 27:73.
560. Rozo M and GK Gronvall (2015). "The reemergent 1977 H1N1 strain and the gain-of-function debate." mBio 6(4): e01013-15.
561. Vogel G (2014). "Bat-filled tree may have been ground zero for the Ebola epidemic." *Science*, 30 December. https://www.science.org/content/article/bat-filled-tree-may-have-been-ground-zero-ebola-epidemic.
562. Wu Z, et al. (2016). "Deciphering the bat virome catalog to better understand the ecological diversity of bat viruses and the bat origin of emerging infectious diseases." *The ISME Journal* 10(3): 609-620.
563. Wallace RG (2009). "Breeding influenza: the political virology of offshore farming." *Antipode* 41(5): 916-951.
564. Gibbs AJ, JS Armstrong and JC Downie (2009). "From where did the 2009 'swine-origin' influenza A virus (H1N1) emerge?" *Virology Journal* 6:207.

565. Nelson MI, et al. (2015). "Global migration of influenza A viruses in swine." *Nature Communications* 6: 6696.

566. Mena I, et al. (2016). "Origins of the 2009 H1N1 influenza pandemic in swine in Mexico." *Elife* 5.pii: e16777.

567. Itani F (2020). "Why did Lebanon let a bomb-in-waiting sit in a warehouse for 6 Years?" *New York Times*, 5 August. https://www.nytimes.com/2020/08/05/opinion/beirut-explosions.html.

568. Andersen K, A Rambaut, WI Lipkin, EC Holmes, and RF Garry (2020). "The proximal origin of SARS-CoV-2." *Nature Medicine* 26: 450-452; Sørensen B, A Dalgleish, and A Susrud (2020). *The Evidence which Suggests that This Is No Naturally Evolved Virus: A Reconstructed Historical Aetiology of the SARS-CoV-2 Spike*. 13 July. https://www.minervanett.no/files/2020/07/13/TheEvidenceNoNaturalEvol.pdf.

569. Latham J and A Wilson (2020). "A proposed origin for SARS-CoV-2 and the COVID-19 pandemic."

570. Ayala FJ (2007). "Darwin's greatest discovery: Design without designer." *Proceedings of the National Academy of the Sciences* 104(S1): 8567– 8573.

571. Dawkins R (1986). *The Blind Watchmaker: Why the Evidence of Evolution Reveals a Universe without Design*. W.W. Norton & Company, New York.

572. Li X, et al. (2020). "Emergence of SARS-CoV-2 through recombination and strong purifying selection." *Science Advances* 6(27): eabb9153.

573. Racaniello V (2020). "SARS-CoV-2 furin cleavage site revisited." *Virology Blog*, 14 May. https://www.virology.ws/2020/05/14/sars-cov-2-furin-cleavage-site-revisited/; Follis KE, J York, and JH Nunberg (2006). "Furin cleavage of the SARS coronavirus spike glycoprotein enhances cell–cell fusion but does not affect virion entry." *Virology* 350(2): 358-369.

574. Zhou H, et al. (2020). "A novel bat coronavirus closely related to SARS-CoV-2 contains natural insertions at the S1/S2 cleavage site of the spike protein." *Current Biology* 30(11): 2196-2203; Li X, et al. (2020). "Genomic feature analysis of betacoronavirus provides insights into SARS and COVID-19 pandemics." *Frontiers in Microbiology* 12: 614494; Lau SKP, et al. (2005) "Severe acute respiratory syndrome coronavirus-like virus in Chinese horseshoe bats." *Proceedings of the National Academy of the Sciences* 102(39): 14040-14045; Ge X-Y, et al. (2013). "Isolation and characterization of a bat SARS-like coronavirus that uses the ACE2 receptor." *Nature* 503: 535-538.

575. Millet JK and GR Whittaker (2014). "Host cell entry of Middle East respiratory syndrome coronavirus after two-step, furin-mediated activation of the spike protein." *Proceedings of the National Academy of the Sciences* 111(42): 15214-15219.

576. Boni MF, et al. (2020). "Evolutionary origins of the SARS-CoV-2 sar-

becovirus lineage responsible for the COVID-19 pandemic." *Nature Microbiology* 5: 1408-1417; Chaw S-M, J-H Tai, S-L Chen, C-H Hsieh, S-Y Chang, et al. (2020). "The origin and underlying driving forces of the SARS-CoV-2 outbreak"; Li X, et al. (2020). "Emergence of SARS-CoV-2 through recombination and strong purifying selection"; Booker TR, BC Jackson, and PD Keightley (2017). "Detecting positive selection in the genome." *BMC Biology,* 15: 98.

577. Boni MF, et al. (2020). "Evolutionary origins of the SARS-CoV-2 sarbecovirus lineage responsible for the COVID-19 pandemic."

578. Chaw S-M, J-H Tai, S-L Chen, C-H Hsieh, S-Y Chang, et al. (2020). "The origin and underlying driving forces of the SARS-CoV-2 outbreak"; Millet JK and GR Whittaker (2014). "Host cell entry of Middle East respiratory syndrome coronavirus after two-step, furin-mediated activation of the spike protein." *Proceedings of the National Academy of the Sciences* 111(42): 15214-15219.

579. Islam MR, et al. (2020). "Genome-wide analysis of SARS-CoV-2 virus strains circulating worldwide implicates heterogeneity." *Scientific Reports* 10: 14004; Morais IJ, et al. (2020). "The global population of SARS-CoV-2 is composed of six major subtypes." *Scientific Reports* 10: 18289; Rochman ND, et al. (2021). "Ongoing global and regional adaptive evolution of SARS-CoV-2." *Proceedings of the National Academy of the Sciences* 118(29): e2104241118.

580. Greenfeld KT (2007) *China Syndrome: The True Story of the 21st Century's First Great Epidemic.* Harper Perennial, New York.

581. Wu Z, et al. (2014). "Novel Henipa-like Virus, Mojiang paramyxovirus, in rats, China, 2012." Emerging Infectious Diseases 20(6): 1064-1066.

582. Slato-Tellez M, E Tan, and B Lim (2005). "ARDS in SARS: cytokine mediators and treatment implications." *Cytokine* 29(2): 92-94; Carotti M, et al. (2020). "Chest CT features of coronavirus disease 2019 (COVID-19) pneumonia: key points for radiologists." *Radiologia Medica* 125(7): 636-646.

583. Sørensen B, A Dalgleish, and A Susrud (2020). *The Evidence which Suggests that This Is No Naturally Evolved Virus: A Reconstructed Historical Aetiology of the SARS-CoV-2 Spike.*

584. Wallace RG (2020). "Midvinter-19."

585. Ibid.

586. Brufsky A and MT Lotze (2020). "DC/L-SIGNs of hope in the COVID-19 pandemic." *Journal of Medical Virology* 92:1396-1398.

587. Boni MF, et al. (2020). "Evolutionary origins of the SARS-CoV-2 sarbecovirus lineage responsible for the COVID-19 pandemic."

588. Ibid.

589. Hou Y, et al. (2010). "Angiotensin-converting enzyme 2 (ACE2) proteins of different bat species confer variable susceptibility to SARS-CoV entry." *Archives of Virology* 155(10): 1563-1569.

590. Fan Y, K Zhao, Z-L Shi, and P Zhou (2019). "Bat coronaviruses in China." *Viruses* 11(3): 210.

591. Frutos R, J Serra-Cobo, T Chen, and CA Devaux (2020). "COVID-19: Time to exonerate the pangolin from the transmission of SARS-CoV-2 to humans."

592. Ibid.

593. Ibid.

594. Cube Plays (2017). "The Death Star blows up Jedha—Star Wars Rogue One—(4K Ultra HD)." YouTube, 14 April. https://www.youtube.com/watch?v=V8EDyD97TZo.

595. Wallace RG (2016). "Homeland"; Garrett L (2011). "The bioterrorist next door." *Foreign Policy*, 15 December. https://foreignpolicy.com/2011/12/15/the-bioterrorist-next-door/#sthash.FbHXLDbC.dpbs; Van Boeckel TP, MJ Tildesley, C Linard, J Halloy, MJ Keeling, and M Gilbert (2013). "The Nosoi commute: a spatial perspective on the rise of BSL-4 laboratories in cities." arXiv 1312 3283v2. https://arxiv.org/abs/1312.3283; Lipsitch M and AP Galvani (2014). "Ethical alternatives to experiments with novel potential pandemic pathogens." *PLoS Medicine* 11(5): e1001646; Lipsitch M (2018). "Why do exceptionally dangerous gain-of-function experiments in influenza?" In Y Yamauchi (ed), *Influenza Virus: Methods and Protocols*. Springer, Cham, pp 589-608.

596. Wallace RG, A Liebman, LF Chaves, and R Wallace (2020). "COVID-19 and circuits of capital." *Monthly Review* 72(1). https://monthlyreview.org/2020/05/01/covid-19-and-circuits-of-capital/.

597. Turner J (2011). "Logic and ontological pluralism." *Journal of Philosophical Logic* 41, 419-448.

The BoJo Strain

598. CBS/AP (2020). "What we know about the new strain of coronavirus in the U.K." 22 December. https://www.cbsnews.com/news/covid-new-strain-uk-what-we-know/; Magome M and A Meldrum (2020). "New strain of COVID-19 is driving South Africa's resurgence". AP News, 21 December. https://apnews.com/article/new-coronavirus-strain-south-africa-31a0d5840a17fa5c82f-2ecd14ba9921b; Kim S (2020). "Hundreds of COVID-Infected mink could have escaped Danish fur farms, spreading new coronavirus strain." *Newsweek*, 1 December. https://www.newsweek.com/coronavirus-mink-escape-fur-farms-denmark-outbreak-1551499.

599. V'kovski P, A Kratzel, S Steiner, H Stalder, and V Thiel (2021). "Coronavirus biology and replication: implications for SARS-CoV-2." *Nature Reviews Microbiology*, 19: 155–170.

600. Russell TW, N Golding, J Hellewell, S Abbott, L Wright, et al. (2020). "Reconstructing the early global dynamics of under-ascertained

COVID-19 cases and infections." *BMC Medicine*, 18: 332 (2020). https://bmcmedicine.biomedcentral.com/articles/10.1186/s12916-020 -01790-9.

601. Levin BR and WL Kilmer (1974). "Interdemic selection and the evolution of altruism: A computer simulation study." *Evolution*, 28(4): 527-545.

602. Messinger SM and A Ostling (2009). "The consequences of spatial structure for the evolution of pathogen transmission rate and virulence." *American Naturalist*, 174(4): 441-454.

603. Freedland J (2020). "This government's incompetence is no accident. It was inevitable." *The Guardian*, 2 October. https://www. theguardian.com/commentisfree/2020/oct/02/incompetence-brexit -johnson-cummings-pandemic.

604. Lipsitch M and ER Moxon (1997). "Virulence and transmissibility of pathogens: what is the relationship?" *Trends in Microbiology*, 5(1):31-37.

605. Boots M and A Sasaki (1999). "'Small worlds' and the evolution of virulence: infection occurs locally and at a distance." *Proceedings of the Royal Society B*, 266(1432): 1933-1938.

606. Rajghatta C (2020). "'Let them eat cake': Americans rage about meager stimulus payment." *Times of India*, 21 December. https://timesofindia. indiatimes.com/world/us/let-them-eat-cake-americans-rage-about- meager-stimulus-payment/articleshow/79843482.cms; Neuburger T (2020). "To save the economy, Biden must first save lives." *Naked Capitalism*, 24 November. https://www.nakedcapitalism.com/2020/11/ to-save-the-economy-biden-must-first-save-lives.html.

607. Richards SE and N Akpan (2020). "Already had the coronavirus? You could get it again." *National Geographic*, 1 December. https:// www.nationalgeographic.com/science/article/why-coronavirus -reinfections-are-happening.

608. Yewdell JW (2021). "Antigenic drift: Understanding COVID-19." *Immunity*, 54(12):2681-2687.

609. Harrison D (2020). "Results from the AstraZeneca/Oxford vaccine trials." 15 December. https://dalewharrison.substack.com/p/ results-from-the-astrazenecaoxford.

610. Fonville JM, SH Wilks, SL James, A Fox, M Ventresca, et al. (2014). "Antibody landscapes after influenza virus infection or vaccination." *Science*, 346(6212): 996-1000.

611. Wallace RG (2020). "Midvinter-19." In *Dead Epidemiologists: On the Origins of COVID-19*. Monthly Review Press, pp 81-97.

612. Wallace RG (2016). "The NAFTA flu." In *Big Farms Make Big Flu: Dispatches on Infectious Disease, Agribusiness, and the Nature of Science*. Monthly Review Press, pp 32-36.

613. Wallace RG. "The Blind Weaponmaker." This volume.

To Live and Die in L.A.

614. Asimov N (2021). "Here's why California has the lowest COVID rate in the nation." *San Francisco Chronicle,* 18 September. https://www.sfchronicle.com/bayarea/article/Here-s-why-California has the-lowest-COVID-rate-16468706.php.

615. New York Times (2021). "Tracking coronavirus in Los Angeles County, Calif." https://www.nytimes.com/interactive/2021/us/los-angeles-california-covid-cases.html.

616. Mossburg C and Waldrop T (2021). "Every 8 minutes, someone in Los Angeles County dies from Covid-19." CNN, 7 January. https://www.cnn.com/2021/01/07/us/los-angeles-county-covid-19-death-every-8-minutes/index.html; Lozano A (2021). "Los Angeles becomes first county to hit 1 million Covid-19 cases." NBC News, 16 January. https://www.nbcnews.com/news/us-news/los-angeles-becomes-first-county-hit-1-million-covid-19-n1254498.

617. Kim C (2020). "New study finds formerly redlined neighborhoods are more at risk for Covid-19." WBUR, 14 September. https://www.wbur.org/hereandnow/2020/09/14/redlined-neighborhoods-coronavirus-study.

618. Bloch M and Cowan J (2021). "In Los Angeles, the virus is pummeling those who can least afford to fall ill." *New York Times*, 29 January. https://www.nytimes.com/interactive/2021/01/29/us/los-angeles-county-covid-rates.html.

619. Rosenfeld D and R Carter (2020). "East San Fernando Valley: A perfect storm for alarming coronavirus spread." *Los Angeles Daily News*, 20 November. https://www.dailynews.com/2020/11/20/east-san-fernando-valley-a-perfect-storm-for-alarming-coronavirus-spread/.

620. Vives R (2020). "San Fernando Valley's Latino neighborhoods staggered by L.A. County virus outbreak." *Los Angeles Times*, 1 December. https://www.latimes.com/california/story/2020-12-01/covid-19-has-hit-las-san-fernando-valley-hard.

621. Ibid.

622. Bloch M and Cowan J (2021). "In Los Angeles, the virus is pummeling those who can least afford to fall ill."

623. Food Chain Workers Alliance (2021). *We Are Not Disposable: Food Workers Organizing on the Covid Frontlines.* https://foodchainworkers.org/wp-content/uploads/2021/02/Food-Workers-Organizing-on-the-COVID-Frontlines-FINAL.pdf.

624. Ibid.

625. COVID-19 Farmworker Study (2020). *Preliminary Data Brief,* 27 July. http://covid19farmworkerstudy.org/survey/wp-content/uploads/2020/08/EN-COFS-Preliminary-Data- Brief_FINAL.pdf.

626. Vives R (2020). "San Fernando Valley's Latino neighborhoods staggered by L.A. County virus outbreak."

627. Smith H (2021). "Unvaccinated people, riskier behavior: What is fueling L.A.'s coronavirus surge?" *Los Angeles Times*, 25 August. https://www.latimes.com/california/story/2021-08-25/whats-fueling-la-covid-surge -how-can-vaccines-help.

628. Rosen J, et al. (2020). *How Do Renters Cope with Unaffordability? Household-Level Impacts of Rental Cost Burdens in Los Angeles.* USC Price Center for Social Innovation, December. https://socialinnovation.usc.edu/rent-burden/.

629. US Census (2021). *Household Pulse Survey, Week 34.* https://www.census.gov/data-tools/demo/hhp.

630. Park J (2020). "Empty bedrooms and overcrowded rentals in Los Angeles." 31st Annual USC-SCAG Demographic Workshop Panel on the Changing Demographic Outlook and Housing Trends, USC Price School of Public Policy, 11 June. https://scag.ca.gov/sites/main/files/file-attachments/junghopark.pdf?1604614104.

631. Chief of Staff Special Projects (2017). *Housing & Health in Los Angeles County: A Snapshot.* Los Angeles County Department of Public Health. http://publichealth.lacounty.gov/centerforhealthequity/PDF/LAC%20Housing%20Health.pdf.

632. Ahmad K, et al. (2020). "Association of poor housing conditions with COVID-19 incidence and mortality across US counties." *PLoS ONE* 15(11): e0241327. https://journals.plos.org/plosone/article?id=10.1371/journal.pone.0241327.

633. Email communication from L.A. housing advocates to the authors.

634. Rihn J (2021). "Eviction moratoriums can't protect the most vulnerable tenants." *Capital & Main*, 2 March. https://capitalandmain.com/eviction-moratoriums-cant-protect-the-most-vulnerable-tenants-0302.

635. Tenants Together, Anti-Eviction Mapping Project, and Hope. (2021). *Tenant COVID-19 Resistance and Experience Oral History Project.* https://hope.xyz/tenantexperienceoralhistoryproject.

636. Tang Y, et al. (2020). "Cytokine storm in COVID-19: The current evidence and treatment strategies." *Frontiers in Immunology*, 11:1708. https://www.frontiersin.org/articles/10.3389/fimmu.2020.01708/full; Melo AKG, et al. (2021). "Biomarkers of cytokine storm as red flags for severe and fatal COVID-19 cases: A living systematic review and meta-analysis." *PLoS ONE*, 16(6): e0253894. https://journals.plos.org/plosone/article?id=10.1371/journal.pone.0253894.

637. Marya R and R Patel (2021). *Inflamed: Deep Medicine and the Anatomy of Injustice.* Farrar Straus and Giroux, New York.

638. Ibid.

639. Bhushan D, et al. (2020). *Roadmap for Resilience: The California Surgeon General's Report on Adverse Childhood Experiences, Toxic Stress, and Health.* Office of the California Surgeon General, 9 December. https://

health.ucdavis.edu/crhd/pdfs/resources/roadmap-for-resilience-ca-surgeon-generals-report-on-aces-toxic-stress-and-health-12092020.pdf.

640. Ibid.

641. UCLA Center for Neighborhood Knowledge. *Los Angeles COVID-19 Vulnerability, Version 1.* https://knowledge.luskin.ucla.edu/maps/.

642. Enochs K and M Tinsay (2021). *Social Determinants: Poverty and Homelessness Coupled with COVID-10 Incidence and Severity. 22* May. University of St. Thomas. Available upon request.

643. L.A. County Dept. of Public Health (2020). *Novel Coronavirus (COVID-19) Guidance for Homeless Service Agencies and Outreach Teams. 27* July. http://publichealth.lacounty.gov/media/Coronavirus/docs/homelessness/GuidanceHomelessServiceAgencies.pdf.

644. Enochs K and M Tinsay (2021). *Social Determinants: Poverty and Homelessness Coupled with COVID-10 Incidence and Severity.* BIOL 474 Senior Seminar in Global Health, University of St Thomas.

645. Kaiser Permanente. *Housing for Health: Thriving Communities Fund.* https://about.kaiserpermanente.org/community-health/improving-community -conditions/housing-security.

646. Benfer E, Leifheit K, Linton S, Pollack C, Schwartz G, and Zimmerman F (2021). "Expiring eviction moratoriums and COVID-19 incidence and mortality." SSRN, 5 August. https://papers.ssrn.com/sol3/papers.cfm?abstract_id=3739576.

647. County of Los Angeles (2021). *Los Angeles County Homelessness & Housing Map.* https://storymaps.arcgis.com/stories/400d7b75f18747c4ae1ad22d662781a3.

648. Smith D. (2021). "L.A. homeless sites 'overwhelmed' by COVID-19: 'These are the toughest times'." *Los Angeles Times,* 3 January. https://www.latimes.com/homeless-housing/story/2021-01-03/homeless-shelters-coronavirus-surge-hospitals.

649. Herr A and A Maloney (2021). "As COVID restrictions lift, green spaces are the front lines in a fight for housing justice." *Grist,* 13 April. https://grist.org/housing/los-angeles-echo-park-homelessness -policing-housing-covid/.

650. Ibid.; Mitchell D (2021). "A late neoliberal holocaust." In DB Monk and M Sorkin (eds), *Between Catastrophe and Revolution: Essays in Honor of Mike Davis.* OR Books, New York, pp 55-77.

651. Herr A and A Maloney (2021). "As COVID restrictions lift, green spaces are the front lines in a fight for housing justice."

652. Chou et al. (2021). "Hundreds pack Echo Park protesting plan to shut area for refurbishment, force homeless to move." *Los Angeles Daily News,* 24 March. https://www.dailynews.com/2021/03/24/hundreds-pack-echo-park-protesting-plan-to-shut-area-for-refurbishment-force-homeless-to-move/.

653. Email communication with the authors.

654. Email communication with the authors.

655. Email communication with the authors.

656. Wagner D. (2021). "Exposed wires, bugs, and eviction notices: Life in an unpermitted LA apartment complex." *LAist*, 2 June. https://laist.com/news/housing-homelessness/unpermitted-housing-illegal-units-pandemic-eviction-los-angeles.

657. Levin S (2020). "California landlords are locking out struggling tenants. A 'tsunami of evictions' may be next." *The Guardian*, 30 July. https://www.theguardian.com/us-news/2020/jul/30/california-covid-19-evictions-landlords-tenants.

658. Email communication to the authors.

659. Bade B, et al. (2021). *Always Essential, Perpetually Disposable: California Farmworkers and the COVID-19 Pandemic.* COVID-19 Farmworker Study, Phase Two Preliminary Report. http://covid19farmworkerstudy.org/survey/wp-content/uploads/2021/03/COFS-_Phase-Two-Preliminary-Report.pdf.

660. Baker M (2020). "Nonrelocatable occupations at increased risk during pandemics: United States, 2018." *American Journal of Public Health* 110(8): 1126-1132. https://ajph.aphapublications.org/doi/10.2105/AJPH.2020.305738.

661. CBS (2021). "COVID study: Food, agriculture, construction workers top list of most at risk of COVID death." CBS SF BayArea, 29 January. https://sanfrancisco.cbslocal.com/2021/01/29/ucsf-covid-study-food-agriculture-construction-workers-death-risk/.

662. Email communication to the authors.

663. Baker M (2020). "Nonrelocatable occupations at increased risk during pandemics: United States, 2018."

664. Bade B et al (2021). *Always Essential, Perpetually Disposable: California Farmworkers and the COVID-19 Pandemic.*

665. Bracha A and MA Burke, M. A. (2018). *The Ups and Downs of the Gig Economy, 2015-2017.* FRB of Boston Working Paper No. 18-12; Anderson M, et al. (2021). "The state of gig work in 2021." Pew Research Center, 8 December. https://www.pewresearch.org/internet/2021/12/08/the-state-of-gig-work-in-2021/; Board of Governors of the Federal Reserve (2021). *Economic Well-Being of U.S. Households in 2020.* Federal Reserve, May 2021. https://www.federalreserve.gov/publications/2021-economic-well-being-of-us-households-in-2020-employment.htm; Pickard-Whitehead G (2021). "COVID and the gig economy." Smallbiztrends.com, 16 November. https://smallbiztrends.com/2021/10/covid-gig-economy-statistics.html; Mitic I (2022). "Gig economy statistics: The new normal in the workplace." Fortunly.com, 17 Feburary. https://fortunly.com/statistics/gig-economy-statistics/#gref.

666. Freelance Forward (2020). https://www.upwork.com/documents/freelance-forward-2020.

667. Jacobs K and M Reich (2019). *The Uber/Lyft Ballot Initiative Guarantees Only $5.64 An Hour.* UC Berkeley Labor Center. https://laborcenter.berkeley.edu/the-uber-lyft-ballot-initiative-guarantees-only-5-64-an-hour-2/.

668. DiSalvo E (2021). "Jobs of desperation: How ridehailing, food delivery workers lose out in the gig economy." *Phoenix Business Journal*, 26 July. https://www.bizjournals.com/phoenix/news/2021/07/26/how-ride-hailing-food-delivery-workers-lose.html.

669. National Employment Law Project (2019). *Rights at Risk: Gig Companies' Campaign to Upend Employment as We Know It.* https://s27147.pcdn.co/wp-content/uploads/Rights-at-Risk-4-2-19.pdf.

670. Mobile Workers' Alliance (2020). *Recap: MWA Statewide COVID-19 Response Call with Assemblymember Lorena Gonzalez.* https://mobile-alliance.org/2020/04/mwa-statewide-covid-call/.

671. Hartmans A (2020). "'This is why people are so angry': Tech giants like Google, Facebook, and Uber built their empires on the backs of contractors." *Business Insider*, 2 April. https://www.businessinsider.com/how-tech-relies-on-contractors-temps-gig-workers-employees-2020-1.

672. UC Berkeley Labor Center, UCLA Labor Center, UCLA LOSH, and UC Berkeley LOHP (2021). *The Fast-Food Industry and COVID-19 in Los Angeles.* https://www.labor.ucla.edu/wp-content/uploads/2021/03/FastFood_Report_2021_Final.pdf.

673. COVID-19 Farmworker Study (2020). Preliminary Data Brief, 27 July.

674. Fu J and S Bloch. "7 ways the Trump administration has deregulated the food system during the Covid-19 pandemic." *The Counter*, 23 July. https://thecounter.org/trump-administration-has-deregulated-the-food-system-covid-19- osha-line-speeds/.

675. Bloch S (2021). "After 10 months of minimal oversight, Biden orders OSHA to get to work." *The Counter*, 26 January. https://thecounter.org/osha-months-minimal-oversight-biden-executive-order-covid-19/; CBS (2021). "COVID study: Food, agriculture, construction workers top list of most at risk of COVID death."

676. Douglas L and Gee G (2021). "A COVID outbreak at a California meat-packing plant started a year ago—and never went away." *Mother Jones*, 16 March. https://www.motherjones.com/food/2021/03/a-covid-outbreak-at-a-california-meatpacking-plant-started-a-year-ago-and-never-went-away/.

677. Bade B et al. (2021). *Always Essential, Perpetually Disposable: California Farmworkers and the COVID-19 Pandemic.*

678. COVID-19 Farmworker Study (2020). Preliminary Data Brief, 27 July.

679. Bade B et al. (2021). *Always Essential, Perpetually Disposable: California Farmworkers and the COVID-19 Pandemic.*

680. Food Chain Workers Alliance (2021). *We Are Not Disposable: Food Workers Organizing on the Covid Frontlines.*

681. UC Berkeley Labor Center, UCLA Labor Center, UCLA LOSH, and UC Berkeley LOHP (2021). *The Fast-Food Industry and COVID-19 in Los Angeles.*

682. Ockenfels-Martinez M (2019). *Driving Away Our Health: The Economic Insecurity of Working for Lyft and Uber.* Human Impact Partners / Gig Workers Rising. https://humanimpact.org/wp- content/uploads/2019/08/DrivingAwayHealthReport_2019.08final-compressed.pdf.

683. Siegrist J and J Li (2017). "Work stress and altered biomarkers: A synthesis of findings based on the effort reward imbalance model." *International Journal of Environmental Research and Public Health* 14(11): 1373.

684. Chandola T and N Zhang (2017). "Re-employment, job quality, health and allostatic load biomarkers: prospective evidence from the UK Household Longitudinal Study." *International Journal of Epidemiology,* 47(1): 47-57.

685. Suler L (2021). "With delta variant fueling COVID surge, concern growing for children not yet eligible for vaccine." *ABC News,* 2 August. https://abc7.com/covid-vaccine-for-kids-fda-vaccines-study-children/10925192/.

686. Choi-Schagrin W (2021). "In the West, a connection between Covid and wildfires." *New York Times,* 13 August. https://www.nytimes.com/2021/08/13/climate/wildfires-smoke-covid.html.

687. County of Los Angeles Public Health (2021). COVID-19 vaccine dashboard, 20 September. http://publichealth.lacounty.gov/media/coronavirus/vaccine/vaccine-dashboard.htm.

688. Dador D (2021). "For first time, Black residents of LA County seeing highest COVID-19 infection rates." *ABC News,* 27 May. https://abc7.com/covid-19-los-angeles-county-black-residents-african-americans-rates-dr-barbara-ferrer/10705961/.

689. Associated Press (2021). "Many unvaccinated Latinos want COVID-19 shot but face barriers, poll finds." *KTLA News,* 13 May. https://ktla.com/news/coronavirus/many-unvaccinated-latinos-want-covid-19-shot-but-face-barriers-poll-finds/.

690. Figueroa M, et al. (2021). "To live and die in Los Angeles: COVID-19, structural stress, and the path to a more resilient health." PReP Neighborhoods, Pandemic Research for the People, 21 September. https://drive.google.com/file/d/1CB_U2dhSWkcP6QFaC2zEuPLG9p35q49n/view.

691. Hurley L and J Wolfe (2021). "US Supreme Court ends CDC's pandemic residential eviction moratorium." *Reuters,* 27 August. https://www.reuters.com/world/us/us-supreme-court-ends-federal-residential-eviction-moratorium-2021-08-27/.

692. Leifheit K, et al. (2021). "Expiring eviction moratoriums and COVID-19 incidence and mortality." *American Journal of Epidemiology,*

kwab196. https://academic.oup.com/aje/advance-article/doi/10.1093/aje/kwab196/6328194.

693. Blankley B (2021). "Landlords sue Los Angeles for $100M over eviction moratorium." *The Center Square*, 12 August. https://www.thecentersquare.com/california/landlords-sue-los-angeles-for-100m-over-eviction-moratorium/article_ae966b5a-fb8e-11eb -8ff8-03c25bea8f27.html.

694. PainterG(2021)."Theevictionmoratoriumwon'tsaverenters—orlandlords." *Politico*, 10 August. https://www.politico.com/news/magazine/2021/08/10/eviction-moratorium-renters-landlord-covid-503352.

695. Levin M, N Duara, and E Yee (2020). "Exclusive: More than 1,600 Californians have been evicted during pandemic." *CalMatters*, 11 August. https://calmatters.org/housing/2020/08/californians-evicted -coronavirus-pandemic/.

696. Levin S (2021). "California promised 100% rent forgiveness for struggling tenants. Most are still waiting." *The Guardian*, 9 August. https://www.theguardian.com/us-news/2021/aug/09/california-promised-100-rent-forgiveness-for-struggling-tenants-most-are-still-waiting.

697. Ibid.

698. McAboy K (2021). "Struggling LA residents describe eviction moratorium as lifesaver during pandemic." *FOX 11 News Los Angeles*, 25 June. https://www.foxla.com/news/struggling-la-residents-describe-eviction-moratorium-as- lifesaver-during-pandemic.

699. LenthangM(2021)."HowCOVID-19vaccinepolicieshavetriggeredlawsuitsand workplace showdowns." *ABC News*, 20 June. https://abcnews.go.com/Business/covid-19-vaccine-policies-triggered-lawsuits-workplace-showdowns/story?id=78204107.

700. Cap Radio (2021). "Law enforcement union pushing back on vaccine requirements." 18 August. https://www.capradio.org/articles/2021/08/18/ california-coronavirus-updates-august-2021/.

701. CBSLA Staff (2021). "Nurses demand better staffing, workplace protections on national day of action." CBS 2 News Los Angeles, 21 July. https://losangeles.cbslocal.com/2021/07/21/nurses-demand-better-staffing-workplace-protections-national-day-of-action/.

702. @ErikaLougheed (2021). "Actual quote from an ER nurse I heard while canvassing this week…"Twitter, 11 Sept https://twitter.com/ErikaLougheed/status/1436840485327417345.

703. National Alliance to End Homelessness (2016). *Housing First Fact Sheet.* https://endhomelessness.org/resource/housing-first/.

704. Moms 4 Housing, https://moms4housing.org/aboutm4h; Poor People's Army (2021). #LivesOverLuxury Press Conference In Support of Housing Takeovers. 29 March https://poorpeoplesarmy.com/#takeovers.

705. Poppe B and National Alliance to End Homelessness (2020). *Responding to Homeless Families' Needs During the COVID-19 Crisis (Version 1).* Framework for an Equitable COVID-19 Homelessness

Response, 16 December. https://endhomelessness.org/wp-content/uploads/2020/12/12-16-2020_Responsing-to-Homeless-Families-Needs-During-the-COVID-19-Crisis_v1.pdf.
706. Ibid.
707. Bloch S (2021). "After 10 months of minimal oversight, Biden orders OSHA to get to work"; Food Chain Workers Alliance (2021). *OSHA's New Emergency COVID Protections Exclude Essential Food Workers*. 10 June. https://foodchainworkers.org/2021/06/oshas-new-emergency-covid-protections-exclude-essential-food- workers/.
708. Advancing Justice—Asian Law Caucus and University of California, Berkeley Labor and Occupational Health Program (2021). *Few Options, Many Risks: Low-Wage Asian and Latinx Workers in the COVID-19 Pandemic*. https://www.advancingjustice-alc.org/news_and_media/covid-workers-report.
709. Park J (2021). "California fast-food workers hold one-day strike over minimum wage, working conditions." *Sacramento Bee*, 18 January. https://www.sacbee.com/article248544970.html.
710. Rathi V (2021). "Epic examples of fast food and retail workers quitting their jobs in protest." *Emergency Worker Organizing*, 12 May. https://workerorganizing.org/3-epic-examples-of-fast-food-and-retail-workers-quitting-their-jobs-in-protest-1957/.
711. Kinder M and L Stateler (2021). "Local COVID-19 hazard pay mandates are doing what Congress and most corporations aren't for essential workers." *The Avenue*, Brookings Institute, 27 January. https://www.brookings.edu/blog/the-avenue/2021/01/27/local-covid-19-hazard-pay-mandates-are-doing-what-congress-and-most-corporations-arent-for-essential-workers/.
712. Food Chain Workers Alliance (2021). *We Are Not Disposable: Food Workers Organizing on the Covid Frontlines*.
713. Mulvaney E and M Allsup (2021). "Millions at stake for gig companies as Prop. 22's reach debated." *Bloomberg Law Daily Labor Report*, 1 July. https://news.bloomberglaw.com/daily-labor-report/millions-at-stake-for-gig-companies-as-prop-22s-reach-debated.
714. Marya R and R Patel (2021). *Inflamed: Deep Medicine and the Anatomy of Injustice*.
715. Ibid.
716. Ibid.
717. Dockray H (2019). "Self-care isn't enough. We need community care to thrive." *Mashable*, 24 May. https://mashable.com/article/community-care -versus-self-care.
718. Marya R and R Patel (2021). *Inflamed: Deep Medicine and the Anatomy of Injustice*.

Homegrown
719. MacFarquhar N (2020). "The coronavirus becomes a battle cry

for U.S. extremists." *New York Times,* 3 May. https://www.nytimes.com/2020/05/03/us/coronavirus-extremists.html.

720. Davis M (1990 [2006]). *City of Quartz: Excavating the Future of Los Angeles.* Verso, New York; Davis M (2002). *Dead Cities: And Other Tales.* The New Press, New York; Chua C (2021). "Lineages of infrastructural power: Los Angeles as a logistical nightmare." In DB Monk and M Sorkin (eds), *Between Catastrophe and Revolution: Essays in Honor of Mike Davis.* OR Books, New York, pp 249-268.

721. Empire Logistics Collective (2020). "The project." http://www.empire-logistics.org/about/the-project/.

722. Wallace R (2016). "Synchronize your barns." In *Big Farms Make Big Flu: Dispatches on Infectious Disease, Agribusiness, and the Nature of Science.* Monthly Review Press, New York, pp 181-191.

723. Zimmer C (2021). "New California variant may be driving virus surge there, study suggests." *New York Times,* 19 January. https://www.nytimes.com/2021/01/19/health/coronavirus-variant-california.html; Corum J and C Zimmer (2021). "Coronavirus variants and mutations." *New York Times,* 4 June. https://www.nytimes.com/interactive/2021/health/coronavirus-variant-tracker.html#epsilon.

724. McCallum M, et al. (2021). "SARS-CoV-2 immune evasion by the B.1.427/B.1.429 variant of concern." *Science,* 373(6555):648-654. https://www.science.org/doi/full/10.1126/science.abi7994.

725. Nguyen TN (2021). "Coronavirus today: Our homegrown triple threat." *Los Angeles Times,* 23 February. https://www.latimes.com/science/newsletter/2021-02-23/california-dominant-strain-triple-threat-coronavirus-today.

726. McCallum M, et al. (2021). "SARS-CoV-2 immune evasion by the B.1.427/B.1.429 variant of concern."

727. Long SW, et al. (2021). "Sequence analysis of 20,453 Severe Acute Respiratory Syndrome Coronavirus 2 genomes from the Houston Metropolitan Area identifies the emergence and widespread distribution of multiple isolates of all major variants of concern." *American Journal of Pathology,* 191(6): 983-992. https://www.ncbi.nlm.nih.gov/pmc/articles/PMC7962948/.

728. Healy M (2021). "California's coronavirus strain looks increasingly dangerous: 'The devil is already here'." *Los Angeles Times,* 23 February. https://www.latimes.com/science/story/2021-02-23/california-homegrown-coronavirus-strain-looks-increasingly-transmissible-and-dangerous.

Mo BoJo

729. Hamblin J (2020). "The mysterious link between COVID-19 and sleep." *The Atlantic,* 21 December. https://www.theatlantic.com/health/archive/2020/12/covid-19-sleep-pandemic-zzzz/617454/.

730. Morrision V (2020). "No More Lockdown." YouTube, 22 October. https://www.youtube.com/watch?v=yUOWS7arfw4.

731. Clapton E and V Morrison (2020). "Stand and Deliver by Eric Clapton—Music from The state51 Conspiracy." YouTube, 18 December. https://www.youtube.com/watch?v=tMkV4vYr_ik; Wikipedia (2020). "Dick Turpin." https://en.wikipedia.org/wiki/Dick_Turpin.

732. Sugden J and S Fidler (2020). "How British scientists tracked down the new Covid-19 variant." *Wall Street Journal*, 23 December 2020. https://www.wsj.com/articles/how-british-scientists-tracked-down-the-new-covid-19-variant-11608750228.

733. Harrison DW (2020). "Results from the AstraZeneca/Oxford Vaccine trials." https://dalewharrison.substack.com/p/results-from-the-astrazenecaoxford.

734. Google Scholar (2020). Search for "Evolution of virulence review." https://scholar.google.com/scholar?hl=en&as_sdt=0%2C24&q=evolution+of+virulence+review&btnG=.

735. Boots M and A Sasaki (1999). "'Small worlds' and the evolution of virulence: infection occurs locally and at a distance." *Proceedings of the Royal Society B*, 266(1432): 1933-1938.

736. Waitzkin H (ed) (2018). *Health Care Under the Knife: Moving Beyond Capitalism for Our Health*. Monthly Review Press, New York

737. Neuburger T (2020). "To save the economy, Biden must first save lives." *Naked Capitalism*, 24 November. https://www.nakedcapitalism.com/2020/11/to-save-the-economy-biden-must-first-save-lives.html.

738. Bermingham F and S Leng (2020). "China trade: exports surge to record levels, as coronavirus lockdowns return to the West." *South China Morning Post*, 7 December. https://www.scmp.com/economy/china-economy/article/3112820/china-trade-exports-sent-rocketing-coronavirus-lockdowns.

739. Anonymous (2020). "New Zealand and Australia play out thrilling draw in front of packed mask-free crowd—in pictures." *The National*, 11 October. https://www.thenationalnews.com/sport/rugby/new-zealand-and-australia-play-out-thrilling-draw-in-front-of-packed-mask-free-crowd-in-pictures-1.1091568.

740. Rambaut A, N Loman, O Pybus, W Barclay, J Barrett, et al. (2020). "Preliminary genomic characterisation of an emergent SARS-CoV-2 lineage in the UK defined by a novel set of spike mutations." COVID Genomics Consortium UK (CoG-UK), December. https://virological.org/t/preliminary-genomic-characterisation-of-an-emergent-sars-cov-2-lineage-in-the-uk-defined-by-a-novel-set-of-spike-mutations/563; Gu H, Q Chen, G Yang, L He, H Fan, et al. (2020). "Adaptation of SARS-CoV-2 in BALB/c mice for testing vaccine efficacy." *Science*, 369(6511):1603-1607.

741. Flower TG, CZ Buffalo, RM Hooy, M Allaire, X Ren, and JH Hurley (2021). "Structure of SARS-CoV-2 ORF8, a rapidly evolving immune evasion protein." *PNAS*, 118(2):e2021785118.

742. Briggs H (2021). "Coronavirus variants and mutations: The sci-

ence explained." BBC News, 6 January. https://www.bbc.com/news/science-environment-55404988.

743. Rambaut A, N Loman, O Pybus, W Barclay, J Barrett, et al. (2020). "Preliminary genomic characterisation of an emergent SARS-CoV-2 lineage in the UK defined by a novel set of spike mutations."

744. Wallace RG. "The BoJo strain." This volume; (2020). Bradley J, S Gebrekidan, and A McCann (2020). "Inside the UK's pandemic spending: waste, negligence." *New York Times,* 17 December.

745. Lover A (2020). "New UK strain of #COVID19 (B1.1.7)." Twitter, 21 December. https://mobile.twitter.com/AndrewALover/status/1341074110953246720.

746. Okamoto KW, V Ong, RG Wallace, R Wallace , LF Chaves (2022). "When might host heterogeneity drive the evolution of asymptomatic, pandemic coronaviruses?" *Nonlinear Dynamics,* https://doi.org/10.1007/s11071-022-07548-7.

747. Ibid.
748. Ibid.
749. Ibid.
750. Ibid.
751. Ibid.

752. Wallace D and R Wallace (2020). *COVID-19 in New York City: An Ecology of Race and Class Oppression.* Springer, Cham.

753. Ibid.

754. Macaskill A and RC Marshall (2021). "The fatal shore: How a coronavirus variant tore through a tiny English island and onto the world stage." Reuters, 26 March. https://www.reuters.com/investigates/special-report/health-coronavirus-uk-variant/?utm_source=pocket-newtab-global-en-GB.

755. Ibid.

756. Okamoto KW, V Ong, RG Wallace, R Wallace, LF Chaves (2020). "When might host heterogeneity drive the evolution of asymptomatic, pandemic coronaviruses?"

757. Wallace D and R Wallace (2020). *COVID-19 in New York City: An Ecology of Race and Class Oppression.*

758. Okamoto KW, V Ong, RG Wallace, R Wallace, LF Chaves (2020). "When might host heterogeneity drive the evolution of asymptomatic, pandemic coronaviruses?"

759. Wallace D and R Wallace (2020). *COVID-19 in New York City: An Ecology of Race and Class Oppression.*

760. Sirota D (2020). "Joe Biden's love of austerity cut the stimulus bill in half." *Jacobin,* 22 December. https://jacobinmag.com/2020/12/joe-biden-austerity-stimulus-bill-cut-in-half-covid-19.

761. Rosenbloom E and S Finegold (2020). "30 original ASCAP songs about the coronavirus pandemic." ASCAP, 13 May. https://www.ascap.com/news-events/articles/2020/05/covid19-original-music.

762. Pop I (2020). "Dirty little virus." BandCamp. https://iggypop.band-camp.com/track/dirty-little-virus.

763. Curren$y and H Fraud (2020). "Curren$y & Harry Fraud—Gold & Chrome." YouTube, 7 August. https://www.youtube.com/watch?v=fiVhSI9qGHk.

Guilty Bystanders

764. Qiu J (2020). "How China's 'Bat Woman' hunted down viruses from SARS to the new coronavirus." *Scientific American*, 1 June. https://www.scientificamerican.com/article/how-chinas-bat-woman-hunted-down-viruses-from-sars-to-the-new-coronavirus1/; Gilbody-Dickerson C (2020). "'Bat woman' warns animals carry more deadly Covid-like viruses that can infect humans," *Mirror*, 5 December. https://www.mirror.co.uk/news/world-news/bat-woman-warns-animals-carry-23121865.

765. Stanway D (2020). "With frozen food clampdown, China points overseas as source of coronavirus." Reuters, 26 November. https://www.reuters.com/article/us-health-coronavirus-china-origin/with-frozen-food-clampdown-china-points-overseas-as-source-of-coronavirus-idUSK-BN2861A2.

766. Cohen J (2020). "Wuhan coronavirus hunter Shi Zhengli speaks out." *Science*, 24 July. https://www.science.org/content/article/trump-owes-us-apology-chinese-scientist-center-covid-19-origin-theories-speaks-out.

767. Guo H, B-J Hu, X-L Yang, L-P Zeng, B Li, S Ouyang, Z-L Shi (2020). "Evolutionary arms race between virus and host drives genetic diversity in bat Severe Acute Respiratory Syndrome-Related Coronavirus Spike genes." *Journal of Virology*, 94(20): e00902-20.

768. Huang Y, C Yang, X-F Xu, W Xu, and S-W Liu (2020). "Structural and functional properties of SARS-CoV-2 spike protein: potential antivirus drug development for COVID-19." *Acta Pharmacologica Sinica*, 41: 1141–1149; Fan Yi, K Zhao, Z-L Shi, and P Zhou (2019). "Bat coronaviruses in China." *Viruses*, 11(3): 210.

769. National Center for Biotechnology Information (2022). "ACE2 angiotensin converting enzyme 2 [Homo sapiens (human)] Gene ID: 59272, updated on 6-Feb-2022." https://www.ncbi.nlm.nih.gov/gene/59272.

770. Guo H, B-J Hu, X-L Yang, L-P Zeng, B Li, S Ouyang, Z-L Shi (2020). Figure 1 in "Evolutionary arms race between virus and host drives genetic diversity in bat Severe Acute Respiratory Syndrome-Related Coronavirus Spike genes." https://www.ncbi.nlm.nih.gov/pmc/articles/PMC7527062/figure/F1/.

771. Guo H, B-J Hu, X-L Yang, L-P Zeng, B Li, S Ouyang, Z-L Shi (2020). "Evolutionary arms race between virus and host drives genetic diversity in bat Severe Acute Respiratory Syndrome-Related Coronavirus Spike genes"; Booker TR, BC Jackson, and PD Keightley (2017). "Detecting positive selection in the genome." *BMC Biology*, 15: 98.

772. Wallace RG. "The blind weaponmaker." This volume; Boni MF, P Lemey, X Jiang, T Tsan-Yuk Lam, BW Perry, TA Castoe, A Rambaut, and DL Robertson (2020). "Evolutionary origins of the SARS-CoV-2 sarbecovirus lineage responsible for the COVID-19 pandemic." *Nature Microbiology*, 5: 1408-1417.
773. Chaw S-M, J-H Tai, S-I. Chen, C-H Hsieh, S-Y Chang, et al. (2020). "The origin and underlying driving forces of the SARS-CoV-2 outbreak." *Journal of Biomedical Science*, 27:73.
774. Wallace RG and D Wallace (2020). "To the Bat Cave." In RG Wallace, *Dead Epidemiologists: On the Origins of COVID-19*. Monthly Review Press, New York, pp 157-175.
775. Wallace RG (2020). "Midvinter-19." In RG Wallace, *Dead Epidemiologists: On the Origins of COVID-19*. Monthly Review Press, New York, pp 81-97.
776. Paschall M (2020). "The lost forest gardens of Europe." Shelterwood Forest Farm, 22 July. https://www.shelterwoodforestfarm.com/blog/the-lost-forest-gardens-of-europe.

Vic Berger's American Public Health
777. Harrison D (2021). "Why the vaccinated need to mask up". Facebook, 25 July. https://www.facebook.com/dale.w.harrison/posts/4583828068303134; Hart R (2021). "Pfizer shot just 39% effective against Delta infection, but largely prevents severe illness, Israel study suggests." *Forbes*, 23 July. https://www.forbes.com/sites/roberthart/2021/07/23/pfizer-shot-just-39-effective-against-delta-infection-but-largely-prevents-severe-illness-israel-study-suggests/?sh=4fbf1f02584f.
778. Zaitchik A (2021). "How Bill Gates impeded global access to Covid vaccines." *The New Republic*, 12 April. https://newrepublic.com/article/162000/bill-gates-impeded-global-access-covid-vaccines.
779. Roberts S (2020). "The Swiss cheese model of pandemic defense." *New York Times*, 5 December. https://www.nytimes.com/2020/12/05/health/coronavirus-swiss-cheese-infection-mackay.html.
780. Yong E (2021). "The fundamental question of the pandemic is shifting." *The Atlantic*, 9 June. https://www.theatlantic.com/health/archive/2021/06/individualism-still-spoiling-pandemic-response/619133/.
781. Cobb J (2021). "Why Republicans are still recounting votes." *The New Yorker*, 3 October. https://www.newyorker.com/magazine/2021/10/11/why-republicans-are-still-recounting-votes.
782. Wallace RG (2016). *Big Farms Make Big Flu: Dispatches on Infectious Disease, Agribusiness, and the Nature of Science*. Monthly Review Press, New York.
783. Di Cesare D (2021). *Immunodemocracy: Capitalist Asphyxia*. MIT Press, Cambridge, MA.
784. Schott B (2021). "Give Amazon and Facebook a seat at the United

Nations." *Bloomberg Opinion*, 3 October. https://www.bloomberg.com/
opinion/articles/2021-10-03/give-amazon-and-facebook-a-seat-at-the
-united-nations.

785. Tooze A (2021). *Shutdown: How Covid Shook the World's Economy*.
Viking, New York.

786. Collins C (2021). "U.S. billionaires got 62 percent richer during pandemic.
They're now up $1.8 trillion." Institute for Policy Studies, 24 August. https://
ips-dc.org/u-s-billionaires-62-percent-richer-during-pandemic/.

787. Cartter E (2021). "Jeff Bezos wore a cowboy hat to space." *GQ*, 20 July.
https://www.gq.com/story/bezos-space-hat.

788. Jameson F (2020). *The Benjamin Files*. Verso, New York.

789. Schlosser D (1997). "Stevens's Lebensweisheitspielerei." *The Explicator*,
55(3): 147-148.

790. Jameson F (2020). *The Benjamin Files*.

791. Bridgers P (2020). "Phoebe Bridgers—I Know the End (Official Video)."
YouTube, 29 July. https://www.youtube.com/watch?v=WJ9-xN6dCW4.

792. Gill J (2021). "Houston doctor treats COVID patients with anti-parasite
drug ivermectin, despite FDA warnings." *Houston Chronicle*, 26 August.
https://www.houstonchronicle.com/news/houston-texas/health/arti-
cle/Houston-doctor-treats-COVID-patients-with-16413955.php.

793. Reis G, et al. (2022). "Effect of early treatment with ivermectin among
patients with Covid-19." *New England Journal of Medicine*, 30 March.
https://www.nejm.org/doi/10.1056/NEJMoa2115869.

794. Anonymous (2021). "Why you should not use ivermectin to treat or
prevent COVID-19." U.S. Food & Drug Administration, 10 December.
https://www.fda.gov/consumers/consumer-updates/why-you-should-
not -use-ivermectin-treat-or-prevent-covid-19.

795. Collins B (2021). "Antivaxx groups on Facebook and Reddit wanted ivermectin . . ." Twitter, 26 August. https://twitter.com/oneunderscore__/
status/1431044495051825155.

796. Passantino J and O Darcy (2020). "Social media giants remove viral
video with false coronavirus claims that Trump retweeted." CNN, 28
July. https://www.cnn.com/2020/07/28/tech/facebook-youtube-coro-
navirus/index.html.

797. Byers P (2021). "Increased poison control calls due to ivermectin inges-
tion and potential toxicity." MS Health Alert Network (HAN) Alert,
Mississippi State Department of Health, 20 August. https://msdh.
ms.gov/msdhsite/_static/resources/15400.pdf.

798. Cummins R (2021). "Ivermectin cures parasites in cows, not COVID-19
in humans." The University of Mississippi Medical Center, 23 August.
https://www.umc.edu/news/News_Articles/2021/08/Ivermectin.html.

799. Collins B (2021). "First off, they really are eating horse dewormer…" Twitter, 26
August. https://twitter.com/oneunderscore__/status/1431041437643247627.

800. Anonymous (2022). "Fraudulent coronavirus disease 2019 (COVID-

19) products." U.S. Food & Drug Administration, 24 February. https://www.fda.gov/consumers/health-fraud-scams/fraudulent-coronavirus-disease-2019-covid-19-products.

801. Cohen L (2021). "Arkansas doctor who prescribed ivermectin to jail detainees for COVID now under investigation by medical board." *CBS News*, 27 August. https://www.cbsnews.com/news/ivermeticin-arkansas-inmates-covid-19-doctor-eva-madison-fda-warnings/.

802. @rdaily (2021). "Putting the microchips in the horse de-wormer was a stroke of genius." Twitter, 29 August. https://twitter.com/rdaily/status/1431975749913874432.

803. Shannon J (2020). "'It's not real': In South Dakota, which has shunned masks and other COVID rules, some people die in denial, nurse says." *USA Today*, 17 November. https://www.usatoday.com/story/news/health/2020/11/17/south-dakota-nurse-jodi-doering-covid-19-patients-denial/6330791002/; @drskyskull (2021). "CNN reporter just quoted a doctor as referring to many COVID patients as 'the talking dead' . . ." Twitter, 28 August. https://twitter.com/drskyskull/status/1431708240396554242.

804. Anonymous (2020). "The Jim Bakker Show." U.S. Food & Drug Administration, 6 March. https://www.fda.gov/inspections-compliance-enforcement-and-criminal-investigations/warning-letters/jim-bakker-show-604820-03062020; TateredVideo (2016). "Pastor Jim Bakker Helps You Prepare for Trump's America." Facebook, 28 November. https://www.facebook.com/TateredVideo/videos/373271109684112.

805. Fakile T (2022). "Ivermectin on its way to becoming available without prescription in Tennessee." WSMV, 8 April. https://www.wsmv.com/2022/04/09/ivermectin-its-way-becoming-available-without-prescription-tennessee/.

806. Bouie J (2021). "Do Republicans Actually Want the Pandemic to End?" *New York Times*, 31 August. https://www.nytimes.com/2021/08/31/opinion/republicans-anti-vax-covid.html.

807. Montemayor S (2021). "GOP candidate Scott Jensen calling for 'civil disobedience' of COVID policies." *Star Tribune*, 10 September. https://www.startribune.com/gop-candidate-scott-jensen-calling-for-civil-disobedience-of-covid-policies/600095847/.

808. Mandavilli A (2021). "The U.S. is getting a crash course in scientific uncertainty." *New York Times*, 22 August. https://www.nytimes.com/2021/08/22/health/coronavirus-covid-usa.html.

809. Ibid.

810. Olson J (2021). "Viral spread in latest Minnesota COVID-19 wave more of a mystery." *Star Tribune*, 21 September. https://www.startribune.com/viral-spread-in-latest-minnesota-covid-19-wave-more-of-a-mystery/600099451/.

811. Wallace RG (2020). "Biden's COVID plan isn't enough." This volume;

Luo E, N Chong, C Erikson, C Chen, S Westergaard, E Salsberg, and P Pittman (2020). "Contact tracing workforce estimator." Fitzhugh Mullan Institute for Health Workforce Equity, George Washington University. https://www.gwhwi.org/estimator-613404.html.

812. Foster JB, B Clark, and H Holleman (2021). "Capital and the ecology of disease." *Monthly Review*, 1 June. https://monthlyreview.org/2021/06/01/capital-and-the-ecology-of-disease/.

813. Olliaro P, E Torreele, and M Vaillant (2021). "COVID-19 vaccine efficacy and effectiveness—the elephant (not) in the room." *The Lancet Microbe* 2(7): e279-e280.

814. Reuters Fact Check (2021). "Fact Check—Why relative risk reduction, not absolute risk eeduction, is most often used in calculating vaccine efficacy." Reuters, 2 June. reuters.com/article/factcheck-thelancet-riskreduction/fact-check-why-relative-risk-reduction-not-absolute-risk-reduction -is-most-often-used-in-calculating -vaccine-efficacy-idUSL2N2NK1XA.

815. Health Desk (2021). "What do the efficacy rates of COVID-19 vaccines mean, and do the efficacy rates impact a population's herd immunity?" *Health Desk*, 31 May. https://health-desk.org/articles/what-do-the-efficacy-rates-of-covid-19-vaccines-mean-and-do-the-efficacy-rates-impact-a-population-s-herd-immunity.

816. Rosenberg ES, et al. (2021). "New COVID-19 cases and hospitalizations among adults, by vaccination status—New York, May 3-July 25, 2021." *Morbidity and Mortality Weekly Report* 70(37): 1306-1311; Ibid.

817. Ramzy A and AC Chien (2021). "Rejecting Covid inquiry, China peddles conspiracy theories blaming the U.S." *New York Times*, 12 October. https://www.nytimes.com/2021/08/25/world/asia/china-coronavirus-covid-conspiracy-theory.html?searchResultPosition=1.

818. Ferere C (2020). "Who you got? A list of Trump-supporting rappers we'll still low-key bump." *Reverie Page*, 6 November. https://www.reveriepage.com/blog/trump-supporting-rappers.

819. Lerner S and M Hvistendahl (2021). "New details emerge about coronavirus research at Chinese lab." *The Intercept*, 6 September. https://theintercept.com/2021/09/06/new-details-emerge-about-coronavirus-research-at-chinese-lab/; Lerner S, M Hvistendahl, and M Hibbett (2021). "NIH documents provide new evidence U.S. funded gain-of-function research in Wuhan." *The Intercept*, 9 September. https://theintercept.com/2021/09/09/covid-origins-gain-of-function-research/; Wallace RG. "The blind weaponmaker." This volume.

820. Žižek S (2011). *Living in the End Times*. Verso, New York.

821. Nair Y (2021). "Stop blaming the unvaccinated." *Yasmin Nair* blog, 26 July. https://yasminnair.com/stop-blaming-the-unvaccinated/.

822. Zengerle P (2021). "U.S. House committee backs $25 billion increase in defense spending." Reuters, 1 September. https://www.reuters.com/

world/us/us-house-committee-backs-25-billion-increase-defense-spending-2021-09-01/.

823. Stephens B (2021). "Another failed presidency at hand." *New York Times*, 7 September. https://www.nytimes.com/2021/09/07/opinion/biden-failed-afghanistan.html.

824. Dear Pandemic (2020). "Those Nerdy Girls." https://dearpandemic.org/the-nerdy-girls/.

825. Dear Pandemic (2021). "New evidence shows mask wearing reduces COVID-19 infections in the community." Instagram, 8 September. https://www.instagram.com/p/CTj5Cufrfbt/.

826. Gilbert M (2021). *Juste un passage au JT.* Editions Luc Pire, Bruxelles, Belgium.

827. Bouffioux M (2020). "Marius Gilbert quitte le celeval: Il explique sa décision." *Paris Match*, 23 September. https://parismatch.be/actualites/societe/431725/marius-gilbert-quitte-le-celeval-il-explique-sa-decision.

828. Eilenberger W (2021). *Time of the Magicians: Wittgenstein, Benjamin, Cassirer, Heidegger, and the Decade that Reinvented Philosophy.* Penguin Press, New York.

829. Hammer MC (2021). "You bore us . . ." Twitter, 22 February. https://twitter.com/mchammer/status1363908982289559553?lang=en.

830. Labatut B (2021). *When We Cease to Understand the World.* NY Review Books, New York.

831. Wallace RG (2020). *Dead Epidemiologists: On the origins of COVID-19.* Monthly Review Press, New York.

832. Patton D (2020). "Flush with cash, Chinese hog producer builds world's largest pig farm." Reuters, 7 December. https://www.reuters.com/article/us-china-swinefever-muyuanfoods-change-s/flush-with-cash-chinese-hog-producer-builds-worlds-largest-pig-farm-idUSKBN28H0MU.

833. Ibid.

834. Ibid.

835. Hudson B (2013). "Undercover video shows alleged mistreatment of Minn. pigs." CBS News, 29 October. https://minnesota.cbslocal.com/2013/10/29/undercover-video-shows-alleged-mistreatment-of-minn-pigs/.

836. Painter KL (2018). "Hormel sells Nebraska pork plant to group of Minnesota, S.D. farmers." *Star Tribune*, 16 August. https://www.startribune.com/hormel-sells-nebraska-pork-plant-to-group-of-minnesota-s-d-farmers/491028371/.

837. Anonymous (2012). "CHS, Land O'Lakes Are Top-Grossing U.S. Co-ops." *Twin Cities Business*, 12 May. https://tcbmag.com/chs-land-olakes-are-top-grossing-u-s-co-ops/.

838. Ibid.

839. Bridgers P (2020). "Phoebe Bridgers—I Know the End (Official Video)."

840. Smith K, et al (2014). "Global rise in human infectious disease outbreaks." *Journal of the Royal Society Interface* 11(101): 20140950.
841. Wallace RG. "The BoJo strain." This volume.
842. Wallace RG (2010). "Do pathogens time travel?" *Farming Pathogens* blog, 12 January. https://farmingpathogens.wordpress.com/2010/01/12/do-pathogens -time-travel/.
843. Wallace RG. "A spray of split seconds." This volume.
844. Stoller M (2021). "Why Joe Biden punched Big Pharma in the nose over Covid vaccines." *BIG by Matt Stoller* blog, 9 May. https://mattstoller.substack.com/p/why-joe-biden-punched-big-pharma?s=r.
845. Watercutter A (2014). "How designers recreated Alan Turing's codebreaking computer for *Imitation Game*." *Wired*, 21 November. https://www.wired.com/2014/11/imitation-game-building-christopher/.
846. Krever M (2021). "UK scientists believe it is 'almost certain' a coronavirus variant will emerge that beats current vaccines." CNN, 1 August. https://www.cnn.com/2021/08/01/health/uk-scientists-covid-variant-beat-vaccines-intl/index.html.
847. Roape (2021). "Third World Network—Africa & ROAPE Webinars: Africa, climate change & the pandemic—crises & radical alternatives." *Review of African Political Economy*, 23 July. https://roape.net/2021/07/23/third-world-network-africa-roape-webinars-africa-climate-change-the-pandemic-interrelated-crises-radical-alternatives/.
848. Mendez R (2021). "WHO extends call for a moratorium on Covid booster disease until the end of the year." CNBC, 8 September. https://www.cnbc.com/2021/09/08/who-extends-call-for-a-moratorium-on-covid-booster-doses-until-the-end-of-the-year.html.
849. Health Justice Initiative (2020). "Who we are." https://healthjusticeinitiative.org.za/.
850. Sisonke Program (2021). "Sisonke2: Protecting healthcare workers." http://sisonkestudy.samrc.ac.za/.
851. Third World Network Africa (2019). "TWN Africa: Equitable transformation in and for Africa." http://twnafrica.org/wp/2017/.
852. Amin S (1990). *Delinking: Towards a Polycentric World.* Zed, London.
853. Flitter E and JB Stewart (2019). "Bill Gates met with Jeffery Epstein many times, despite his past." *New York Times,* 12 October. https://www.nytimes.com/2019/10/12/business/jeffrey-epstein-bill-gates.html.
854. The International Institute of Social History. "Collections." https://iisg.amsterdam/en/collections.
855. Morton T (2019). *Humankind: Solidarity with Non-Human People.* Verso, New York.
856. Wark M (2021). *Capital Is Dead: Is this Something Worse?* Verso, New York.
857. Dendinger R (2021). "Vector or value Chains?" *Monthly Review*

Online, 24 September. https://mronline.org/2021/09/24/vectors-or-value-chains/; Suwandi I (2019). *Value Chains: The New Economic Imperialism*. Monthly Review Press, New York.

858. Eisenstein, C (2021). "Mob morality and the unvaxxed." *Charles Eisenstein* blog, 1 August. https://charleseisenstein.substack.com/p/mob-morality-and-the-unvaxxed?s=r.

859. Bratton B (2021). "Agamben WTF, or how philosophy failed the pandemic." Verso blog, 28 July. https://www.versobooks.com/blogs/5125-agamben-wtf-or-how-philosophy-failed-the-pandemic; Foster JB (2020). *The Return of Nature: Socialism and Ecology*. Monthly Review Press, New York.

860. Aratani L (2021). "99.2% of US Covid deaths in June were unvaccinated, says Fauci." *The Guardian*, 8 July. https://www.theguardian.com/us-news/2021/jul/08/fears-of-new-us-covid-surge-as-delta-spreads-and-many-remain-unvaccinated.

861. Antona D, et al. (2013). "Measles elimination efforts and 2008-2011 outbreak, France." *Emerging Infectious Diseases*, 19(3):357; Smith PJ, et al. (2015). "Children and adolescents unvaccinated against measles: Geographic clustering, parents' beliefs, and missed opportunities." *Public Health Reports*, 130(5): 485-504.

862. Di Cesare D (2021). *Immunodemocracy: Capitalist Asphyxia*. MIT Press, Cambridge, MA.

863. Rivoli D (2021). "Protestors outside City Hall slam COVID-19 vaccine requirement." Spectrum News NY 1, 25 August. https://www.ny1.com/nyc/all-boroughs/news/2021/08/26/protesters-outside-city-hall-slam-covid-19-vaccine-requirement; Lonas L (2021). "Anti-vaccine protesters tear down COVID-19 testing site in New York City." *The Hill*, 5 October. https://thehill.com/homenews/state-watch/575379-anti-vaccine-protesters-tear-down-covid-19-testing-site-in-new-york-city.

864. Meyer R (2021). "Congress is slashing a $30 billion plan to fight the next pandemic." *The Atlantic*, 2 August. https://www.theatlantic.com/science/archive/2021/08/congress-slashing-plan-end-pandemics/619640/.

865. Lang A, M Warren, and L Kulman (2018). "A funding crisis for public health and safety: State-by-state public health funding and key health facts 2018." Trust for America's Health, March. https://www.tfah.org/wp-content/uploads/2019/03/InvestInAmericaRpt-FINAL.pdf.

866. Chicago Tribune Staff (2021). "Illinois launches online site for residents to check COVID-19 vaccination status." *Chicago Tribune*, 12 August. https://www.chicagotribune.com/coronavirus/vaccine/ct-illinois-vaccination-status-app-20210812-7czhh6l3z5ejllep3brjejwupe-story.html.

867. Yong E (2021). "How the pandemic now ends." *The Atlantic*, 12 August. https://www.theatlantic.com/health/archive/2021/08/delta-has-changed -pandemic-endgame/619726/.

868. Dear Pandemic (2020). "Those Nerdy Girls." https://dearpandemic.
     org/the-nerdy-girls/.
869. Von Dassow E, et al (2021). "U has botches its vaccine mandate." *Star
     Tribune*, 17 August. https://www.startribune.com/u-has-botched-its-
     vaccine-mandate/600088702/; Osterholm M and M Oakes (2021).
     "Counterpoint: Vaccine mandate at U would be counterproductive."
     Star Tribune, 22 June. https://www.startribune.com/counterpoint-vac-
     cine-mandate-at-u-would-be-counterproductive/600070928/.
870. Faircloth R (2021). "University of Minnesota to require COVID vaccina-
     tions for students once shots receive FDA approval." *Star Tribune*, 9 August.
     https://www.startribune.com/university-of-minnesota-to-require-covid-
     vaccinations-for-students-once-shots-receive-fda-approval/600086330/.
871. Pabst Y (2020). "Coronavirus: 'Agribusiness would risk millions of
     deaths.'" Marx21, 11 March. https://www.marx21.de/coronavirus-agri-
     businesswould-risk-millions -of-deaths/.
872. Miller Z and M Balsamo (2021). "'Great day for America': Vaccinated can
     largely ditch masks." *Associated Press*, 13 May. https://apnews.com/article/
     coronavirus-masks-cdc-guidelines-9d10c8b5f80a4ac720fa1df2a4fb93e5.
873. Ahluwalia S and L Priya (2021). "U.S. Covid-19 death toll hits 700,000."
     Reuters, 1 October. https://www.reuters.com/world/us/us-covid-
     19-death-toll-hits-700000-2021-10-01/; Our World in Data (2021).
     "Weekly confirmed COVID-19 cases." https://ourworldindata.org/
     grapher/weekly-covid-cases?tab=chart&country=~USA.
874. Tolj B (2021). "'The talking dead': Nurse details grim reality of Covid
     ICU." Yahoo News, 31 August. https://au.news.yahoo.com/the-talking-
     dead-nurse-details-grim-reality-of-covid-icu-082201652.html .
875. Efird CR and AF Lightfoot (2020). "Missing Mayberry: How white-
     ness shapes perceptions of health among white Americans in a rural
     Southern community." *Social Science & Medicine*, 253: 112967.
876. Zaitchik A (2021). "How Bill Gates impeded global access to Covid
     vaccines." *The New Republic*, 12 April. https://newrepublic.com/
     article/162000/bill-gates-impeded-global-access-covid-vaccines.
877. Lane A (2020). "The heart sick hilarity of John Berryman's letters." *The New
     Yorker*, 12 October. https://www.newyorker.com/magazine/2020/10/19/
     the-heartsick-hilarity-of-john-berrymans-letters.
878. Hatfield A (2020). "P.O.S. shares apology following abuse allegations,
     is 'stepping away from music'." *BrooklynVegan* blog, 16 July. https://
     www.brooklynvegan.com/p-o-s-shares-apology-following-abuse-alle-
     gations-is-stepping-away-from-music/.
879. Maber P (2008). " 'So-called black': Reassessing John Berryman's black-
     face minstrelsy." *Arizona Quarterly: A Journal of American Literature,
     Culture, and Theory*, 64(4): 129-149; Johnson K (2020). "Stanzas: John
     Berryman." *The Sewanee Review*, April. https://thesewaneereview.com/
     articles/stanzas-john-berryman.

880. di Prima D (2005). *Revolutionary Letters*. "Last Gasp of San Francisco," San Francisco.

881. Dickinson T (2021). "Minneapolis police caught on video 'hunting' activists." *Rolling Stone*, 13 October. https://www.rollingstone.com/politics/politics-features/minneapolis-police-video-hunting-activists-jaleel-stallings-1241227/.

882. di Prima D (2005). *Revolutionary Letters*.

883. University of Minnesota Institute on the Environment (2016). "Current Supporters." http://environment.umn.edu/support/current-supporters/.

884. Harrison D (2021). "Immune protection from vaccination vs natural infection." Facebook, 5 September. https://www.facebook.com/dale.w.harrison/posts/4711629128856360; Caniels T.G., et al. (2021). "Emerging SARS-CoV-2 variants of concern evade humoral immune responses from infection and vaccination." *Science Advances*, 7(36): eabj5365.

885. Yang M (2021). "Milk crate challenge has doctors warning it's 'worse than falling from a ladder.'" *The Guardian*, 25 August. https://www.theguardian.com/technology/2021/aug/25/milk-crate-challenge-tiktok-doctors-warnings.

886. Zdechlik M and W Matuska (2021). "State Fair won't mandate masks, receives pushback." MPR News, 18 August. https://www.mprnews.org/story/2021/08/18/no-blanket-face-mask-requirement-for-the-state-fair.

887. Rahming D (2021). "Fewer than 300 COVID transmissions linked to State Fair." Kare 11 News, 21 September. https://www.kare11.com/article/news/local/fewer-than-300-covid-transmissions-linked-to-state-fair/89-a8e68fcc-d746-4ce8-b84c-700641a9aa4e.

888. WCCO-TV Staff (2021). "COVID in Minnesota: COVID Cases in ICU reach peaks not seen since last winter." CBS News, 14 September. https://minnesota.cbslocal.com/2021/09/14/covid-in-minnesota-covid-cases-in-icu-reach-peaks-not-seen-since-last-winter/.

889. Anonymous (2022). "Eviction Moratorium Phaseout Info & FAQ." Home Line MN, 24 February. https://homelinemn.org/phaseout/.

890. Lilley S, et al. (2012). *Catastrophism: The Apocalyptic Politics of Collapse and Rebirth*. PM Press, Oakland, CA.

891. Srnicek N and A Williams (2015). "*Inventing the Future: Postcapitalism and a World Without Work*," with Nick Srnicek and Alex Williams. Discussion at Housmans Bookshop, London, 28 October. https://www.versobooks.com/events/1259-inventing-the-future-postcapitalism-and-a-world-without-work-with-nick-srnicek-and-alex-williams.

892. Wallace RG (2019). "It's unfortunate I'm receiving their screenshots secondhand." Facebook, 18 September. https://www.facebook.com/rob.wallace.3133/posts/10219334429532019.

893. Marx, K (1842). "Proceedings of the Sixth Rhine Province Assembly. Third Article. Debates on the Law on Thefts of Wood." *Rheinische Zeitung*,

25 October. https://www.marxists.org/archive/marx/works/download/
Marx_Rheinishe_Zeitung.pdf; Marx K and F Engels (1845; 1932). *The
German Ideology.* Marx-Engels Institute, Moscow; Marx K (1847; 1939).
Grundrisse. Marx-Engels Institute, Moscow; Marx K (1867). *Capital: A
Critique of Political Economy,* vol. 1. Progress Publishers, Moscow; Marx
K (1875; 1970). *Critique of the Gotha Programme.* Progress Publishers,
Moscow; Marx K (1894; 1993). *Capital: A Critique of Political Economy,*
vol. 3. Penguin, New York.

894. Foster JB (2016). "Marx as a food theorist." *Monthly Review,* 68(7):
1-22.

895. Ross K (2015). *Communal Luxury: The Political Imaginary of the
Paris Commune.* Verso, London; Foster JB (2000). *Marx's Ecology:
Materialism and Nature.* Monthly Review Press, New York; Saito K
(2017). *Karl Marx's Ecosocialism: Capital, Nature, and the Unfinished
Critique of Political Economy.* Monthly Review Press, New York.

896. Hobsbawm EJ (1964). "Introduction." In Marx K, *Pre-Capitalist
Economic Formations.* International Publishers, New York.

897. Ajl, M (2021). *A People's Green New Deal.* Pluto Press, London.

898. Yong E (2021). "We're already barreling toward the next pandemic."
The Atlantic, 29 September. https://www.theatlantic.com/health/
archive/2021/09/america-prepared-next-pandemic/620238/.

899. Edelman M (2021). "Why, in this otherwise excellent article, is there no
mention of industrial poultry and hog farms…" Twitter, 29 September.
https://twitter.com/MarcEdelmanNYC/status/1443192097117462535.

900. Wallace RG. "Bidenfreude" This volume.

901. Sheppard E (2020). "What's next? Trump, Johnson, and globalizing
capitalism." *Environment and Planning A: Economy and Space* 52(4):
679-687.

902. Shear MD and B Mueller (2021). "Biden promised to follow the science. But sometimes, he gets ahead of the experts." *New York Times,* 24
September. https://www.nytimes.com/2021/09/24/us/politics/biden-
science-boosters-vaccine.html.

903. Editorial Board (2021). "Biden's unforced COVID miscues." *Star
Tribune,* 22 September. https://www.startribune.com/bidens-unforced-
covid-miscues /600099832/.

904. Phillips M (2016). "The Newsroom—America is not the greatest country in the world anymore. (explicit)." YouTube, 5 December.

905. Wallace R (2020). "How the enemy gets a vote: Fog-of-war, fic-
tion, and the cultural riverbanks of the Clausewitz landscape." *The
Journal of Defense Modeling and Simulation* 18(4): 349-363; Wallace
RG (2019). "Redwashing capital: Left tech bros are honing Marx
into a capitalist tool." *Uneven Earth,* 11 July. http://unevenearth.
org/2019/07/redwashing-capital/; BreakThrough News (2021).
"Marxist epidemiologist calls bullsh*t on antivaxxers, details COVID's

capitalist roots." YouTube, 18 September. https://www.youtube.com/watch?v=pIhKzUnWEas.

906. Chaves LF, et al. "What is 'land'?" This volume; Figueroa M, et al. (2021). "To live and die in L.A." This volume.

907. Chaves LF, et al. (2021). "Trade, uneven development and people in motion: Used territories and the initial spread of COVID-19 in Mesoamerica and the Caribbean." *Socio-economic Planning Sciences*: 101161; Santos M (2017). *Toward an Other Globalization: From the Single Thought to Universal Conscience*, vol. 12. Springer, Cham; Amin S (2017). *Capitalism in the Age of Globalization: The Management of Contemporary Society*. Zed Books Ltd, London.

908. Wallace RG and F Pitta (2021). "Capitalismo, agronegócio e pandemia." Discussion with Fórum Popular da Natureza, Zoom, 14 October. https://www.facebook.com/forumpopulardanatureza/posts/402312641263144.

909. Environmental Quality Board (2019). "Minnesota State Agency Report: Emerald Ash Borer in Minnesota 2019." https://www.eqb.state.mn.us/sites/default/files/documents/2019%20Minnesota%20State%20Agency%20Emerald%20Ash%20Borer%20Report.pdf.

910. Iverson L, et al. (2016). "Potential species replacements for Black Ash (*Fraxinus nigra*) at the confluence of two threats: Emerald Ash Borer and a changing climate." *Ecosystems* 19: 248–270.

911. Mahamu F and J Walsh (2017). "Minneapolis and St. Paul are losing thousands of trees to emerald ash borer." *Star Tribune*, 9 May. https://www.startribune.com/minneapolis-and-st-paul-are-losing-thousands-of-trees-to-emerald-ash-borer/421687683/.

912. Dunens E, et al. (2012). "Facing the emerald ash borer in Minnesota: Stakeholder understandings and their implications for communication and engagement."

913. Prather S (2020). "Which Twin Cities neighborhoods can use more trees? A new data-driven mapping tool can help." *Star Tribune*, 8 June. https://www.startribune.com/which-twin-cities-neighborhoods-can-use-more-trees-a-new-data-driven-mapping-tool-can-help/571087242/.

914. Fox 9 Minneapolis-St. Paul (2021). "Group planting trees in St. Paul too close gap in tree inequalities." YouTube, 9 October. https://www.youtube.com/watch?v=V81fFjgIYfk.

915. Baker MG, N Wilson, and A Anglemyer (2020). "Successful elimination of Covid-19 transmission in New Zealand." *New England Journal of Medicine* 383(8): e56.

916. Frost N (2021). "Battling Delta, New Zealand abandons its Zero-Covid ambitions." *New York Times*, 4 October. https://www.nytimes.com/2021/10/04/world/australia/new-zealand-covid-zero.html.

917. Hale T, et al. (2022). "Chinese provincial government responses to Covid-19." *Blavatnik School of Government*; Garrison C (2021). "Panama approaching herd immunity against COVID-19, president

says." Reuters, 23 September. https://finance.yahoo.com/news/panama-approaching-herd-immunity-against-165832235.html.

918. Brisley A (2020). "Coronavirus and Capitalist Realism." Medical Anthropology at UCL, 27 March. https://medanthucl.com/2020/03/27/coronavirus-and-capitalist-realism/.

919. Frost N (2021). "Battling Delta, New Zealand abandons its Zero-Covid ambitions."

920. Han BC (2021). *Capitalism and the Death Drive.* Polity Press, Cambridge, UK.

921. Figueroa M, et al. (2021). "To live and die in Los Angeles." PRePNeighborhoods, Pandemic Research for the People, Dispatch 8, 21 September. https://drive.google.com/file/d/1CB_U2dhSWkcP6QFaC2zEuPLG9p35q49n/view.

922. NBC News (2021). "Biden discusses CDC lifting mask restrictions for fully vaccinated people." YouTube, 13 May. https://www.youtube.com/watch?v=qnTEeD7ddG8; Covert B (2021). "No, the unvaccinated aren't all just being difficult." *New York Times,* 6 August. https://www.nytimes.com/2021/08/06/opinion/covid-delta-vaccines-unvaccinated.html; Data Futures Platform. "Global dashboard for vaccine equity." https://data.undp.org/vaccine-equity/.

923. Frost N (2021). "Battling Delta, New Zealand abandons its Zero-Covid ambitions."

924. Ibid.

925. Ehrenreich B (2021). *Desert Notebooks: A Road Map for the End of Time.* Catapult, New York.

926. Wallace RG. "A spray of split seconds." This volume.

927. Táíwò OO (2022). *Elite Capture: How the Powerful Took Over Identity Politics (and Everything Else).* Haymarket Books, Chicago.

928. Gadson R (2021). "'There's No There There': Keeanga-Yamahtta Taylor on the Future of the Left." *Public Books,* 6 October. https://www.publicbooks.org/theres-no-there-there-keeanga-yamahtta-taylor-on-the-future-of-the-left/.

929. Anonymous. "Purdue awarded $10 million for #DiverseCornBelt project." Purdue University College of Agriculture, 6 October. https://ag.purdue.edu/stories/purdue-awarded-10-million-for-diversecorn-belt-project/ .

930. Midwest Health Ag (2020). "About." https://midwesthealthyag.org/about-our-work.

931. Okamoto KW, A Liebman, and RG Wallace (2020). "At what geographic scales does agricultural alienation amplify foodborne disease outbreaks? A statistical test for 25 US states, 1970-2000." *MedRxiv:* 2019-12.

932. Godelier M (2012). *The Mental and the Material.* Verso, New York.

933. Lindisfarne N and J Neale (2021). "Afghanistan: The End of the Occupation." Anne Bonny Pirate, 17 August. https://annebonnypirate.org/2021/08/17/afghanistan-the-end-of-the-occupation/.

934. Kessler G (2021). "Biden's claim that nation-building in Afghanistan 'never made any sense to me'." *The Washington Post*, 23 August. https://www.washingtonpost.com/politics/2021/08/23/bidens-claim-that-nation-building-afghanistan-never-made-any-sense/.
935. Fernandez B (2021). "Women's rights and the US's 'civilising' mission in Afghanistan." *Al Jazeera*, 21 August. https://www.aljazeera.com/opinions/2021/8/21/white-women-washing-the-uss-civilising-mission-in-afghanistan.
936. Beaumont H (2021). "Revealed: pipeline company paid Minnesota police for arresting and surveilling protesters." *The Guardian*, 5 October. https://www.theguardian.com/uk-news/2021/oct/05/line-3-pipeline-enbridge-paid-police-arrest-protesters.
937. Jemison NK (2017). *The Stone Sky*. Orbit, London.
938. Bennett S (2021). "American Indians have the highest Covid vaccination rate in the US." Nova Next by PBS, 6 July. https://www.pbs.org/wgbh/nova/article/native-americans-highest-covid-vaccination-rate-us/.

Puzzled Patients

939. Biswas S (2021). "Mucormycosis: The 'black fungus' maiming Covid patients in India." BBC News, 9 May. https://www.bbc.com/news/world-asia-india-57027829.
940. Stone N, N Gupta, and I Schwartz (2021). "Mucormycosis: time to address this deadly fungal infection." *The Lancet Microbe* 2(8): e343-e344
941. Elliott L (2021). "Chile detects first case of Covid 'black fungus'." *The Times*, 3 June. https://www.thetimes.co.uk/article/chile-detects-first-case-of-covid-black-fungus-j87dkshb0; Regional Office for the Eastern Mediterranean (2021). "Black fungus a reemerging infection." Weekly Epidemiological Monitor, 20 June/ World Health Organization. https://applications.emro.who.int/docs/EPI/2021/2224-4220-2021-1425-eng.pdf?ua=1.
942. Wang C (2020). "Grand challenges in the research of fungal interactions with animals." *Frontiers in Fungal Biology* 1:602032.
943. Mahalaxmi I, et al. (2021). "Mucormycosis: An opportunistic pathogen during COVID-19." *Environmental Research* 201: 111643.
944. Ibid.
945. Pal R, et al. (2021). "COVID-19-associated mucormycosis: An updated systematic review of literature." *Mycoses* 64(12):1452-1459; Dutta S (2021). "India reported over 45,000 black fungus cases so far, says Mandaviya in RS." *Hindustan Times*, 20 July. https://www.hindustantimes.com/india-news/india-reported-over-45-000-black-fungus-cases-so-far-says-mandaviya-in-rs-101626781531292.html.
946. Dasgupta R (2021). "Doctors have been blamed for the rise in black fungus in India, but the COVID treatment guidelines could be contributing." *The Conversation*, 3 June. https://theconversation.com/

doctors-have-been-blamed-for-the-rise-in-black-fungus-in-india-but-the-covid-treatment-guidelines-could-be-contributing-161507.

947. Seyedmousavi S, et al. (2018). "Fungal infections in animals: a patchwork of different situations." *Medical Mycology* 56(S1): S165-S187.

948. Liebman A and RG Wallace (2019). "A factory farm fungus among us." *Seed & Hatchet*, 10 April. Agroecology and Rural Economics Research Corps. https://arerc.wordpress.com/2019/04/10/a-factory-farm-fungus-among-us/; Barnagarwala T and S Ahsan (2021). "Explained: Why there is shortage of black fungus drug in India." *The Indian Express*, 2 June. https://indianexpress.com/article/explained/shortage-of-black-fungus-drug-cases -india-7330327/.

949. Henriksson PJG, et al. (2018). "Unpacking factors influencing antimicrobial use in global aquaculture and their implications for management: a review from a systems perspective." *Sustainability Science* 13: 1105-1120; Doron A and A Broom (2019). "The spectre of superbugs: Waste, structural violence and antimicrobial resistance in India." *Worldwide Waste* 2(1): 1–10.

950. Singer M (2009). *Introduction to Syndemics: A Critical Systems Approach to Public and Community Health*. Jossey-Bass, San Francisco, CA; Singer M, N Bulled, B Ostrach, and E Mendenhall (2017). "Syndemics and the biosocial concept of health." *The Lancet* 389: 941-950.

951. De Rossi A, et al. (1991). "Reciprocal activation of human T-lymphotropic viruses in HTLV I-transformed cells superinfected with HIV-1." *Journal of Acquired Immune Deficiency Syndromes* 4(4): 380-385; Singer M (2010). "Pathogen-pathogen interaction: A syndemic model of complex biosocial processes in disease." *Virulence* 1(1): 10-18.

952. Wallace R (1988). "A synergism of plagues: 'Planned Shrinkage,' contagious housing destruction, and AIDS in the Bronx." Environmental Research 47: 1-33; Wallace R (1990) "Urban desertification, public health and public order: Planned shrinkage, violent death, substance abuse and AIDS in the Bronx." *Social Science Medicine* 31(7): 801-813; Singer M and S Clair (2003). "Syndemics and public health: Reconceptualizing disease in bio-social context." *Medical Anthropology Quarterly* 17(4): 423-441.

953. Wallace RG and R Wallace (eds). *Neoliberal Ebola: Modeling Disease Emergence from Finance to Forest and Farm*. Springer International Publishing; Wallace R, LF Chaves, LR Bergmann, C Ayres, L Hogerwerf, R Kock, and RG Wallace (2018). *Clear-Cutting Disease Control: Capital-Led Deforestation, Public Health Austerity, and Vector-Borne Infection*. Springer International Publishing, Cham.

954. Nokukhanya Msomi N, R Lessells, K Mlisana, and T de Oliveira (2021). "Africa: tackle HIV and COVID-19 together." *Nature* 600: 33-36.

955. Karim F, et al. (2021)."Persistent SARS-CoV-2 infection and intra-host evolution in association with advanced HIV infection." medRxiv, 4 June.

https://www.medrxiv.org/content/10.1101/2021.06.03.21258228v1; Voloch CM (2021). "Intra-host evolution during SARS-CoV-2 prolonged infection." *Virus Evolution* 7(2): veab078.

956. Mukherjee J, H Abbasi, and M Morse (2022). "Global vaccine inequity led to the COVID-19 Omicron variant: It's time for collective action." *Health Affairs*, 26 January. https://www.healthaffairs.org/do/10.1377/forefront.20220124.776516/.

957. Hickel J (2012). "Neoliberal plague: The political economy of HIV transmission in Swaziland." *Journal of Southern African Studies* 38(3): 513-529; Mendenhall E (2016). "Beyond comorbidity: A critical perspective of syndemic depression and diabetes in cross-cultural contexts." *Medical Anthropology Quarterly* 30(4): 462-478.

958. Venkatakrishnan AJ, et al. (2021). "Omicron variant of SARS-CoV-2 harbors a unique insertion mutation of putative viral or human genomic origin." OSF Preprints, 2 December. 10.31219/osf.io/f7txy.

959. Musuuza JS, et al. (2021). "Prevalence and outcomes of co-infection and superinfection with SARS-CoV-2 and other pathogens: A systematic review and meta-analysis." *PLoS One*16: e0251170.

960. Wallace R and RG Wallace (2002). "Immune cognition and vaccine strategy: Beyond genomics." *Microbes and Infection* 4(4): 521-527; Wallace R, D Wallace, and RG Wallace (2003). "Toward cultural oncology: The evolutionary information dynamics of cancer." *Open systems & Information Dynamics* 10(2): 159-181; Wallace R, D Wallace, and RG Wallace (2004). "Coronary heart disease, chronic inflammation, and pathogenic social hierarchy: A biological limit to possible reductions in morbidity and mortality." *Journal of the National Medical Association* 96(5): 609-619; Marya R and R Patel (2021). *Inflamed: Deep Medicine and the Anatomy of Injustice.* Farrar Straus and Giroux, New York.

961. Wallace RG, R Kock, L Bergmann, M Gilbert, L Hogerwerf, C Pittiglio, R Mattioli, and R Wallace (2016). "Did neoliberalizing West African forests produce a new niche for Ebola?" *International Journal of Health Services* 46(1): 149-165.

962. Reche PA (2020). "Potential cross-reactive immunity to SARS-CoV-2 from common human pathogens and vaccines." *Frontiers in Immunology* 1:586984.

963. Nikiphorou E, D Alpizar-Rodriguez, A Gastelum-Strozzi,M Buch,and I Peláez-Ballestas (2021). "Syndemics & syndemogenesis in COVID-19 and rheumatic and musculoskeletal diseases: old challenges, new era." *Rheumatology* 60(5): 2040-2045.

964. Pai M and A Olatunbosun-Alakija (2021). "Vax the world." *Science* 374(6571): 1031.

965. Xia W, J Hughes, D Robertson, and X Jiang, (2021). "How one pandemic led to another: Asfv, the disruption contributing to Sars-Cov-2

emergence in Wuhan." *Preprints* 2021020590. https://www.preprints. org/manuscript/202102.0590/v1.

966. Wallace RG. "The blind weaponmaker." This volume.
967. Wallace RG (2016). "The axis of viral." In *Big Farms Make Big Flu: Dispatches on Infectious Disease, Agribusiness, and the Nature of Science*. Monthly Review Press, New York, pp 140–144; Tucker C, et al. (2021). "Parallel pandemics illustrate the need for One Health solutions." *Frontiers in Microbiology* 12:718546.
968. Chaves L, et al. "Syndemic geographies: Learning from COVID-19 and Vector-Borne diseases in the Americas." Manuscript submitted for publication.
969. Ibid.
970. Wallace RG (2016). "We can think ourselves into a plague." In *Big Farms Make Big Flu: Dispatches on Infectious Disease, Agribusiness, and the Nature of Science*. Monthly Review Press, New York, pp 90–94; Wallace RG (2016). "Alien vs. Predator." In *Big Farms Make Big Flu: Dispatches on Infectious Disease, Agribusiness, and the Nature of Science*, pp 126-130.

Omicron Prime

971. Wallace RG. "A Spray of Split Seconds." This volume; Wallace RG. "Vic Berger's American Public Health." This volume; Wallace RG. "Biden's COVID plan isn't enough." This volume.
972. Maxmen A (2021). "The US records more Covid deaths this year than last." Twitter, 23 November. https://twitter.com/amymaxmen/status/1463377722718101513.
973. Klein M (1997). *Envy and Gratitude and Other Works 1946-1963*. Vintage, London.
974. Schapira LL (1988). *The Cassandra Complex: Living with Disbelief*. Inner City Books, Toronto.
975. Wallace RG (2021). "Information underload." Patreon, 13 November. https://www.patreon.com/posts/58647472; Wallace RG. "Mo BoJo." This volume.
976. Bedford T (2021). "There have been a number of overview threads on the emerging variant designated as @PangoNetwork lineage B.1.1.529, @nextstrain clade 21K and @WHO Variant of Concern Omicron." Twitter, 26 November. https://twitter.com/trvrb/status/1464353224417325066; GISAID Initiative. https://www.gisaid.org/.
977. De Oliveira T (2021). "Busy day on B.1.1.529—a variant of great concern—The world should provide support to South Africa and Africa and not discriminate or isolate it!" Twitter, 25 November. https://twitter.com/Tuliodna/status/1463911554538160130; Malan M (2021). "[Thread] What is the potential impact of the new B.1.1.529 #COVID19 variant?" Twitter, 25 November. https://twitter.com/miamalan/status/1463846528578109444.

978. Bedford T (2021). "There have been a number of overview threads on the emerging variant designated as @PangoNetwork lineage B.1.1.529, @nextstrain clade 21K and @WHO Variant of Concern Omicron."

979. Zimmer C (2021). "New virus variant stokes concern but vaccines still likely to work." *New York Times*, 26 November. https://www.nytimes.com/2021/11/26/health/omicron-variant-vaccines.html.

980. Pai M (2021). "Maybe this makes more sense after #Omicron?" Twitter, 26 November. https://twitter.com/paimadhu/status/1464396435730927622.

981. Pai M and A Olatunbosun-Alakija (2021). "Vax the world." *Science* 374(6571): 1031.

982. Ibid.

983. Ibid.

984. Wallace RG (2021). "Information underload."

985. Pai M (2021). "How to NOT deal with a pandemic: Big panic over a new variant that's not fully understood yet & punishing countries for reporting it." Twitter, 26 November. https://twitter.com/paimadhu/status/1464272234504065028; Maxmen A (2021). "'Instead of solving the problem by vaccinating the world & cutting off new variants, rich countries seem prepared to fork over more money for boosters, & live in a state of endless fear,' Achal Prabhala told me back in JULY." Twitter, 25 November. https://twitter.com/amymaxmen/status/1463980514923085825.

986. Brown G (2021). "A new Covid variant is no surprise when rich countries are hoarding vaccines." *The Guardian*, 26 November. https://www.theguardian.com/commentisfree/2021/nov/26/new-covid-variant-rich-countries-hoarding-vaccines.

987. Wallace RG. "A Spray of Split Seconds." This volume.

988. Ibid.

989. Wallace RG, T Hormeku-Ajei, M Richter, and F Chipato (2021). "Webinar One: Vaccine imperialism: scientific knowledge, capacity and production in Africa." Third World Network-Africa & ROAPE Webinars, 5 August. https://roape.net/2021/07/23/third-world-network-africa-roape-webinars-africa-climate-change-the-pandemic-interrelated-crises-radical-alternatives/.

990. Wallace RG. "A Spray of Split Seconds." This volume.

991. Wallace RG, R Kock, L Bergmann, M Gilbert, L Hogerwerf, C Pittiglio, R Mattioli, and R Wallace (2016). "Did neoliberalizing West African forests produce a new niche for Ebola?" *International Journal of Health Services* 46(1): 149-165.

992. Cortez MF and A Thomson (2021). "China, isolated from the world, is now the last major country still pursuing a 'Zero COVID' strategy." *Time*, 6 October. https://time.com/6104303/china-zero-covid/.

993. Kissler SM, C Tedijanto, E Goldstein, YH Grad, and M Lipsitch (2020). "Projecting the transmission dynamics of SARS-CoV-2 through the postpandemic period." *Science* 368(6493): 860-868.

994. Aberth J (2020). *The Black Death: A New History of the Great Mortality in Europe, 1347–1500.* Oxford University Press, Oxford.

995. Yong E (2021). "Even health-care workers with Long COVID are being dismissed." *The Atlantic,* 24 November. https://www.theatlantic.com/health/archive/2021/11/health-care-workers-long-covid-are-being-dismissed/620801/.

996. Mackey R (2021). "Jen Psaki accidentally tells the truth about how expensive Covid rapid tests are in U.S." *The Intercept,* 7 December. https://theintercept.com/2021/12/07/jen-psaki-cant-explain-americans-dont-get-free -home-covid-tests/.

Corrupted Software

997. Wallace RG (2016). "Two gentlemen of Verona." In *Big Farms Make Big Flu: Dispatches on Infectious Disease, Agribusiness, and the Nature of Science.* Monthly Review Press, New York, pp 160-166.

998. Wallace RG. "A Spray of Split Seconds." This volume.

999. Husseini S (2020). "Peter Daszak's EcoHealth Alliance has hidden almost $40 Million in Pentagon funding and militarized pandemic science." *Independent Science News,* 16 December. https://www.independentsciencenews.org/news/peter-daszaks-ecohealth-alliance-has-hidden-almost-40-million-in-pentagon-funding/.

1000. Wallace RG (2020). "Midvinter-19." In *Dead Epidemiologists: On the Origins of COVID-19.* Monthly Review Press, pp 81-97.

1001. Cohen J (2021). "Prophet in purgatory: EcoHealth Alliance's Peter Daszak is fighting accusations that his pandemic prevention work helped spark COVID-19." *Science,* 17 November. https://www.science.org/content/article/we-ve-done-nothing-wrong-ecohealth-leader-fights-charges-his-research-helped-spark-covid-19; Spence M, (2021). "The rise and fall of British virus hunter Peter Daszak." *The Sunday Times,* 26 June. https://www.thetimes.co.uk/article/the-rise-and-fall-of-british-virus-hunter-peter-daszak-05q8brpz7; Browne E (2021). "Peter Daszak, who sought U.S. funds for Wuhan lab and aided cover-up, faces calls to quit." *Newsweek,* 6 October. https://www.newsweek.com/peter-daszak-u-s-funds-wuhan-institute-virology-aided-cover-faces-calls-quit-ecohealth-alliance-1636103.

1002. Harrison NL (2021). "Peter Daszak—the Elizabeth Holmes of pandemic prevention?" Medium, 26 November. https://medium.com/@leftback45/peter-daszak-the-elizabeth-holmes-of-pandemic-prevention-adfe0b841d71.

1003. Wallace RG (2020). *Dead Epidemiologists: On the Origins of COVID-19.* Monthly Review Press, New York; Mackey R (2021). "Rand Paul's attack on Anthony Fauci chills scientific debate over gain-of-function research." *The Intercept,* 27 July. https://theintercept.com/2021/07/27/covid-anthony-fauci-rand-paul-research/.

1004. Harrison NL (2021). "Peter Daszak—the Elizabeth Holmes of pandemic prevention?"

1005. Ibid.

1006. Ibid.

1007. Cohen J (2021). "Fights over confidentiality pledge and conflicts of interest tore apart COVID-19 origin probe." *Science,* 18 October. https://www.science.org/content/article/fights-over-confidentiality-pledge-and-conflicts-interest-tore-apart-covid-19-origin-probe.

1008. Lerner S, M Hvistendahl, and M Hibbett (2021). "NIH documents provide new evidence U.S. funded gain-of-function research in Wuhan." *The Intercept,* 9 September. https://theintercept.com/2021/09/09/covid-origins-gain-of-function-research/; Jacobsen R (2021). "How Dr. Fauci and other officials withheld information on China's coronavirus experiments." *Newsweek,* 22 November. https://www.newsweek.com/how-dr-fauci-other-officials-withheld-information-chinas-coronavirus-experiments-1652002.

1009. Husseini S (2020). "Peter Daszak's EcoHealth Alliance has hidden almost $40 Million in Pentagon funding and militarized pandemic science."

1010. Franz DR and J Miller (2020). "A biosecurity failure: America's key lab for fighting infectious disease has become a Pentagon backwater." *City Journal,* 21 March. https://www.city-journal.org/biosecurity-failure-usamriid.

1011. Ratiliff E (2020). "We can protect the economy from pandemics: Why didn't we?" *Wired,* 16 June. https://www.wired.com/story/nathan-wolfe-global-economic-fallout-pandemic-insurance/.

1012. Preston P (2013). "Reporter? Secret agent? It's hard to tell with spies like us." *The Guardian,* 7 September. https://www.theguardian.com/media/2013/sep/08/reporter-secret-agent-spies-like-us; T Vanden Brook (2013). "System failure: anthropologists on the battlefield." *USA Today,* 11 August. https://www.usatoday.com/story/nation/2013/08/11/human-terrain-system-afghanistan-war-anthropologists/2640297/; Wallace RG (2010). "Imperial storm scientists." *Farming Pathogens* blog, 21 August. https://farmingpathogens.wordpress.com/2010/08/21/imperial-storm-scientists/; Wallace RG (2014). "Merican Mengele." *Farming Pathogens* blog, 21 December. https://farmingpathogens.wordpress.com/2014/12/21/merican-mengele/.

1013. Patel R (2013). "The Long Green Revolution." *Journal of Peasant Studies,* 40(1): 1-63.

1014. Wallace RG, L Bergmann, R Kock, M Gilbert, L Hogerwerf, R Wallace, and M Holmberg (2015). "The dawn of Structural One Health: A new science tracking disease emergence along circuits of capital." *Social Science & Medicine* 129: 68-77; Wallace RG (2016). "The virus and the virus." In In *Big Farms Make Big Flu: Dispatches on Infectious Disease,*

Agribusiness, and the Nature of Science. Monthly Review Press, New York, pp 280-286.

1015. Attewell W (2015). "Ghosts in the Delta: USAID and the historical geographies of Vietnam's 'other' war." *Environment and Planning A* 47(11): 2257-2275.

1016. Roche B [@BenRocheGroup] (2020). "Very proud that the opening of our International Joint Laboratory #ELDORADO on the link between biodiversity and pathogens has been done with @ PeterDaszak." Twitter, 12 March. https://twitter.com/BenRocheGroup/status/1238084225041076226; Dirección General de Comunicación Social (2021). "Con su potencial científico y technológico, La UNAM participial en inciviativa mundial para prevenir pandemias." Boletín UNAM-DGCS-560, Ciudad Universitaria, 3 July. https://www.dgcs.unam.mx/boletin/bdboletin/2021_560.html; El Dorado (2021). "Financiadores." https://lmi-eldorado.org/financiadores/.

1017. El Dorado (2021). "Laboratorio Mixto Internacional El Dorado." https://lmi-eldorado.org/projectos_laboratorio-mixto-internacional-el-dorado/.

1018. GRAIN (2020). "The misnamed 'Mayan Train': Multimodal land grabbing." 3 March. https://grain.org/en/article/6423-the-misnamed-mayan-train-multimodal-land-grabbing; Hernandez E (2022). "Se 'suben' 53 empresas hidalguenses para construir 42 vagones del Tren Maya." Milenio, 14 March. https://www-milenio-com.translate.goog/politica/organismos/empresas-hidalguenses-suman-proyecto-tren-maya?_x_tr_sl=es&_x_tr_tl=en&_x_tr_hl=en&_x_tr_pto=sc; Quintanilla AG, et al. (2020). *Observaciones a la Manifestación de Impacto Ambiental Modalidad Regional (MIA-R). Tren Maya Fase 1 Palenque-Izamal.* https://geopolitica.iiec.unam.mx/sites/geopolitica.iiec.unam.mx/files/2021-01/Observaciones%20MIA-R%20para%20SEMARNAT%20.pdf; Sexta Grietas del Norte (2020). "Statement of solidarity with the struggle against the Maya Train, a megaproject of death." 15 April. https://sextagrietasdelnorte.org/our-word/statement-of-solidarity-with-the-struggle-against-the-maya-train-a-megaproject-of-death/.

1019. Abi-Habib M (2022). "Over caves and over budget, Mexico's train project barrels toward disaster." *New York Times*, 28 August. https://www.nytimes.com/2022/08/28/world/americas/maya-train-mexico-amlo.html.

1020. GRAIN (2020). "The misnamed 'Mayan Train': Multimodal land grabbing."

1021. Ibid; Manning C and J Bender (2020). "Dispatches from resistant Mexico #7: Maya Train: Eye of the storm (2020, 23:55, bilingual)." Caitlin Manning Films, 17 November. https://resistanceshorts.wordpress.com/2020/11/17/dispaches-from-resistant-mexico-7-maya-train-eye-of-the-storm-2020-2355-bilingual/.

1022. Manning C and J Bender (2020). "Dispatches from resistant Mexico #7: Maya Train: Eye of the storm (2020, 23:55, bilingual)"; Quintanilla AG, et al. (2020). *Observaciones a la Manifestación de Impacto Ambiental Modalidad Regional (MIA-R)*. *Tren Maya Fase 1 Palenque-Izamal*; Redacción (2020). "MIA del Tren Maya sin valoración suficiente sobre impacto: expertos." *La Jornada*, 30 July. https://www.jornada.com.mx/ultimas/politica/2020/07/30/mia-del-tren-maya-sin-valoracion-suficiente-sobre-impacto-expertos-9545.html.

1023. Anonymous (2022). " 'Es el dinero': López Obrador dice que empresarios y EE.UU. financian las acciones de organizaciones para frenar las obras de un tramo del Tren Maya." RT, 29 April. https://actualidad.rt.com/actualidad/428432-lopez-obrador-empresarios-eeuu-tren-maya.

1024. Abi-Habib M (2022). "Over caves and over budget, Mexico's train project barrels toward disaster."

1025. Ibid.

1026. Ibid.

1027. Anonymous (2022). " 'Es el dinero': López Obrador dice que empresarios y EE.UU. financian las acciones de organizaciones para frenar las obras de un tramo del Tren Maya."

1028. Manning C and J Bender (2020). "Dispatches from resistant Mexico #7: Maya Train: Eye of the storm (2020, 23:55, bilingual)."

1029. GRAIN (2020). "The misnamed 'Mayan Train': Multimodal land grabbing."

1030. Ibid.

1031. Ibid.; Wallace RG, M Figueroa, K Enouchs, M Tinsay, T Kerssen, A Henry, F Ramirez, D Bond, and J Gulick. "Homegrown." This volume.

1032. Radwin M (2022). "Full steam ahead for Tren Maya project as lawsuits hit judicial hurdles." *Mongbay*, 28 January. https://news.mongabay.com/2022/01/full-steam-ahead-for-tren-maya-project-as-lawsuits-hit-judicial-hurdles/.

1033. Secretaría de Relaciones Exteriores (2021). "Mexican Foreign Ministry—French Ministry for Europe and Foreign Affairs joint declaration." Gobierno de México, 1 July. https://www.gob.mx/sre/prensa/mexican-foreign-ministry-french-ministry-for-europe-and-foreign-affairs-joint-declaration.

1034. Ibid.

1035. Weatherford J (1988). *Indian Givers: How the Indians of the Americas Transformed the World*. Crown Publishers, New York.

1036. Redacción 24 Horas (2021). "¡Qué elegancia! Con dormitorios y restaurante, así serán por dentro los convoyes del Tren Maya." *24 Horas El Diario Sin Límites*, 28 May. https://www.24-horas.mx/2021/05/28/que-elegancia-con-dormitorios-y-restaurante-asi-seran-por-dentro-los-convoyes-del-tren-maya/.

1037. Wallace RG. "A spray of split seconds." This volume; Wallace R (2021).

"How policy failure and power relations drive COVID-19 pandemic waves: A control theory perspective." HAL Open Science, 2 May. https://hal.archives-ouvertes.fr/hal-03214718.

1038. Wallace RG. "Bidenfreude" This volume; Wallace RG. "Biden's COVID plan isn't enough." This volume; Maxmen A (2021). "The US records more Covid deaths this year than last." Twitter, 23 November. https://twitter.com/amymaxmen/status/1463377722718101513.

1039. Faria NR, MA Suchard, A Rambaut, and P Lemey (2011). "Towards a quantitative understanding of viral phylogeography." *Current Opinion in Virology* 1(5):423-429; Wallace RG (2021). "Even as the U.S. serves as home to some of the world's top phylogeographers, it doesn't actually put such work into public health practice." Twitter, 29 November. https://twitter.com/FarmingPathogen/status/1465449540257939457.

1040. Maxmen A (2020). "The race to unravel the biggest coronavirus outbreak in the United States." *Nature*, 6 March. https://www.nature.com/articles/d41586-020-00676-3.

1041. Chappell B (2021). "The omicron variant was in Europe a week before South Africa reported it." NPR, 30 November. https://www.npr.org/2021/11/30/1060025081/omicron-variant-netherlands-europe-south-africa.

1042. Florko N (2021). "Biden's new Covid plan: more boosters, free home testing, and 'monoclonal antibody strike teams.'" *STAT*, 2 December. https://www.statnews.com/2021/12/02/757561/.

1043. McNeil DG (2020). "Inside China's all-out war on the coronavirus." *New York Times*, 4 March. https://www.nytimes.com/2020/03/04/health/coronavirus-china-aylward.html.

1044. O'Connell A (2022). "Emergency bans on evictions and other tenant protections related to coronavirus." NOLO, 17 January. https://www.nolo.com/evictions-ban.

1045. Boesler M, J Deaux, and K Dmitrieva (2021). "Fattest profits since 1950 debunk wage-inflation story of CEOs." Bloomberg News, 30 November. https://www.bloomberg.com/news/articles/2021-11-30/fattest-profits-since-1950-debunk-inflation-story-spun-by-ceos.

1046. Mitchell TS (2021). "Nearly 100 new people achieved billionaire status in the US during the pandemic." *Insider*, 29 October. https://www.insider.com/100-us-newcomers-join-musk-bezos-zuckerberg-gates-as-billionaires-2021-10; Backman M (2021). "3.3 Million Americans fell into poverty during the pandemic." *The Ascent*, 17 November. https://www.fool.com/the-ascent/personal-finance/articles/33-million-americans-fell-into-poverty-during-the-pandemic/.

1047. Tozzi J, Emma Court, and A Peebles (2021). "Omicron lands in U.S. with hospitals still battered by Covid." Bloomberg News, 2 December. https://www.bloomberg.com/news/articles/2021-12-02/omicron-lands-in-u-s-with -hospitals-already-battered-by-covid.

1048. Figueroa M, K Enochs, M Tinsay, T Kerssen, A Henry, F Ramirez, D Bond, J Gulick, and RG Wallace. "To live and die in Los Angeles." This volume.

1049. Daszak P (2011). "Smart surveillance: Analyzing environmental drivers of emergence to predict and prevent pandemics." *EcoHealth* 7:S12-S13; Roche B (2020). "Very proud that the opening of our International Joint Laboratory #ELDORADO on the link between biodiversity and pathogens has been done with @PeterDaszak." Twitter, 12 March. https://twitter.com/BenRocheGroup/status/1238084225041076226.

Station Ten

1050. Wallace RG. "The Blind Weaponmaker." This volume.

1051. Latham J and A Wilson (2021). "Why China and the WHO will never find a zoonotic origin for the COVID-19 pandemic virus." *Independent Science News*, 16 February. https://www.independentsciencenews.org/commentaries/why-china-and-the-who-will-never-find-a-zoonotic-origin-for-the-covid19-pandemic-virus/; Xie E, J Cai, and G Rui (2020). "Why wild animals are a key ingredient in China's coronavirus outbreak." *South China Morning Post*, 22 January. https://www.scmp.com/news/china/society/article/3047238/why-wild-animals-are-key-ingredient-chinas-coronavirus-outbreak; Bossons M (2020). "No, you won't find 'wild animals' in most of China's wet markets." *Radii*, 25 Feburary. https://radiichina.com/wet-markets-wild-animals-china/.

1052. Fan Y, K Zhao, Z-L Shi, and P Zhou (2019). "Bat coronaviruses in China." *Viruses* 11(3): 210; Wallace RG (2020). "Midvinter-19." In *Dead Epidemiologists: On the Origins of COVID-19.* Monthly Review Press, New York, pp 81-97.

1053. Latham J and A Wilson (2021). "Why China and the WHO will never find a zoonotic origin for the COVID-19 pandemic virus."

1054. Ibid.

1055. Menachery VD, et al. (2015). "A SARS-like cluster of circulating bat coronaviruses shows potential for human emergence." *Nature Medicine* 21(12): 1508-13; Wallace RG. "The guilty bystanders" This volume.

1056. Editorial Board (2022). "Another potential Covid-19 lab leak clue." *Wall Street Journal*, 17 Feburary. https://www.wsj.com/articles/another-potential-covid-19-lab-leak-clue-china-11644615472; Csaba I, K Papp, D Visontai, J Stéger, and N Solymosi (2022). "Unique Sars-Cov-2 variant found in public sequence data of antarctic soil samples collected in 2018-2019." Research Square, 23 December. https://assets.researchsquare.com/files/rs-1177047/v1_covered.pdf?c=1640220418; Csabai I and N Solymosi (2022). "Host genomes for the unique SARS-CoV-2 variant leaked into antarctic soil metagenomic sequencing data." Research Square, 7 February. https://www.researchsquare.com/article/rs-1330800/v1.

1057. Csaba I, K Papp, D Visontai, J Stéger, and N Solymosi (2022). "Unique Sars-Cov-2 variant found in public sequence data of antarctic soil samples collected in 2018-2019."

1058. Wang Q, R Zhu, Y Zheng, T Bao, and L Hou (2019). "Effects of sea animal colonization on the coupling between dynamics and activity of soil ammonia-oxidizing bacteria and archaea in maritime Antarctica." *Biogeosciences* 16: 4113-4128; Dai H-T, R-B Zhu, B-W Sun, C-S Che, and L-J Hou (2020). "Effects of sea animal activities on tundra soil denitrification and nirs- and nirk-encoding denitrifier community in maritime Antarctica." *Frontiers in Microbiology* 11: 2537.

1059. Csaba I, K Papp, D Visontai, J Stéger, and N Solymosi (2022). "Unique Sars-Cov-2 variant found in public sequence data of antarctic soil samples collected in 2018-2019"; Csabai I and N Solymosi (2022). "Host genomes for the unique SARS-CoV-2 variant leaked into antarctic soil metagenomic sequencing data."

1060. Ibid.

1061. Admin (2018). "Principle and workflow of Illumina next-generation sequencing." CD Genomics Blog, 17 October. https://www.cd-genomics.com/blog/principle-and-workflow-of-illumina-next-generation-sequencing/.

1062. Csabai I and N Solymosi (2022). "Host genomes for the unique SARS-CoV-2 variant leaked into antarctic soil metagenomic sequencing data."

1063. Bloom J (@jbloom_lab) (2022). "I'd like to add my preliminary thoughts…" Twitter, 9 February. https://twitter.com/jbloom_lab/status/1491297779855278082; Kumar S (2021). "An evolutionary portrait of the progenitor SARS-CoV-2 and its dominant offshoots in COVID-19 pandemic." *Molecular Biology and Evolution* 38(8): 3026-3059.

1064. Bloom J (@jbloom_lab) (2022). "I'd like to add my preliminary thoughts…"; Editorial Board (2022). "Another potential Covid-19 lab leak clue."

1065. Wallace RG (2020). "Notes on a novel coronavirus." *MROnline*, 29 January. https://mronline.org/2020/01/29/notes-on-a-novel-coronavirus/.

1066. Pekar J, et al. (2022). "SARS-CoV-2 emergence very likely resulted from at least two zoonotic events." Zenodo, 26 Feburary. https://zenodo.org/record/6342616#.YkkQKUBOlPY.

1067. Worobey M, et al. (2022). "The Huanan market was the epicenter of SARS-CoV-2 emergence." Zenodo, 26 Feburary. https://zenodo.org/record/6299600#.YknL7kBOlPY.

1068. Wallace RG. "The blind weaponmaker." This volume.

1069. Xiao X, C Newman, CD Buesching, DW Macdonald, and Z-M Zhou (2021). "Animal sales from Wuhan wet markets immediately prior to the COVID-19 pandemic." *Scientific Reports* 11: 11898.

1070. Wannian L, et al. (2021). *WHO-Convened Global Study of Origins of SARS-CoV-2: China Part.* World Health Organization, https://www.

who.int/publications/i/item/who-convened-global-study-of-origins
-of sars-cov-2-china-part.

1071. Pekar J, et al. (2022). "SARS-CoV-2 emergence very likely resulted
from at least two zoonotic events"; Bloom J (2021). "Recovery of
deleted deep sequencing data sheds more light on the early Wuhan
SARS-CoV-2 epidemic." bioRxiv, 22 June. https://www.biorxiv.org/con
tent/10.1101/2021.06.18.449051v1.full.pdf.

1072. Kumar S (2021). "An evolutionary portrait of the progenitor SARS-
CoV-2 and its dominant offshoots in COVID-19 pandemic." *Molecular
Biology and Evolution* 38(8): 3046-3059.

1073. Pekar J, et al. (2022). "SARS-CoV-2 emergence very likely resulted
from at least two zoonotic events."

1074. Worobey M, et al. (2022). "The Huanan market was the epicenter of
SARS-CoV-2 emergence."

1075. Pekar J, et al. (2022). "SARS-CoV-2 emergence very likely resulted
from at least two zoonotic events."

1076. Wannian L, et al. (2021). *WHO-Convened Global Study of Origins of
SARS-CoV-2: China Part.*

1077. Liu WJ, et al. (2022). "Surveillance of SARS-CoV-2 in the environment
and animal samples of the Huanan Seafood Market." Research Square,
25 February. https://www.researchsquare.com/article/rs-1370392/v1.

1078. Cohen J (2022). "Do three new studies add up to proof of COVID-
19's origin in a Wuhan animal market?" *Science*, 28 February. https://
www.science.org/content/article/do-three-new-studies-add-proof-
covid-19-s-origin-wuhan-animal-market.

1079. Liu WJ, et al. (2022). "Surveillance of SARS-CoV-2 in the environment
and animal samples of the Huanan Seafood Market."

1080. Ibid.

1081. Ibid.

1082. Wallace RG. "Guilty bystanders." This volume.

1083. Liu WJ, et al. (2022). "Surveillance of SARS-CoV-2 in the environment
and animal samples of the Huanan Seafood Market."

1084. Worobey M, et al. (2022). "The Huanan market was the epicenter of
SARS-CoV-2 emergence."

1085. Cohen J (2022). "Do three new studies add up to proof of COVID-19's
origin in a Wuhan animal market?"

1086. Eban K (2022). "'This shouldn't happen': Inside the virus-hunting non-
profit at the center of the lab-leak controversy." *Vanity Fair*, 31 March.
https://www.vanityfair.com/news/2022/03/the-virus-hunting-non-
profit-at-the-center-of-the-lab-leak-controversy.

1087. Bloom J (2021). "Recovery of deleted deep sequencing data sheds more
light on the early Wuhan SARS-CoV-2 epidemic."

1088. Cohen J (2022). "Do three new studies add up to proof of COVID-19's
origin in a Wuhan animal market?"

1089. Eban K (2022). "'This shouldn't happen': Inside the virus-hunting non-profit at the center of the lab-leak controversy."

1090. Eban K (2022). "'This shouldn't happen': Inside the virus-hunting nonprofit at the center of the lab-leak controversy"; Bloom J (2021). "Recovery of deleted deep sequencing data sheds more light on the early Wuhan SARS-CoV-2 epidemic."

1091. Ibid.

1092. Ibid.

1093. Pekar J, et al. (2022). "SARS-CoV-2 emergence very likely resulted from at least two zoonotic events"; Wallace RG, A Liebman, LF Chaves, and R Wallace (2020). "COVID-19 and circuits of capital." *Monthly Review* 72(1). https://monthlyreview.org/2020/05/01/covid-19-and-circuits-of-capital/; Wallace Wallace RG (2020). "Midvinter-19."

1094. Boni MF, et al. (2020). "Evolutionary origins of the SARS-CoV-2 sarbecovirus lineage responsible for the COVID-19 pandemic." *Nature Microbiology* 5: 1408-1417; Chaw S-M, J-H Tai, S-L Chen, C-H Hsieh, S-Y Chang, et al. (2020). "The origin and underlying driving forces of the SARS-CoV-2 outbreak." *Journal of Biomedical Science* 27:73; Singh D and SV Yi (2021). "On the origin and evolution of SARS-CoV-2." *Experimental and Molecular Medicine* 53: 537-547; Voskarides K (2022). "SARS-CoV-2: tracing the origin, tracking the evolution." *BMC Medical Genomics* 15: 62.

1095. Voskarides K (2022). "SARS-CoV-2: tracing the origin, tracking the evolution."

1096. Worobey M, et al. (2008). "Direct evidence of extensive diversity of HIV-1 in Kinshasa by 1960." *Nature* 455(7213): 661-664.

1097. Sánchez CA, H Li, KL Phelps, C Zambrana-Torrelio, L-F Wang, KJ Olival, and P Daszak (2021). "A strategy to assess spillover risk of bat SARS-related coronaviruses in Southeast Asia." MedRxiv, 14 September. https://www.medrxiv.org/content/10.1101/2021.09.09.21263359v1.

1098. Ibid.

1099. Wallace RG, L Bergmann, R Kock, M Gilbert, L Hogerwerf, R Wallace, and M Holmberg (2015). "The dawn of Structural One Health: A new science tracking disease emergence along circuits of capital." *Social Science & Medicine* 129: 68-77; Wallace RG, A Liebman, LF Chaves, and R Wallace (2020). "COVID-19 and circuits of capital." *Monthly Review*, 1 May. https://monthlyreview.org/2020/05/01/covid-19-and-circuits-of-capital/; Ceddia MG (2020). "The super-rich and cropland expansion via direct investments in agriculture." *Nature Sustainability* 3(4): 312-318; Chaves L, et al. "What is 'land'?" This volume.

1100. Eban K (2022). "'This shouldn't happen': Inside the virus-hunting non-profit at the center of the lab-leak controversy."

1101. Ibid.

1102. Wallace RG (2016). "Two gentlemen of Verona." In *Big Farms Make Big*

Flu: Dispatches on Infectious Disease, Agribusiness, and the Nature of Science. Monthly Review Press, New York, pp 160-166.

1103. Lerner S, M Hvistendahl, and M Hibbett (2021). "NIH documents provide new evidence U.S. funded gain-of-function research in Wuhan." *The Intercept,* 9 September. https://theintercept.com/2021/09/09/covid-origins-gain-of-function-research/; Lerner S and M Hibbett (2021). "EcoHealth Alliance conducted risky experiments on MERS virus in China." *The Intercept,* 21 October. https://theintercept.com/2021/10/21/virus-mers-wuhan-experiments/; Lerner S and M Hvistendahl (2021). "NIH officials worked with EcoHealth Alliance to evade restrictions on coronavirus experiments." *The Intercept,* 3 November. https://theintercept.com/2021/11/03/coronavirus-research-ecohealth-nih-emails/; Lerner S (2022). "NIH sent *The Intercept* 292 fully redacted pages related to virus research in Wuhan." *The Intercept,* 20 February. https://theintercept.com/2022/02/20/nih-coronavirus-research-wuhan-redacted/.

1104. Wallace RG (2020). "Midvinter-19."; Husseini S (2020). "Peter Daszak's EcoHealth Alliance has hidden almost $40 Million in Pentagon funding and militarized pandemic science." *Independent Science News,* 16 December. https://www.independentsciencenews.org/news/peter-daszaks-ecohealth-alliance-has-hidden-almost-40-million-in-pentagon-funding/.

1105. Chaves L, et al. "What is 'land'?" This volume.

1106. Levins R and R Lewontin (1985). *The Dialectical Biologist.* Harvard University Press, Cambridge, MA.

1107. Latham J and A Wilson (2021). "Phylogeographic mapping of newly discovered coronaviruses pinpoints the direct progenitor of SARS-CoV-2 as originating from Mojiang, China." *Independent Science News,* 2 August. https://www.independentsciencenews.org/commentaries/phylogeographic-mapping-of-newly-discovered-coronaviruses-pinpoints-direct-progenitor-of-sars-cov-2-as-originating-from-mojiang/.

1108. Dellicour S, et al. (2020). "Epidemiological hypothesis testing using a phylogeographic and phylodynamic framework." *Nature Communications* 11: 5620; Dellicour S, et al. (2021). "Relax, keep walking—A practical guide to continuous phylogeographic inference with BEAST." *Molecular Biology and Evolution* 38(8): 3486-3493; Blokker T, G Baele, P Lemey, and S Dellicour (2022). "Phycova—a tool for exploring covariates of pathogen spread." *Virus Evolution* 8(1): veac015.

1109. Lemey P, et al. (2020). "Accommodating individual travel history and unsampled diversity in Bayesian phylogeographic inference of SARS-CoV-2." *Nature Communications* 11: 5110.

1110. Latham J and A Wilson (2020). "A proposed origin for SARS-CoV-2 and the COVID-19 pandemic." *Independent Science News,* 15 July. https://www.independentsciencenews.org/commentaries/a-proposed-origin-for-sars-cov-2-and-the-covid-19-pandemic/; Wallace RG. "The blind weaponmaker." This volume.

1111. Wallace RG and WM Fitch (2008). "Influenza A H5N1 immigration is filtered out at some international borders." *PLoS One* 3(2): e1697.

1112. Sánchez CA, H Li, KL Phelps, C Zambrana-Torrelio, L-F Wang, KJ Olival, and P Daszak (2021). "A strategy to assess spillover risk of bat SARS-related coronaviruses in Southeast Asia."

1113. Latham J and A Wilson (2021). "Phylogeographic mapping of newly discovered coronaviruses pinpoints the direct progenitor of SARS-CoV-2 as originating from Mojiang, China."

1114. Worobey M, et al. (2022). "The Huanan market was the epicenter of SARS-CoV-2 emergence."

1115. Latham J and A Wilson (2021). "Phylogeographic mapping of newly discovered coronaviruses pinpoints the direct progenitor of SARS-CoV-2 as originating from Mojiang, China."

1116. Lytras S, et al. (2022). "Exploring the natural origins of SARS-CoV-2 in the light of recombination." *Genome Biology and Evolution* 14(2): evac018.

1117. Ibid.

1118. Temmam S, et al. (2022). "Bat coronaviruses related to SARS-CoV-2 and infectious for human cells." *Nature*, 16 February. https:// doi.org/10.1038/s41586-022-04532-4.

1119. Ibid.

1120. Martin DP, et al. (2022). "Selection analysis identifies clusters of unusual mutational changes in Omicron lineage BA.1 that likely impact Spike function." *Molecular Biology and Evolution*, msac061, https://doi.org/10.1093/molbev/msac061.

1121. Latham J and A Wilson (2021). "Phylogeographic mapping of newly discovered coronaviruses pinpoints the direct progenitor of SARS-CoV-2 as originating from Mojiang, China."

1122. Wallace RG. "Guilty bystanders." This volume.

1123. MacLean OA, et al. (2021). "Natural selection in the evolution of SARS-CoV-2 in bats created a generalist virus and highly capable human pathogen." *PLoS Biol* 19(3): e3001115.

1124. Olson SH, et al. (2014). "Sampling strategies and biodiversity of Influenza A subtypes in wild birds." PLoS One 9(3): e90826; Gass JD, et al. (2022). "Global dissemination of Influenza A virus is driven by wild bird migration through arctic and subarctic zones." Preprint manuscript. https://bibbase.org/network/publication/gass-dusek-hall-hallgrimsson-halldorsson-vignisson-ragnarsdottir-jonsson-etal-glo-baldisseminationofinfluenzaavirusisdrivenbywildbirdmigrationthro-ugharcticandsubarcticzones-2022.

1125. MacLean OA, et al. (2021). "Natural selection in the evolution of SARS-CoV-2 in bats created a generalist virus and highly capable human pathogen."

1126. Krebs C and J Myers (2022). "On replication in ecology." *Ecological Rants* blog, 7 April. https://www.zoology.ubc.ca/~krebs/ecological_rants/ on replication-in-ecology/.

1127. Frutos R, et al. (2022). "Origin of COVID-19: Dismissing the Mojiang mine theory and the laboratory accident narrative." *Environmental Research* 204: 112141.

1128. Brenner N and S Ghosh (2022). "Between the colossal and the catastrophic: Planetary urbanization and the political ecologies of emergent infectious disease." *Environment and Planning A,* 4 April. https://doi.org/10.1177/0308518X221084313.

1129. Frutos R (2022). "There is no 'origin' to SARS-CoV-2." *Environmental Research* 207: 112173.

Don't Look Up . . . COVID's Infectious Period

1130. Centers for Disease Control and Prevention (2022). "COVID data tracker: Variant proportions." US Department of Health and Human Services, 7 March. https://covid.cdc.gov/covid-data-tracker/#variant-proportions.

1131. Ortiz J, J Bacon, and C Tebor (2022). "Nation averaging 550,000 reported infections per day; Biden tells vaccinated people: 'You are highly protected': COVID updates." *USA Today,* 5 January. https://www.usatoday.com/story/news/health/2022/01/04/covid-omicron-cases-biden -vaccines-tests/9084898002/.

1132. Wallace RG. "Omicron Prime." This volume.

1133. Zimmer C and A Ghorayshi (2021). "Studies suggest why Omicron is less severe: It spares the lungs." *New York Times,* 31 December. https://www.nytimes.com/2021/12/31/health/covid-omicron-lung-cells.html.

1134. Yong E (2021). "The fundamental question of the pandemic is shifting." *The Atlantic,* 9 June. https://www.theatlantic.com/health/archive/2021/06/individualism-still-spoiling-pandemic-response/619133/.

1135. Nebehay S (2021). "Omicron cases doubling in 1.5 to 3 days in areas with local spread—WHO." Reuters, 18 December. https://www.reuters.com/business/healthcare-pharmaceuticals/omicron-cases-doubling-15-3-days-areas-with-local-spread-who-2021-12-18/.

1136. Ritchie H, et al (2020). "Coronavirus pandemic (COVID-19)." *OurWorldinData,* 6 January. https://ourworldindata.org/covid-deaths.

1137. Centers for Disease Control and Prevention (2022). "COVID-19 Forecasts: Deaths." US Department of Health and Human Services, 2 March. https://www.cdc.gov/coronavirus/2019-ncov/science/forecasting/forecasting-us.html.

1138. Planas D, et al. (2021). "Considerable escape of SARS-CoV-2 variant Omicron to antibody neutralization (preprint)."

1139. Natario N (2021). "UTMB study shows unvaccinated, natural immunity offers little protection against omicron." ABC 13, 23 December. https://abc13.com/houston-coronavirus-utmb-research-omicron-variant-protecting-against/11372883/.

1140. Wang R, J Chen, and GW Wei (2021). "Mechanisms of SARS-CoV-2 evolution revealing vaccine-resistant mutations in Europe and America." *The Journal of Physical Chemistry Letters* 12(49): 11850-11857.

1141. @Patricia_Ann_E (2021). "I'll say it again: Don't use euphemisms like 'hospital beds' when what you actually mean is nursing staff." Twitter, 11 December. https://twitter.com/Patricia_Ann_E/status/1469677786659016705.

1142. Centers for Disease Control and Prevention (2022). "COVID data tracker: State-issued prevention measures at the county-level." US Department of Health and Human Services, 7 March. https://covid.cdc.gov/covid-data-tracker/#county-level-covid-policy.

1143. Cullen K (2021). "In the last three months, five conservative talk show hosts have died from COVID." *Boston Globa,* 21 October. https://www.bostonglobe.com/2021/10/21/metro/dying-an-audience/.

1144. Devine A (2021). "'Don't let me die': Life and death inside Tallahassee Memorial HealthCare's COVID unit." *Tallahassee Democrat,* 2 September. https://www.tallahassee.com/story/news/2021/08/27/tallahassee-memorial-healthcare-covid-unit-behind-curtain-life-death/8240656002/.

1145. Miranda G (2021). "'I don't have COVID': Doctor says some COVID patients deny virus, decry vaccines from their deathbed." *USA Today,* 25 September. https://www.usatoday.com/story/news/nation/2021/09/25/dr-matthew-trunsky-says-some-dying-covid-patients-deny-virus/5866695001/.

1146. @oneunderscore_ (2021). "First off, they really are eating horse dewormer…" Twitter, 26 August. https://twitter.com/oneunderscore__/status/1431041437643247627.

1147. @tomaskenn (2021). "Ron DeSantis shut down all state-operated COVID testing sites…" Twitter, 31 December. https://twitter.com/tomaskenn/status/1476938187490562051; Gillespie R (2021). "Florida doesn't plan to open COVID testing sites amid surge, Orange County official says." *Orlando Sentinel,* 29 December. https://www.orlandosentinel.com/coronavirus/os-ne-coronavirus-fdoh-demings-omicron-20211230-zh4mpc74xzacbljz5khyqchqzy-story.html.

1148. Anonymous (2022). "Coronavirus in the US: Latest map and case count." *New York Times,* 7 March. https://www.nytimes.com/interactive/2021/us/covid-cases.html.

1149. Wallace RG (2018). "Black mirror." https://antipodeonline.org/wpcontent/uploads/2018/01/book-review_wallace-on-richards1.pdf.

1150. Guse C (2021). "NYU team gets $4M grant to study COVID's toll on MTA workers." New York Daily News, 27 September. https://www.nydailynews.com/new-york/ny-nyu-study-mta-covid-pandemic-deaths-20210927-lhu5pdygv5h6bnog4xwnsrphby-story.html; Funk J (2021). "At least 59,000 U.S. meat workers caught COVID-19 in 2020, 269 died." PBS News Hour, 27 October. https://www.pbs.org/newshour/health/at-least-59000-u-s-meat-workers-caught-covid-19-in 2020-269-died.

1151. FunkJ(2021)."Atleast59,000U.S.meatworkerscaughtCOVID-19in2020,269 died." PBS News Hour, 27 October. https://www.pbs.org/newshour/health/at-least-59000-u-s-meat-workers-caught-covid-19-in-2020-269-died.

1152. Wallace R (2021). "How policy failure and power relations drive COVID-19 pandemic waves: A control theory perspective." *Hal Open Science*: hal-03214718.

1153. Baker MG (2020). "Nonrelocatable Occupations at Increased Risk During Pandemics: United States, 2018." *American Journal of Public Health* 110(8): 1126-1132.

1154. Hurley KJ (2021). *Stuck in Stockholm: Examining Sexual Harassment and Covid-19 Related Factors as Predictors of Stockholm Syndrome in the Workplace.* Dissertation, The University of West Florida. https://www.proquest.com/openview/3f97b9c10e4afc7bff142f727c528291/1?pq-origsite=gscholar&cbl=18750&diss=y.

1155. U.S. Department of Labor. "Sick Leave." https://www.dol.gov/general/topic/workhours/sickleave.

1156. Goodman PS (2021). "On the slaughterhouse floor, fear and anger remain." *New York Times*, 29 December. https://www.nytimes.com/2021/12/29/business/meat-factories-covid.html.

1157. Anonymous (2016). "Illness as indicator." *The Economist*, 19 November. https://www.economist.com/united-states/2016/11/19/illness-as-indicator.

1158. Efird CR and AF Lightfoot (2020). "Missing Mayberry: How whiteness shapes perceptions of health among white Americans in a rural Southern community." *Social Science & Medicine*, 253: 112967.

1159. Feldman S and C Morris (2021). "Year in Review: 2021 with the pandemic." *Ipsos*, 23 December. https://www.ipsos.com/en-us/news-polls/year-in-review-with-the-pandemic.

1160. Simmons-Duffin S (2021). "Confused by CDC's latest mask guidance? Here's what we've learned." MPR News, 15 May. https://www.npr.org/sections/health-shots/2021/05/14/996879305/confused-by-cdcs-latest-mask-guidance-heres-what-weve-learned.

1161. Merelli A (2021). "The White House is blaming the wrong people for the coming Covid-19 wave." Quartz, 20 December. https://qz.com/2104281/the-white-house-is-wrong-to-blame-the-unvaccinated-for-omicron/.

1162. Olson J (2021). "Breakthrough infections rise in Minnesota, but unvaccinated at greatest COVID-19 risk." *Star Tribune*, 12 November. https://www.startribune.com/breakthrough-infections-rise-in-minnesota-but-unvaccinated-at-greatest-covid-19-risk/600115932/.

1163. Scharringa S, et al. (2021). "Vaccination and their importance for lung transplant recipients in a COVID-19 world." *Expert Review of Clinical Pharmacology* 14(11): 1413-1425.

1164. Anthes E (2021). "Booster protection wanes against symptom-

atic Omicron infections, British data suggest." *New York Times*, 23
December. https://www.nytimes.com/2021/12/23/health/booster-pro-
tection-omicron.html.

1165. Eban K (2021). "The Biden administration rejected an October proposal for 'Free Rapid Tests for the Holidays'." *Vanity Fair*, 23 December.
https://www.vanityfair.com/news/2021/12/the-biden-administration-
rejected-an-october-proposal-for-free-rapid-tests-for-the-holidays.

1166. Ibid.

1167. Edmondson C (2021). "Senate passes $768 billion defense bill, send-
ing it to Biden." *New York Times*, 15 December. https://www.nytimes.
com/2021/12/15/us/politics/defense-spending-bill.html.

1168. Wallace A (2021). "Just mail covid tests to everyone? Absolutely. My
government does it." *The Washington Post*, 9 December. https://www.
washingtonpost.com/outlook/2021/12/09/coronavirus-test-rapid
-free-psaki/.

1169. Anthes E (2021). "Affordable coronavirus tests are out there, if you look."
New York Times, 16 December. https://www.nytimes.com/2021/12/16/
health/coronavirus-testing-holidays.html.

1170. @fingerblaster (2022). "wild that the most unhinged republican president in history sent us $2000 checks…" Twitter, 3 January. https://
twitter.com/fingerblaster/status/1478027433089536000.

1171. Casselman B (2022). "Child tax credit's extra help ends, just as Covid
surges anew." *New York Times*, 2 January. https://www.nytimes.
com/2022/01/02/business/economy/child-tax-credit.html.

1172. Dorn S and R Gordon (2021). "The Catastrophic Cost of Uninsurance:
COVID-19 Cases and Deaths Closely Tied to America's Health
Coverage Gaps." FamiliesUSA: The Voice for Health Care Consumers,
4 March. https://familiesusa.org/resources/the-catastrophic-cost-of-
uninsurance-covid-19-cases-and-deaths-closely-tied-to-americas-
health-coverage-gaps/; McLaughlin JM, et al. (2021). "County-level
predictors of coronavirus disease 2019 (COVID-19) cases and deaths
in the United States: What happened, and where do we go from here?"
Clinical Infectious Disease 73(7): e1814-e1821.

1173. Leifheit KM, et al. (2021). "Expiring eviction moratoriums and COVID-
19 incidence and mortality." *American Journal of Epidemiology* 190(12):
2503-2510.

1174. del Rio C, H Ting, and E Bastian (2021). "Delta Letter to CDC." Delta
Air Lines, Inc., 21 December. https://news.delta.com/sites/default/
files/2021-12/delta-letter-to-cdc-december-21-2021.pdf.

1175. Yang W and J Shaman (2022). "Viral replication dynamics could critically modulate vaccine effectiveness and should be accounted for when
assessing new SARS-CoV-2 variants." *Influenza and Other Respiratory
Viruses* 16(2): 366.

1176. Cui L, et al. (2021). "Dynamic Zero-Covid strategy curtails mutagenesis and emergence of new variants of the SARS-CoV-2." Preprint from Research Square, 28 Dec 2021, https://europepmc.org/article/ppr/ppr436586.

1177. Pulliam JRC, et al. (2021). "Increased risk of SARS-CoV-2 reinfection associated with emergence of the Omicron variant in South Africa." *Science* 376(6593): eabn4947.

1178. Bartha FA, et al. (2021). "Potential severity, mitigation, and control of Omicron waves depending on pre-existing immunity and immune evasion (preprint)." *medRxiv*.

1179. Ankel S (2021). "WHO warns that coronavirus variants are spreading faster than vaccines can stop them." *Insider*, 4 July. https://www.businessinsider.com/who-speed-up-covid-19-vaccine-rollout-variants-catch-up-2021-7.

1180. Lee S (2020). "JetBlue's founder helped fund a Stanford study that said the coronavirus wasn't that deadly." *Buzzfeed*, 15 May. https://www.buzzfeednews.com/article/stephaniemlee/stanford-coronavirus-neeleman-ioannidis-whistleblower.

1181. Brueck H and A Bendix (2021). "CDC director fights back tears as she warns of soaring COVID-19 cases: 'Right now I'm scared'." Yahoo News, 29 March. https://news.yahoo.com/cdc-director-fights-back-tears-172155352.html.

1182. Park A (2022). "CDC Director Rochelle Walensky faces a surging virus—and a crisis of trust." *TIME*, 5 January. https://time.com/6132792/rochelle-walensky-covid-19-cdc-profile/.

1183. Wallace RG (2016). "Made in Minnesota." In *Big Farms Make Big Flu: Dispatches on Infectious Disease, Agribusiness, and the Nature of Science.* Monthly Review Press, New York, pp 347-358.

1184. Anonymous (2021). "Reactions to 'Not letting COVID-19 take my shifts' CDC ad are less than positive." *God*, 31 December. https://god.dailydot.com/reactions-covid-cdc-ad/.

1185. @CDCgov (2021). "Hospital stay can be expensive, but COVID-19 vaccines are free." Twitter, 27 December. https://twitter.com/CDCgov/status/1475529419812974595.

1186. Tankersley J (2021). "Rising prices, once seen as temporary, threaten Biden's agenda." *New York Times*, 26 October. https://www.nytimes.com/2021/10/26/business/economy/biden-inflation.html.

1187. Briefing Room (2021). "Press briefing by White House COVID-19 response team and public health officials." The White House, 17 December. https://www.whitehouse.gov/briefing-room/press-briefings/2021/12/17/press-briefing-by-white-house-covid-19-response-team-and-public-health-officials-74/.

1188. Centers for Disease Control and Prevention (2021). "CDC updates operational strategy for K-12 schools to reflect new evidence on physical distance in classrooms." CDC Newsroom, 19 March. https://www.

cdc.gov/media/releases/2021/p0319-new-evidence-classroom-physi-cal-distance.html.

1189. Politi D (2021). "CDC admits the coronavirus is airborne, can be transmitted more than 6 feet away." *Slate*, 8 May. https://slate.com/news-and-politics/2021/05/cdc-coronavirus-airborne-infection-six-feet.html.

1190. Panchal U, et al. (2021). "The impact of COVID-19 lockdown on child and adolescent mental health: systematic review." *European Child & Adolescent Psychiatry*, 18 Aug. https://link.springer.com/article/10.1007/s00787-021-01856-w.

1191. España G, et al. (2021). "Impacts of K-12 school reopening on the COVID-19 epidemic in Indiana, USA." *Epidemics* 37: 100487.

1192. Wu LL (2021). "CPR on a COVID patient: Not a moment to waste looking for PPE." *MedPage Today*, 14 October. https://www.medpage-today.com/emergencymedicine/emergencymedicine/95038.

1193. @rob_sheridan (2021). "I want you to die working at Jamba Juice so the Dow Jones can increase by .3%." Instagram, 28 December. https://www.instagram.com/p/CYCbK2TvhB8/.

1194. @zak_toscani (2021). "CDC recommends splitting up your quarantine over your two 15min breaks." Twitter, 27 December. https://twitter.com/zak_toscani/status/1475614666567008256/.

1195. @eduwonkette_jen (2021). "I guess I missed the rewriting of the Hippocratic Oath: first, do no harm to bars and restaurants." Twitter, 24 September. https://twitter.com/eduwonkette_jen/status/1441432043200528391.

1196. @roywoodjr (2021). "CDC just said you only need to quarantine if you are on a ventilator . . ." Twitter, 28 December. https://twitter.com/roywoodjr/status/1475882203582189568.

1197. @ProducedByTip (2021). "Y'all keep talking about the CDC, the CDC, the CDC…" Twitter, 27 December. https://twitter.com/ProducedByTip/status/1475669051376648200.

1198. @alexanderchee (2021). "If you have to deploy the military to support hospitals…" Twitter, 22 December. https://twitter.com/alexanderchee/status/1473656680827269121.

1199. @gnarlotte (2021). "CDC okays pull-out method as "eh, good enough"." Twitter, 28 December. https://twitter.com/gnarlotte/status/1476026896966062086.

1200. Lau YC, et al. (2021). "Joint estimation of generation time and incubation period for coronavirus disease 2019." *The Journal of Infectious Diseases* 224(10): 1664-1671.

1201. Laerd Statistics. "Measures of Central Tendency." https://statistics.laerd.com/statistical-guides/measures-central-tendency-mean-mode-median.php.

1202. Park A (2022). "CDC Director Rochelle Walensky faces a surging virus—and a crisis of trust." *TIME*, 5 January. https://time.com/6132792/rochelle-walensky-covid-19-cdc-profile/.

1203. Spectrum News Staff (2021). "Health expert warns Omicron could be as transmissible as measles." Spectrum News NY 1, 17 December. https://www.ny1.com/nyc/all-boroughs/news/2021/12/18/health-expert-warns-omicron-could-be-as-transmissible-as-measles.

1204. Edwards E (2022). "CDC clarifies isolation guidance to include testing, if possible." NBC News, 4 January. https://www.nbcnews.com/health/health-news/cdc-clarifies-isolation-guidance-include-testing-possible-rcna10864.

1205. @JoeBiden (2020). "We're eight months into this pandemic, and Donald Trump still doesn't have a plan to get this virus under control..." Twitter, 15 October. https://twitter.com/joebiden/status/1316894374500962305?lang=en.

1206. @JoeBiden (2020). "I am alarmed by the surge in reported COVID-19 infections, hospitalizations, and fatalities..." Twitter, 13 November. https://twitter.com/joebiden/status/1327418359848300545?lang=en.

1207. @beingrealmac (2021). "Joe Biden on covid: 'There is no federal solution. This gets solved at a state level.'" Twitter, 27 December. https://web.archive.org/web/20211227165611/https://twitter.com/beingrealmac/status/1475509915607351300; Woodall C, G McGrath, and B Gordon (2021). "As COVID wanes, state legislatures are limiting governors' emergency powers. Why it matters." GoErie, 7 June. https://www.goerie.com/story/news/2021/06/07/covid-states-limiting-governors-emergency-powers/7512483002/.

1208. @RaviHVJ (2022). "It is simply false that 'everyone will catch Omicron.'" Twitter, 3 January. https://twitter.com/RaviHVJ/status/1478093936736546816.

1209. Normile D (2021). "'Zero COVID' is getting harder—but China is sticking with it." Science, 17 November. https://www.science.org/content/article/zero-covid-getting-harder-china-sticking-it.

1210. Anonymous (2022). "A cluster of Covid-19 cases in China prompts a citywide lockdown." The Economist, 1 January. https://www.economist.com/china/a-cluster-of-covid-19-cases-in-china-prompts-a-citywide-lockdown/21806929.

1211. Bloomberg News (2022). "China's locked-down city thrown into chaos after Covid app crash." Bloomberg, 4 January. https://www.bloomberg.com/news/articles/2022-01-05/china-s-health-code-app-crashes-in-xi-an-spiking-lockdown-chaos; @SecondRingSZN (2021). "Free grocery delivered to residents in Xi'an during lockdown." Twitter, 29 December. https://twitter.com/SecondRingSZN/status/1476085796918734849.

1212. Wallace R (2021). "How policy failure and power relations drive COVID-19 pandemic waves: A control theory perspective."

1213. Bedford T, et al. (2020). "Cryptic transmission of SARS-CoV-2 in Washington State." Science 370(6516): 571-575.

1214. Roberts S (2020). "The swiss cheese model of pandemic defense."

New York Times, 5 December. https://www.nytimes.com/2020/12/05/health/coronavirus-swiss-cheese-infection-mackay.html.

1215. Eban K (2021). "The Biden administration rejected an October proposal for 'Free Rapid Tests for the Holidays'. "

1216. Harrison DW (2021). "The risks of at-home Covid tests." *Dale Harrison* blog, 22 August. https://dalewharrison.substack.com/p/the-risks-of-at-home-covid-tests?s=r; Harrison D (2021). "COVID testing – Part II." Facebook, 27 December. https://www.facebook.com/dale.w.harrison/posts/5097459370273332.

1217. Eban K (2021). "The Biden Administration rejected an October proposal for 'Free Rapid Tests for the Holidays'. "

1218. Harrison D (2021). "COVID testing—Part III." Facebook, 27 December. https://www.facebook.com/dale.w.harrison/posts/5097459370273332.

1219. Wallace RG. "Vic Berger's American public health." This volume.

1220. Wallace RG. "Biden's COVID plan isn't enough." This volume.

1221. Wallace RG, A Liebman, LF Chaves, and R Wallace (2020). "COVID-19 and circuits of capital." *Monthly Review*, 1 May. https://monthlyreview.org/2020/05/01/covid-19-and-circuits-of-capital/.

1222. Mays GP and SA Smith (2011). "Evidence links increases in public health spending to declines in preventable deaths." *Health Affairs* 30(8): 1585-1593.

1223. Lang A, M Warren, and L Kulman (2018). "A Funding Crisis for Public Health and Safety: State-by-State Public Health Funding and Key Health Facts 2018." Trust for America's Health, March. https://www.tfah.org/wp-content/uploads/2019/03/InvestInAmericaRpt-FINAL.pdf.

1224. Alfonso YN, et al. (2021). "US public health neglected: Flat or declining spending left states ill equipped to respond to COVID-19: Study examines US public health spending." *Health Affairs* 40: 664-671.

1225. Yong E (2021). "Why health-care workers are quitting in droves." *The Atlantic*, 16 November. https://www.theatlantic.com/health/archive/2021/11/the-mass-exodus -of-americas-health-care-workers/620713/.

1226. Empire without Emperor. "Systemic cycles of accumulation of capital." https://empirewithoutemperor.wordpress.com/world-system-theory/ii-3-systemic-cycles-of-accumulation-of-capital/.

1227. Shalal A, J Mason, and D Lawder (2021). "U.S. reverses stance, backs giving poorer countries access to COVID vaccine patents." Reuters, 5 May. https://www.reuters.com/business/healthcare-pharmaceuticals/biden-says-plans-back-wto-waiver-vaccines-2021-05-05/; Zaitchik A (2021). "How Bill Gates Impeded Global Access to Covid Vaccines." *The New Republic*, 12 April. https://newrepublic.com/article/162000/bill-gates-impeded-global-access-covid-vaccines.

1228. @MorePerfectUS (2021). "Bill Gates opposes sharing COVID vaccine patents with less wealthy nations so they can manufacture it themselves..." Twitter, 27 April. https://twitter.com/MorePerfectUS/status/1387106780833067026.

1229. Prabhala A and A Alsalhani (2021). "Pharmaceutical manufacturers across Asia, Africa and Latin America with the technical requirements and quality standards to manufacture mRNA vaccines." AccesssIBSA project, December 10. https://accessibsa.org/mrna/.

1230. Anonymous (2021). "Experts identify 100 plus firms to make Covid-19 mRNA vaccines." Human Rights Watch, 15 December. https://www.hrw.org/news/2021/12/15/experts-identify-100-plus-firms-make-covid -19-mrna-vaccines#.

1231. Nolen S (2021). "Here's why developing countries can make mRNA Covid vaccines." New York Times, 22 October. https://www.nytimes.com/interactive/2021/10/22/science/developing-country-covid-vaccines.html.

1232. @MGSchmelzer (2021). "The global concentration of capital is extreme..." Twitter, 7 December. https://twitter.com/MGSchmelzer/status/1468152818397851649.

1233. @4TaxFairness (2022). "BREAKING: America's billionaires got $1 Trillion richer in 2021..." Twitter, 4 January. https://twitter.com/4TaxFairness/status/1478403006186012674.

1234. Califano J (2021). ""COVID has been a perfect illustration . . ." Twitter, 16 December. https://br.ifunny.co/picture/jack-califano-jackcalifano-covid-has-been-a-perfect-illustration-of-1zjnvCVA9.

1235. Fullilove M et al (2021). "Learning from Covid: A Community-Based Approach to Pandemic Planning." Pandemic Thinktank. https://drive.google.com/file/d/1bPzCcw0PEFIb0AAujsdmFDgQ8Jjgtn-w/view.

1236. @s_j_prins (2021). "Turns out lots of blue check public health experts moonlight as pandemic profiteers." Twitter, 28 December. https://mobile.twitter.com/s_j_prins/status/1475861271316684802.

1237. @EpiEllie (2021). "Honestly baffled by people who claim the COVID plan..." Twitter, 21 December. https://mobile.twitter.com/EpiEllie/status/1473290134036652033.

1238. Feldman J (2021). "A year in, how has Biden done on pandemic response?" Medium, 14 May. https://jmfeldman.medium.com/a-year-in-how-has-biden-done-on-pandemic-response-88452c696f2. Feldman J. (2021). " 'There's 'a lot to unpack' about how the only substantive criticism . . .'" Twitter, 23 December. https://twitter.com/jfeldman_epi/status/1474218257368248322.

1239. @economicexile (2021). "I'm an intensivist and have been taking care of COVID patients..." Twitter, 27 December. https://twitter.com/economicexile/status/1475629298342141953.

1240. @luckytran (2022). "We are not 'learning to live with COVID'. " Twitter, 1 January. https://twitter.com/luckytran/status/1477384454704357387.

1241. MarchforScience (2021). Repost of Bree Newsome Bass's (@

BreeNewsome) tweet on the out-of-pocket costs of at-home Covid-19 tests. Instagram, 20 December. https://www.instagram.com/p/CXuGg6OrQS3/.

1242. Wallace RG (2020). "Biden's COVID plan isn't enough"; Wallace RG (2021). "Bidenfreude"; Wallace RG (2020). *Dead Epidemiologists: On the Origins of COVID-19.* Monthly Review Press, New York.

1243. HOLC. "You're a wizard, Harry." T shirt. TeePublic. https://www.teepublic.com/t-shirt/3667898-youre-a-wizard-harry-santa-claus.

1244. Kissler SM, et al. (2020). "Projecting the transmission dynamics of SARS-CoV-2 through the postpandemic period." *Science* 368(6493): 860-868.

1245. Badiou A (2018). *Can Politics Be Thought?* Duke University Press, Durham, NC.

1246. Becker C and D Bloom (1998). "The demographic crisis in the former Soviet Union: Introduction." *World Development* 26(11): 1913-1919; Venkataramani AS, R O'Brien, and AC Tsai (2021). "Declining life expectancy in the United States: the need for social policy as health policy." *Journal of the American Medical Association* 325(7): 621-622.

Governance Is Key

1247. An BY, S Porcher, S-Y Tang, and EE Kim (2021). "Policy design for COVID-19: Worldwide evidence on the efficacies of early mask mandates and other policy interventions." *Public Administration Review* 81(6): 1157-1182.

1248. Gerrish PJ, F Saldaña, B Galeota-Sprung, A Colato, EE Rodriguez, and JXV Hernández (2021). "How unequal vaccine distribution promotes the evolution of vaccine escape." medRxiv. https://www.medrxiv.org/content/10.1101/2021.03.27.21254453v3.

1249. Rosenberg ES, V Dorabawila, D Easton, UE Bauer, J Kumar, et al. (2022). "Covid-19 vaccine effectiveness in New York State." *New England Journal of Medicine* 386: 116-127.

1250. Gerrish PJ, F Saldaña, B Galeota-Sprung, A Colato, EE Rodriguez, and JXV Hernández (2021). "How unequal vaccine distribution promotes the evolution of vaccine escape."

1251. Engbert R, MM Rabe, R Kliegl, and S Reich (2021). "Sequential data assimilation of the stochastic SEIR epidemic model for regional COVID-19 dynamics." *Bulletin of Mathematical Biology* 83(1): 1-16.

1252. Diekmann O, JAP Heesterbeek, and JA Metz (1990). "On the definition and the computation of the basic reproduction ratio R_0 in models for infectious diseases in heterogeneous populations." *Journal of Mathematical Biology* 28(4): 365-382.

1253. Hale T, J Anania, N Angrist, T Boby, E Cameron-Blake, M Di Folco, L Ellen, R Goldszmidt, L Hallas, B Kira, M Luciano, S Majumdar, R Nagesh, A Petherick, T Phillips, H Tatlow, S Webster, A Wood, and

Y Zhang (2021). "Variation in government responses to COVID-19." Version 12.0. Blavatnik School of Government Working Paper. www.bsg.ox.ac.uk/covidtracker.

1254. Emanuel E and M Osterholm (2022). "China's Zero-Covid policy is a pandemic waiting to happen." *New York Times*, 25 January. https://www.nytimes.com/2022/01/25/opinion/china-covid-19.html.

1255. Hallas L, A Hatibie, R Koch, S Majumdar, M Pyarali, A wood, and T Hale (2021). "Variation in US states' COVID-19 policy responses." BSG-WP-2020/034 Version 3.0. 7 May. www.bsg.ox.ac.uk/covidtracker.

1256. Gerrish PJ, F Saldaña, B Galeota-Sprung, A Colato, EE Rodriguez, and JXV Hernández (2021). "How unequal vaccine distribution promotes the evolution of vaccine escape."

1257. Wallace R (2021). "How policy failure and power relations drive COVID-19 pandemic waves: A control theory perspective." https://hal.archives-ouvertes.fr/hal-03214718/document.

1258. Chaves LF, MD Friberg, LA Hurt, RM Rodríguez, D O'Sullivan, and LR Bergmann (2021). "Trade, uneven development and people in motion: Used territories and the initial spread of COVID-19 in Mesoamerica and the Caribbean." *Socio-Economic Planning Sciences*. Corrected proof. https://www.sciencedirect.com/science/article/pii/S0038012121001531.

1259. Wallace R, LF Chaves, LR Bergmann, C Ayres, L Hogerwerf, R Kock, and RG Wallace (2018). *Clear-Cutting Disease Control: Capital-Led Deforestation, Public Health Austerity, and Vector-Borne Infection.* Springer International Publishing, Cham.

1260. Chaves LF, MD Friberg, LA Hurt, RM Rodríguez, D O'Sullivan, and LR Bergmann (2021). "Trade, uneven development and people in motion: Used territories and the initial spread of COVID-19 in Mesoamerica and the Caribbean"; Wallace R, LF Chaves, LR Bergmann, C Ayres, L Hogerwerf, R Kock, and RG Wallace (2018). *Clear-Cutting Disease Control: Capital-Led Deforestation, Public Health Austerity, and Vector-Borne Infection.*

1261. Wallace R and RG Wallace (2016). "Introducing pandemic control theory." In RG Wallace and R Wallace (eds), *Neoliberal Ebola: Modeling Disease Emergence from Finance to Forest and Farm.* Springer International Publishing, Cham, pp 69-79; Galea S, SM Abdalla, and JL Sturchio (2020). "Social determinants of health, data science, and decision-making: Forging a transdisciplinary synthesis." *PLoS Medicine* 17: e1003174.

1262. Spiegel JM, J Breilh, and A Yassi (2015). "Why language matters: insights and challenges in applying a social *determination* of health approach in a North-South collaborative research program." *Globalization and Health* 11: 9.

1263. Okamoto K, V Ong, RG Wallace, R Wallace, and L Fernando Chaves

(2022). "When might host heterogeneity drive the evolution of asymptomatic, pandemic coronaviruses?" *Nonlinear Dynamics*, in press.

1264. Levins R and C Lopez (1999). "Toward an ecosocial view of health." *International Journal of Health Services* 29(2): 261-293.

What Is "Land"?

1265. Zhuangzi (2009). *Zhuangzi: The Essential Writings with Selections from Traditional Commentaries*. Brook Ziporyn (translator). Hackett Pub. Co., Indianapolis.

1266. Levins R and R Lewontin (1980). "Dialectics and reductionism." *Synthese* 43: 47-78.

1267. Simpson LB (2021). *A Short History of the Blockade: Giant Beavers, Diplomacy, and Regeneration in Nishnaabewin*. University of Alberta Press; Simpson LB (2017). *As We Have Always Done: Indigenous Freedom Through Radical Resistance*. University of Minnesota Press, Minneapolis.

1268. Marx K (1857; 1965). *Pre-Capitalist Economic Formations*. International Publishers, New York; Wood EM (1999; 2002). *The Origins of Capitalism: A Longer View*. Verso, New York; Perelman M (2000). *The Invention of Capitalism*. Duke University Press, Durham, NC; Arrighi G (1994; 2010). *The Long Twentieth Century: Money, Power and the Origins of Our Times*. Verso, London; Van Bavel BJP (2010). *Manors and Markets: Economy and Society in the Low Countries 500-1600*. Oxford University Press, Oxford, UK.

1269. Wolfe ND, P Daszak, AM Kilpatrick, and DS Burket (2005). "Bushmeat hunting, deforestation, and prediction of zoonotic disease." *Emerging Infectious Diseases* 11(12): 1822-1827; Pimentel D, et al. (2007). "Ecology of infectious diseases: Population growth and environmental degradation." *Human Ecology* 35: 653-668; Quammen D (2012). *Spillover: Animal Infections and the Next Human Pandemic*. W.W. Norton and Co, New York; Li HY, et al. (2020). "A qualitative study of zoonotic risk factors among rural communities in southern China." *Int Health* 12(2): 77-85.

1270. Weinstock JA (1983). "Rattan: Ecological balance in a Borneo rainforest swidden." *Economic Botany* 37: 58-68; Denevan WM, et al. (1988). *Swidden-Fallow Agroforestry in the Peruvian Amazon*. Advances in Economic Botany Vol. 5. New York Botanical Garden Press, New York; Coomes OT, Y Takasaki, and JM Rhemtulla (2017). "What fate for swidden agriculture under land constraint in tropical forests? Lessons from a long-term study in an Amazonian peasant community." *Journal of Rural Studies* 54: 39-51; Altieri MA (2018). *Agroecology: The Science of Sustainable Agriculture*. Second Edition. CRC Press, Boca Raton.

1271. Marx K and F Engels (1998). *The German Ideology: Including Theses on Feuerbach and Introduction to The Critique of Political Economy*. Prometheus Books, Amherst, NY.

1272. Santos M (2000). *Por uma outra globalização: do pensamento único à consciência universal*. Record, Rio de Janeiro.
1273. Levins R (2010). "Why programs fail." *Monthly Review* 61(10): 43–9.
1274. Xiong VC (1999). "The land-tenure system of Tang China: a study of the equal-field system and the turfan documents." *T'oung Pao* 85: 328–390.
1275. Villa Rojas A (1961). "Notas sobre la tenencia de la tierra entre los mayas de la antigüedad." *Estudios de Cultura Maya* 1(1): 21–46; Caso A (1963). "Land tenure among the ancient Mexicans." *American Anthropologist* 65(4): 863–878.
1276. Zurbach J (2013). "The formation of Greek city-states: Status, class, and land tenure systems." *Annales* 68(4): 615–657.
1277. Pliny the Elder (1938). *Natural History*. Harvard University Press, Cambridge, MA.
1278. Marx K (1949). *El Capital (Critica de la Economia Politica)*. Fondo de Cultura Economica, Mexico; Saito K (2017). *Karl Marx's Ecosocialism: Capital, Nature, and the Unfinished Critique of Political Economy*. Monthly Review Press, New York.
1279. Fairbairn M (2020). *Fields of Gold: Financing the Global Land Rush*. Cornell University Press, Ithaca, NY.
1280. Foster JB, B Clark, and R York (2010). *The Ecological Rift: Capitalism's War on the Earth*. Monthly Review Press, New York; Liberti S (2013). *Land Grabbing: Journeys in the New Colonialism*. Verso, New York; Li TM (2014). "What is land? Assembling a resource for global investment." *Transactions of the Institute of British Geographers* 39(4): 589–602; Seufert P, ML Mendonça, and F Pitta (2019). *When Land Becomes a Global Financial Asset: The MATOPIBA Case in Brazil*. https://www.righttofoodandnutrition.org/files/3._eng_when_land_becomes_a_global_financial_asset.pdf.
1281. Celli A (1933). *The History of Malaria in the Roman Campagna from Ancient Times*. John Bale, Sons & Danielsson, Ltd., London.
1282. Chaves LF (2013). "The dynamics of latifundia formation." *PLOS ONE* 8(12): e82863.
1283. Glaser V (2001). "Zoonotic diseases—An interview with Karl M. Johnson, M.D." *Vector-Borne and Zoonotic Diseases* 1(3): 243–248.
1284. Johnson KM (2008). "Infection and ecology: *Calomys callosus*, Machupo virus, and acute hemorrhagic fever." In RS Ostfeld, F Kessing, and VT Eveiner (eds), *Infectious Disease Ecology*. Princeton University Press; Princeton, pp 404–422.
1285. Kuns ML (1965). "Epidemiology of Machupo Virus Infection: II. Ecological and control studies of hemorrhagic fever." *American Journal of Tropical Medicine and Hygiene* 14(5): 813–816; Johnson KM (1965). "Epidemiology of Machupo Virus Infection: III. Significance of virological observations in man and animals." *American Journal of Tropical Medicine and Hygiene* 14(5): 816–818.

1286. Johnson KM (2008). "Infection and ecology: *Calomys callosus*, Machupo virus, and acute hemorrhagic fever."

1287. Kuns ML (1965). "Epidemiology of Machupo Virus Infection: II. Ecological and control studies of hemorrhagic fever."

1288. Johnson KM (2008). "Infection and ecology: *Calomys callosus*, Machupo virus, and acute hemorrhagic fever."

1289. Glaser V (2001). "Zoonotic diseases—An interview with Karl M. Johnson, M.D."

1290. Tesh RB, ML Wilson, R Salas, et al. (1993). "Field studies on the epidemiology of Venezuelan Hemorrhagic Fever: Implication of the cotton rat *Sigmodon alstoni* as the probable rodent reservoir." *American Journal of Tropical Medicine and Hygiene* 49(2): 227-235.

1291. Ibid.

1292. Ibid.

1293. Santos M (2017). *Toward an Other Globalization: From the Single Thought to Universal Conscience*. Translated by Lucas Melgaco and Tim Clarke. Springer, Cham.

1294. Celli A (1900). "The new prophylaxis against malaria: an account of experiments in Latium." *The Lancet* 156(4031): 1603-1606; Chaves LF, M Ramírez Rojas, S Delgado Jiménez, M Prado, and R Marín Rodríguez (2020). "Housing quality improvement is associated with malaria transmission reduction in Costa Rica." *Socio-Economic Planning Sciences* 2020: 100951.

1295. Chaves LF, JE Calzada, C Rigg, A Valderrama, NL Gottdenker, and A Saldaña A (2013). "Leishmaniasis sand fly vector density reduction is less marked in destitute housing after insecticide thermal fogging." *Parasites & Vectors* 6(1): 164; Pérez J, et al. (2014). "Species composition and seasonal abundance of sandflies (Diptera: Psychodidae: Phlebotominae) in coffee agroecosystems." *Memórias do Instituto Oswaldo Cruz*, 109: 80-86.

1296. Archibald S, W Bond, W Stock, and D Fairbanks (2005). "Shaping the landscape: fire–grazer interactions in an African savanna." *Ecological Applications* 15(1): 96-109.

1297. Tesh RB, ML Wilson, R Salas, et al. (1993). "Field studies on the epidemiology of Venezuelan Hemorrhagic Fever: Implication of the cotton rat *Sigmodon alstoni* as the probable rodent reservoir."

1298. Perfecto I, J Vandermeer,and SM Philpott SM (2014). "Complex ecological interactions in the coffee agroecosystem." *Annual Review of Ecology, Evolution, and Systematics* 45(1): 137-158; Vandermeer J and I Perfecto (2019). "Hysteresis and critical transitions in a coffee agroecosystem." *Proceedings of the National Academy of Sciences* 116(30): 15074-15079; Vandermeer J, I Armbrecht, A de la Mora, et al. (2019). "The community ecology of herbivore regulation in an agroecosystem: Lessons from complex systems." *BioScience* 69(12): 974-996.

1299. Scorza J, M Valera, E Moreno, and R Jaimes (1983). "Epidemiologic survey of cutaneous leishmaniasis: an experience in Mérida, Venezuela." *Bulletin of the Pan American Health Organization* 17(4): 361-374; Scorza JV, and E Rojas (1988). "Caficultura y leishmaniasis tegumentaria en Venezuela." *Boletín de la Dirección de Malariologia y Saneamiento Ambiental* 28: 114-127; Warburg A, J Montoya-Lerma, C Jaramillo, AL Cruz-Ruiz, and K Ostrovska (1991). "Leishmaniasis vector potential of *Lutzomyia* spp. in Colombian coffee plantations." *Medical and Veterinary Entomology* 5(1): 9-16; Alexander B, LA Agudelo, F Navarro F, et al. (2001). "Phlebotomine sandflies and leishmaniasis risks in Colombian coffee plantations under two systems of cultivation." *Medical and Veterinary Entomology* 15(4): 364-373; Alexander B, EBD Oliveria, E Haigh, and LLD Almeida (2002). "Transmission of Leishmania in coffee plantations of Minas Gerais, Brazil." *Memórias do Instituto Oswaldo* 97: 627-630.

1300. Liebman A, T Jonas, I Perfecto, L Kelly, et al. (2020). "Can agriculture stop COVID-21, -22, and -23? Yes, but not by greenwashing agribusiness." Pandemic Research for the People. Dispatch 6, December 10. https://drive.google.com/file/d/1M-yW7JakFwSV_ZFUNZdQLdYWhlbn_L6D/view.

1301. Ibid.

1302. Ceddia MG (2020). "The super-rich and cropland expansion via direct investments in agriculture." *Nature Sustainability* 3(4): 312-318.

1303. Wallace RG, L Bergmann, R Kock, M Gilbert, L Hogerwerf, R Wallace, and M Holmberg (2015). "The dawn of Structural One Health: A new science tracking disease emergence along circuits of capital." *Social Science & Medicine* 129: 68-77.

1304. Birn A-E, Y Pillay, and TH Holtz (2017). "Health equity and the social determinants of health." In A-E Birn, Y Pillay, and TH Holtz (eds), *Textbook of Global Health*. Oxford University Press, New York, pp 285-334; Morand S and C Lajaunie (2021). "Outbreaks of vector-borne and zoonotic diseases are associated with changes in forest cover and oil palm expansion at global scale." *Frontiers in Veterinary Science*, 24 March. https://doi.org/10.3389/fvets.2021.661063.

1305. Chiappero MB, MAF Piacenza, MAC Provensal, GE Calder, CN Gardenal, and JJ Polop (2018). "Effective population size differences in *Calomys musculinus*, the host of Junin Virus: Their relationship with the epidemiological history of Argentine hemorrhagic fever." *American Journal of Tropical Medicine and Hygiene* 99(2): 445-450.

1306. Santos M (2017). "The return of the territory." In L Melgaço and C Prouse (eds), *Milton Santos: A Pioneer in Critical Geography from the Global South*. Springer, Cham, pp 25-31.

1307. Robbins J (2012). "The ecology of disease." *New York Times*, 14 July. https://www.nytimes.com/2012/07/15/sunday-review/the-ecology-of-disease.html?pagewanted=1&emc=eta1%22.

1308. White B (1973). "Demand for labor and population growth in colonial Java." *Human Ecology* 1(3): 217-236; Franke R. (1987). "The effects of colonialism and neocolonialism on the gastronomic patterns of the Third World." In *Food and Evolution: Toward a Theory of Human Food Habits.* Temple University Press, Philadelphia, pp 455-479.

1309. Peluso NL and P Vandergeest (2001). "Genealogies of the political forest and customary rights in Indonesia, Malaysia, and Thailand." *The Journal of Asian Studies* 60(3): 761-812.

1310. Afiff S (2016). "REDD, land management and the politics of forest and land tenure reform with special reference to the case of Central Kalimantan province." In JF McCarthy and K Robinson (eds), *Land and Development in Indonesia: Searching for the People's Sovereignty.* ISEAS-Yusof Ishak Institute.

1311. Kelley LC, NL Peluso, KM Carlson, and S Afiff (2020). "Circular labor migration and land-livelihood dynamics in Southeast Asia's concession landscapes." *Journal of Rural Studies,* 73: 21-33.

1312. Shiva V (2004). "The future of food: countering globalisation and recolonisation of Indian agriculture." *Futures* 36(6-7): 715-732; Shiva V (ed) (2016). *Seed Sovereignty, Food Security: Women in the Vanguard of the Fight Against GMOs and Corporate Agriculture.* North Atlantic Books, Berkeley, CA.

1313. Card K and T Castle (2021). "Geographies of racial capitalism with Ruth Wilson Gilmore." Antipode Foundation. https://antipodeonline. org/geographies-of-racial-capitalism/; Gilmore RW (2021). *Change Everything: Racial Capitalism and the Case for Abolition.* Haymarket Books, Chicago.

1314. Schaffer R and N Smith (1986). "The gentrification of Harlem?" *Annals of the Association of American Geographers* 76(3): 347-65; Niedt C (2006). "Gentrification and the grassroots: Popular support in the revanchist suburb." *Journal of Urban Affairs* 28(2): 99-120; Lloyd JM (2016). "Fighting redlining and gentrification in Washington, DC: The Adams-Morgan organization and tenant right to purchase." *Journal of Urban History* 42(6): 1091-1109.

1315. Amin S (1973). *Le développement inégal. Essai sur les formations sociales du paitalisme périphérique.* Les Editions de Minuit, Paris.

1316. Rodney W (1981). *How Europe Underdeveloped Africa.* Howard University Press, Washington DC; Suwandi I (2019). *Value Chains: The New Economic Imperialism.* Monthly Review Press, New York; Liebman A, T Jonas, I Perfecto, L Kelly, et al. (2020). "Can agriculture stop COVID-21, -22, and -23? Yes, but not by greenwashing agribusiness." Pandemic Research for the People.

1317. Daszak P (2021). "Welcome and recap day 2." Systematizing the One Health Approach in Preparedness and Response Efforts for Infectious Disease Outbreaks: A Virtual Workshop, February

23-25, 2021. https://www.nationalacademies.org/event/02-25-2020/systematizing-the-one-health-approach-in-preparedness-and-response-efforts-for-infectious-disease-outbreaks-a-workshop

1318. Wallace RG (2016). "Two gentlemen of Verona." In *Big Farms Make Big Flu: Dispatches on Infectious Disease, Agribusiness, and the Nature of Science.* Monthly Review Press, New York, pp 160 166.

1319. Husseini S (2021). "Peter Daszak's EcoHealth Alliance has hidden almost $40 Million in Pentagon funding and militarized pandemic science." *Independent Science News,* 16 December. https://www.independentsciencenews.org/news/peter-daszaks-ecohealth-alliance-has-hidden-almost-40-million-in-pentagon-funding/.

1320. Terry M (2020). "NIH awards EcoHealth Alliance $7.5 million grant despite political furor." *BioSpace,* 28 August. https://www.biospace.com/article/1nih-awards-ecohealth-alliance-7-5-million-grant-despite-political-furor/.

1321. Arrighi G (1994 [2010]). *The Long Twentieth Century: Money, Power and the Origins of Our Times.*

1322. Patel R (2013). "The Long Green Revolution." *The Journal of Peasant Studies* 40(1): 1-63.

1323. Matchaba P (2021). "The COVID recovery needs to be green: A Capitals approach to tackling global health challenges." Capitals Coalition, 3 March. https://capitalscoalition.org/the-covid-recovery-needs-to-be-green-a-capitals-approach-to-tackling-global-health-challenges-by-patrice-matchaba/.

1324. Wallace RG (2020). "Midvinter-19." In *Dead Epidemiologists: On the Origins of COVID-19.* Monthly Review Press, New York; Patel R and R Marya (2021). "Against philanthropy: The role of foundations in colonising the food system." ORFC Global 2021 Session. https://www.youtube.com/watch?v=oekGymm1rYg.

1325. Napier SJ (2000). *Anime from Akira to Princess Mononoke: Experiencing Contemporary Japanese Animation.* Palgrave, New York; Wegner PE (2010). "An unfinished project that was also a missed opportunity": Utopia and alternate history in Hayao Miyazaki's *My Neighbor Totoro. ImageTexT: Interdisciplinary Comics Studies* 5(2).

1326. Kropotkin PA (1939). *Mutual Aid: A Factor of Evolution.* Penguin Books Ltd., Harmondsworth, England; Foster JB (2020). *The Return of Nature: Socialism and Ecology.* Monthly Review Press, New York.

1327. Levins R (2008). "Living the 11th thesis." *Monthly Review* 59(8): 29-37.

1328. Teicher JG (2020). "The Revolution will not be 'Green.'" *Uneven Earth,* 7 July. https://unevenearth.org/2020/07/the-revolution-will-not-be-green/.

Index

CPSIA information can be obtained
at www.ICGtesting.com
Printed in the USA
JSHW060109311222
35571JS00005B/12